# Handbook of Pediatric Otolaryngology

A Practical Guide for Evaluation and Management of Pediatric Ear, Nose, and Throat Disorders

# Handbook of Pediatric Otolaryngology

## A Practical Guide for Evaluation and Management of Pediatric Ear, Nose, and Throat Disorders

**Nina L. Shapiro, MD**
*University of California, Los Angeles, USA*

*Editor*

World Scientific

NEW JERSEY • LONDON • SINGAPORE • BEIJING • SHANGHAI • HONG KONG • TAIPEI • CHENNAI

*Published by*

World Scientific Publishing Co. Pte. Ltd.
5 Toh Tuck Link, Singapore 596224
*USA office:* 27 Warren Street, Suite 401-402, Hackensack, NJ 07601
*UK office:* 57 Shelton Street, Covent Garden, London WC2H 9HE



**British Library Cataloguing-in-Publication Data**
A catalogue record for this book is available from the British Library.

**HANDBOOK OF PEDIATRIC OTOLARYNGOLOGY**
**A Practical Guide for Evaluation and Management of Pediatric Ear, Nose, and Throat Disorders**



ISBN-13 978-981-4282-05-5
ISBN-10 981-4282-05-7

Typeset by Stallion Press
Email: enquiries@stallionpress.com

Printed by FuIsland Offset Printing (S) Pte Ltd Singapore

# Contents

# Contributors

**Elliot Abemayor, MD, PhD**
Professor of Surgery
Department of Otolaryngology-Head and Neck Surgery
David Geffen School of Medicine at UCLA
10833 Le Conte Ave
Los Angeles, CA 90095, USA

**Gerald Berke, MD**
Professor and Chief
Division of Head and Neck Surgery
University of California, Los Angeles School of Medicine
10833 Le Conte Avenue, 62-132 CHS
Los Angeles, CA 90095, USA

**Prabhat K. Bhama, MD**
Resident, Research Fellow
Department of Otolaryngology-Head and Neck Surgery
University of Washington School of Medicine
1959 NE Pacific Street, Box 356515
BB 1165 OTOHNS
Seattle, WA 98195, USA

**Emily F. Boss, MD, MPH**
Pediatric Otolaryngology
Department of Otolaryngology-Head and Neck Surgery
Johns Hopkins University School of Medicine
601 N. Caroline St., 6th Floor
Baltimore, MD 21287, USA

**Matthew T. Brigger, MD, MPH**
LCDR MC USN
Adjunct Assistant Professor
F. Edward Hebert School of Medicine/Uniformed Services University of the Health Sciences
Department of Otolaryngology-Head and Neck Surgery
Naval Medical Center San Diego
34800 Bob Wilson Drive
San Diego, CA 92134, USA

**Dinesh K. Chhetri, MD**
Associate Professor, Head and Neck Surgery
Voice, Airway, and Swallowing Disorders
University of California, Los Angeles School of Medicine
200 Medical Plaza, Suite 550
Los Angeles, CA 90095, USA

**Sukgi S. Choi, MD, FACS, FAAP**
Professor of Otolaryngology and Pediatrics
The George Washington University School of Medicine
Vice Chief, Division of Pediatric Otolaryngology
Children's National Medical Center
111 Michigan Ave NW
Washington, DC 20010, USA

**Michael J. Cunningham, MD**
Professor, Department of Otology and Laryngology
Harvard Medical School

Chief, Department of Otolaryngology and Communication Enhancement
Children's Hospital Boston
300 Longwood Avenue, Lo-367
Boston, MA 02115, USA

**Craig S. Derkay, MD, FACS, FAAP**
Professor and Vice-Chairman
Department of Otolaryngology-Head and Neck Surgery
Eastern Virginia Medical School
Director, Pediatric Otolaryngology
Children's Hospital of the King's Daughters
2nd Floor, Pediatric Otolaryngology
601 Children's Lane
Norfolk, VA 23507, USA

**Daniel DeUgarte, MD, FACS, FAAP**
Assistant Professor, Division of Pediatric Surgery
David Geffen School of Medicine at UCLA
10833 Le Conte Avenue, Box 709818
Los Angeles, CA 90095-7098, USA

**Joseph E. Dohar, MD, MS, FAAP, FACS**
Associate Professor of Otolaryngology
University of Pittsburgh School of Medicine
Children's Hospital of Pittsburgh of UPMC
4401 Penn Avenue, floor 3
Pittsburgh, PA 15224, USA

**Christopher J. Hartnick, MD, M.Epi**
Associate Professor
Department of Otology and Laryngology
Harvard Medical School
Massachusetts Eye and Ear Infirmary
243 Charles St.
Boston, MA 02114, USA

**Thomas S. Higgins, MD, MPH**
Resident Physician
Department of Otolaryngology-Head and Neck Surgery
Eastern Virginia Medical School
Norfolk, VA 23507, USA

**Richard W. Hong, MD**
Assistant Clinical Professor
Chief of Obstetrical Anesthesiology
David Geffen School of Medicine at UCLA
757 Westwood Plaza Suite 3325
Los Angeles, CA 90095-7404, USA

**N. Scott Howard, MD, MBA**
Major
Chief, Eyes-Ears-Nose-Throat Clinic
Dwight D. Eisenhower Army Medical Center
Room 2J-11
Fort Gordon, GA 30905, USA

**Anita Jeyakumar, MD**
Assistant Professor
Department of Otolaryngology-Head and Neck Surgery
Saint Louis University School of Medicine
Cardinal Glennon Children's Medical Center
1465 S. Grand, Suite B824
St Louis, MO 63104, USA

**Jodi L. P. Jones, MD, FRCSC**
Pediatric Otolaryngologist
Assistant Professor
Department of Otolaryngology
University of Manitoba
GB 421 820 Sherbrook Street
Winnipeg, Manitoba R3A 1R9, Canada

**Deborah S. F. Kacmarynski, MD, MS**
Pediatric Otolaryngologist
Co-Director Cleft and Craniofacial Service
Clinical Assistant Professor
Department of Otolaryngology-Head and Neck Surgery
University of Iowa
200 Hawkins Drive, 21262 PFP
Iowa City, IA 52242-1078, USA

**Amy S. Ketcham, MD**
Resident Physician
Department of Otolaryngology-Head and Neck Surgery
Eastern Virginia Medical School
Norfolk, VA 23507, USA

**Peter J. Koltai, MD**
Professor and Chief
Division of Pediatric Otolaryngology
Stanford University School of Medicine
801 Welch Road
Stanford, CA 94305-5739, USA

**Ontario D. Lau, MD**
3rd Medical Group
5955 Zeamer Avenue
Elmendorf Airforce Base
AK 99506, USA

**Sofia Lyford-Pike, MD**
Department of Otolaryngology-Head and Neck Surgery
Johns Hopkins University School of Medicine
601 N. Caroline St., 6th Floor
Baltimore, MD 21287, USA

**Raymond C. Maguire, DO**
Assistant Professor Otolaryngology
University of Pittsburgh School of Medicine
Children's Hospital of Pittsburgh of UPMC
4401 Penn Avenue, floor 3
Pittsburgh, PA 15224, USA

**Scott C. Manning, MD**
Chief, Division of Pediatric Otolaryngology
Children's Hospital Seattle
Professor, Department of Otolaryngology
University of Washington
W-7771, 4800 Sand Point Way NE
Seattle, WA 98105, USA

**Brian F. McGettigan, MD**
Department of Otolaryngology-Head and Neck Surgery
Thomas Jefferson University School of Medicine
1020 Walnut Street
Philadelphia, PA 19107, USA

**Anna K. Meyer, MD, FAAP**
Assistant Professor
Division of Pediatric Otolaryngology-Head and Neck Surgery
Department of Otolaryngology-Head and Neck Surgery
University of California, San Francisco
2330 Post St., 3rd Floor
San Francisco, CA 94115, USA

**Ron B. Mitchell, MD**
Professor of Otolaryngology and Pediatrics
Department of Otolaryngology-Head and Neck Surgery
Director of Pediatric Otolaryngology
Saint Louis University School of Medicine
Cardinal Glennon Children's Medical Center
1465 S. Grand, Suite B824
St Louis, MO 63104, USA

**T. J. O-Lee, MD**
Assistant Professor of Surgery
Department of Otolaryngology-Head and Neck Surgery
University of Nevada School of Medicine
2040 W. Charleston Boulevard, Suite 601
Las Vegas, NV 89102, USA

**Swati Patel, MD**
Clinical Professor
Chief, Division of Pediatric Anesthesiology
Department of Anesthesiology
David Geffen School of Medicine at UCLA
Mattel Children's Hospital UCLA
Ronald Reagan-UCLA Medical Center
757 Westwood Plaza
Los Angeles, CA 90095-7403, USA

**Seth M. Pransky, MD**
Clinical Professor of Surgery
University of California, San Diego
Division of Otolaryngology
Director, Pediatric Otolaryngology
Rady Children's Specialist Medical Foundation
3030 Children's Way #402
San Diego, CA 92123, USA

**Diego A. Preciado, MD, PhD**
Assistant Professor of Otolaryngology, Pediatrics, and Integrative Systems Biology
The George Washington University School of Medicine
Fellowship Program Director
Division of Pediatric Otolaryngology
Children's National Medical Center
111 Michigan Ave NW
Washington, DC 20010, USA

**Kristina W. Rosbe, MD, FAAP, FACS**
Associate Professor
Director, Division of Pediatric Otolaryngology-Head and Neck Surgery
Department of Otolaryngology-Head and Neck Surgery
University of California, San Francisco
2330 Post St., 3rd Floor
San Francisco, CA 94115, USA

**Andrew R. Scott, MD**
Divisions of Pediatric Otolaryngology and Facial Plastic and Reconstructive Surgery
Floating Hospital for Children, Tufts Medical Center
Assistant Professor of Otolaryngology and Pediatrics
Tufts University School of Medicine
800 Washington St., #850
Boston, MA 02111, USA

**Udayan K. Shah, MD, FACS, FAAP**
Associate Professor
Otolaryngology-Head and Neck Surgery and Pediatrics
Thomas Jefferson University School of Medicine
Director, Fellow and Resident Education in Pediatric Otolaryngology
Division of Pediatric Otolaryngology
Nemours/Alfred I DuPont Hospital for Children
1600 Rockland Road
Wilmington, DE 19803, USA

**Nina L. Shapiro, MD, FACS, FAAP**
Associate Professor of Surgery
Director of Pediatric Otolaryngology
Division of Head and Neck Surgery
David Geffen School of Medicine at UCLA
UCLA Surg-Hd and NK
Box 951624, 62-158A CHS
Los Angeles, CA 90095-1624, USA

**Douglas Sidell, MD**
Division of Head and Neck Surgery
David Geffen School of Medicine at UCLA
UCLA Surg-Hd and NK
Box 951624, 62-158 CHS
Los Angeles, CA 90095-1624, USA

**Kathleen C. Y. Sie, MD**
Professor, Department of Otolaryngology-Head and Neck Surgery
University of Washington School of Medicine
Clinical Director, Childhood Communications Center
Co-Director, Pediatric Cochlear Implant Program
Seattle Children's Hospital
4800 Sand Point Way N.E.
Seattle, WA 98105, USA

**Lawrence M. Simon, MD**
Assistant Professor of Clinical Otolaryngology
Louisiana State University Health Sciences Center
533 Bolivar Street, Suite 566
New Orleans, LA 70112, USA
Pediatric Otolaryngologist
Co-director, Vascular Anomalies Center
The Regional Medical Center for Children
200 Henry Clay Avenue, Suite 4119
New Orleans, LA 70118, USA

**Yvonne S. Sininger, PhD**
Professor in Residence, Head and Neck Surgery
David Geffen School of Medicine at UCLA
62-132 Center for Health Sciences, Box 951624
Los Angeles, CA 90095-1624, USA

**Maie A. St. John, MD, PhD**
Assistant Professor, Department of Surgery
Division of Head and Neck Surgery
Jonsson Comprehensive Cancer Center

David Geffen School of Medicine at UCLA
Chief, Department of Otolaryngology-Head and Neck Surgery
Harbor-UCLA Medical Center
10833 Le Conte Ave
Los Angeles, CA 90095, USA

**Betty S. Tsai, MD**
Clinical Fellow, The Otology Group of Vanderbilt
Department of Otolaryngology-Head and Neck Surgery
Vanderbilt University Medical Center
7209 Medical Center East, South Tower
1215 21st Avenue, South
Nashville, TN 37232-8605, USA

**Jennifer Veraldi, MD**
Resident
Department of Otolaryngology-Head and Neck Surgery
Saint Louis University School of Medicine
Cardinal Glennon Children's Medical Center
1465 S. Grand, Suite B824
St Louis, MO 63104, USA

**Samuel H. Wald, MD**
Clinical Professor, Pediatric Anesthesiology
Department of Anesthesiology
David Geffen School of Medicine at UCLA
757 Westwood Plaza, Suite 3304
Los Angeles, CA 90095, USA

**Keren Ziv, MD**
Associate Clinical Professor
Department of Anesthesiology
David Geffen School of Medicine at UCLA
Ronald Reagan-UCLA Medical Center
757 Westwood Plaza
Los Angeles, CA 90095-7403, USA

# Preface

The subspecialty of pediatric otolaryngology has undergone tremendous evolution over the last several decades. In its initial years, it consisted of groups of otolaryngologists with an interest in pediatric issues who met for study sessions, where challenging cases would be presented and discussed. Over the last 25 years, it has developed into a large subspecialty, with fellowship training and many national and international societies. With the growth of the subspecialty, there has been more need for up-to-date reference tools for the busy clinician.

This text is geared toward the clinician at all levels of training and experience — from the medical student with an interest in the specialty, to the established pediatric otolaryngologist with a need for a comprehensive, yet concise book. It contains all of the critical areas of pediatric otolaryngology, and is enhanced by including areas from relevant pediatric subspecialists such as audiologists, anesthesiologists, and pediatric surgeons. General otolaryngologists will benefit from this book, as a large portion of the general otolaryngologist's practice involves treatment of children. Residents and fellows will be able to use this book as a study source as well as a reference guide for both common and complex pediatric otolaryngologic disorders.

I wish to thank all of the authors of this book, who have produced up-to-date information in their respective areas of expertise. To them I am indebted, and I feel lucky to be in a field with such collegiality and mutual support. I am sure that I speak for all of the authors when I thank our patients and their families, who put their child's welfare in our hands, and from whom we learn so much.

I would also like to thank my many mentors who have given me guidance and wisdom in the lifelong process of the practice of medicine. I have had many wonderful teachers and guides over the years, but most notably I thank Drs. Stanley Shapiro, Adam Shapiro, Marshall Strome, Marvin Fried, Michael Cunningham, Roland Eavey, Allan Seid, and Seth Pransky. Last but certainly not least, I thank my family, who have given unconditional support in this and other endeavors — my husband, Dr. Elliot Abemayor, who supports me in every way, and my children, Alessandra and Charles.

Nina L. Shapiro, MD
Editor
Associate Professor
Pediatric Otolaryngology
UCLA School of Medicine

# OTOLOGY

# 1

# Acute and Chronic Otitis Media

*Betty S. Tsai, Anna K. Meyer and Kristina W. Rosbe*

## INTRODUCTION

Otitis media is one of the most common illnesses for which preschool-age children visit their pediatrician, accounting for more than US $3 billion in expenditures annually.[1,2] Up to 80% of children under the age of six will experience at least one ear infection.[3] Children with acute otitis media typically present with otalgia or pulling of the ears, irritability, and fever, and it is often associated with a viral upper respiratory infection.[4] Chronic otitis media with effusion, on the other hand, is defined as fluid in the middle ear for at least three months and typically presents without signs of acute inflammation. Within the first year of life, at least 50% of children will experience otitis media with effusion, and while most resolve spontaneously, 30%–40% will persist, with 5%–10% of the episodes lasting at least one year.[5]

## ANATOMY

The ear can be separated into three compartments: the outer ear, the middle ear, and the inner ear. The tympanic membrane serves as the boundary between the outer ear and middle ear whereas the

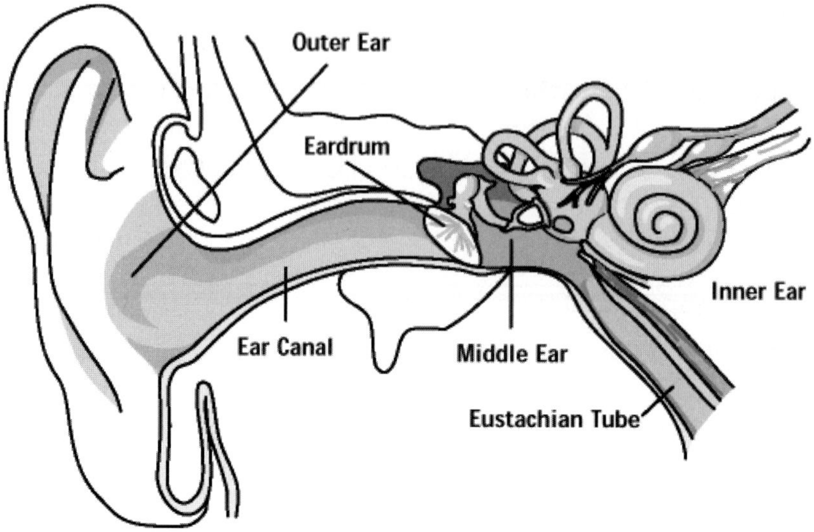


**Fig. 1.** The basic structure of the ear. (Reprinted with permission from the New York State Department of Health.)

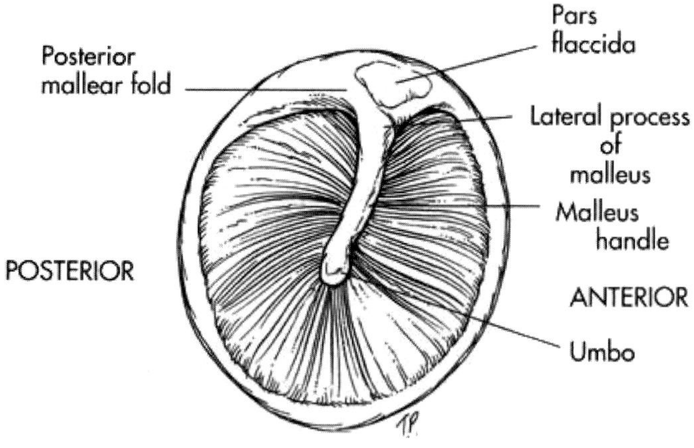


**Fig. 2.** Tympanic membrane. (Reprinted with permission from *Cummings Otolaryngology: Head and Neck Surgery*, 2010, Figure 8–4.)[6]

oval window between the stapes and cochlea distinguishes the middle ear from the inner ear (Fig. 1).

The tympanic membrane (Fig. 2) is an oval-shaped structure which is divided into two parts, pars tensa and pars flaccida. Centrally, there is a depression where the tympanic membrane is attached to the malleus. Along the superior aspect, a triangular portion of the tympanic membrane, the pars flaccida, lacks support of radial and circular fibers, making it more vulnerable to retraction pockets and the formation of cholesteatoma. The pars tensa, on the other hand, is completely surrounded by a bony groove, known as the sulcus, and contains radial and circular fibers, providing additional support for the membrane.

The middle ear is an air-filled space through which sound is conducted. A chain of three ossicles (malleus, incus, and stapes) connect the tympanic membrane to the oval window and in the process, amplify sound that enters through the outer ear. Pathology within the middle ear space can lead to hearing loss through various mechanisms. The presence of fluid within the middle ear space dampens the vibrations of the ossicles resulting in decreased amplification of sound reaching the inner ear. Complications of otitis media, such as cholesteatoma can impede the movement of the ossicles or even erode the ossicular chain, resulting in a conductive hearing loss.

The incidence of otitis media is significantly higher in infants compared to older children, and is related to changes in eustachian tube anatomy as a child ages.[7] The eustachian tube is a mucosa-lined structure with a lumen connecting the middle ear to the nasopharynx. This tube has an osseous (middle ear) and cartilaginous portion, with the most narrow segment in the mid-portion (Fig. 3). While the osseous segment is open at all times, the cartilaginous segment is closed at rest and opens during Valsalva maneuvers, swallowing, yawning or sneezing and permits equalization of middle-ear and atmospheric pressures.[8] In young children, the eustachian tube is located at 10° from the Frankfort horizontal plane, whereas in adults, it is at 45° (Fig. 3).[9] Children also have a shorter eustachian tube[10] with decreased stiffness and mass.[11]

Although the exact mechanism of eustachian tube dilation is controversial, it is associated with four muscles: the tensor veli palatini, the levator veli palatini, the salpingopharyngeus, and the tensor tympani. The tensor veli palatini muscle, which is less efficient in the

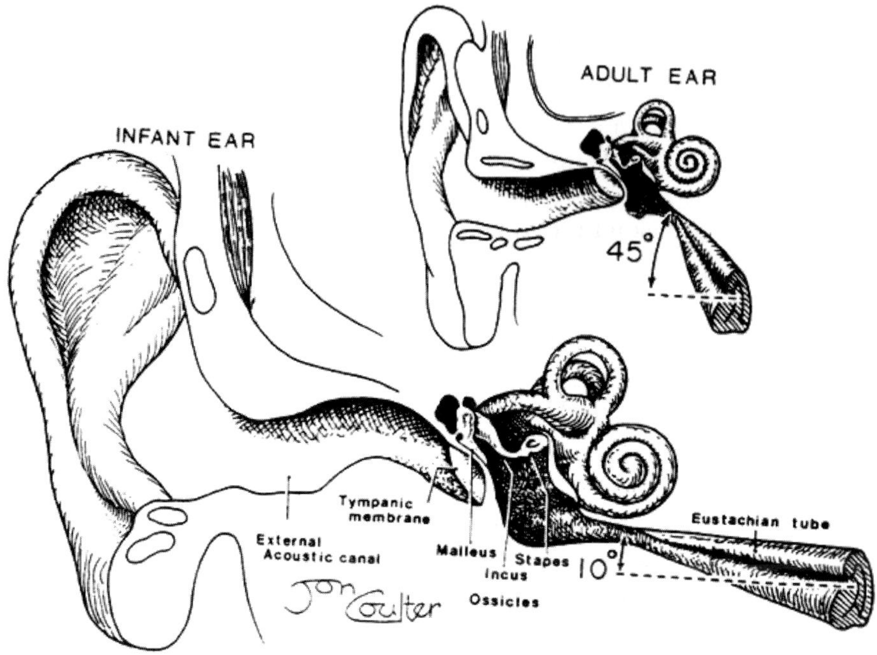


**Fig. 3.** Eustachian tube anatomy differences between a child and an adult. (Reprinted with permission from Corbeel, 2007.)[7]

infant, is believed to be the primary dilator of the eustachian tube.[8,12] The levator veli palatini also makes a contribution to eustachian tube dilation, whereas the salpingopharyngeus muscle and tensor tympani muscle assist in maintaining the physiologic state of the middle ear by controlling the opening of the eustachian tube.[13]

## RISK FACTORS AND PATHOPHYSIOLOGY

Eustachian tube dysfunction is often the cause of otitis media. As outlined (see Anatomy), the anatomical variance between children and adults leads to a higher incidence of otitis media in young children. Additionally, children with abnormal anatomy in proximity to the eustachian tube, such as cleft palate or other craniofacial disorders, are at higher risk for otitis media.[14]

The eustachian tube is lined with respiratory mucosa that is contiguous with the pharynx and inflammatory responses in the nasopharynx, including environmental and/or food allergies, upper respiratory tract infections, gastroesophageal reflux, and adenoid hypertrophy, have all been shown to contribute to the development of otitis media.[8,15] It is believed that edema and congestion of the eustachian tube and middle ear mucosa result in a narrowed lumen that increases negative middle-ear pressure allowing for an influx of pathogens from the nasopharynx when the tube opens. The subsequent inflammatory response recruits neutrophils and lymphocytes into the middle-ear space, worsening the obstruction and ventilation of the middle ear.[14]

Additionally, the status of the immune system can determine the susceptibility to developing otitis media. Infants and toddlers have immature immune systems and therefore are more likely to develop infection.[16] Those with congenital or acquired immunocompromised states are at higher risk. Immunodeficiencies associated with a higher risk for otitis media include: IgA deficiency, B-cell deficiencies such as hypogammaglobulinemia, T-cell deficiences such as DiGeorge syndrome, and complement deficiencies.

The pathogens most commonly identified in acute otitis media include *Streptococcus pneumoniae, Haemophilus influenza, Moraxella catarrhalis,* and group A streptococci.[14,17] However, up to 20% of the time, gram-negative enteric bacteria and *Staphylococcus aureus* are found.[16] Over recent years, there have been increasing numbers of *β*-lactamase *Haemophilus influenza* and resistant streptococci.[18] Prior to the introduction of vaccines, the highly-aggressive strain of *Haemophilus influenza* type B (HiB) accounted for nearly all the disease attributed to *Haemophilus influenza,* including bacterial meningitis as a complication of otitis media.[19] Following the widespread use of the HiB vaccine, various strains of pneumococcus are typically the more virulent pathogens in otitis media, although nontypable *Haemophilus* still is relatively common.[20] The subsequent introduction of the heptavalent conjugated pneumococcal vaccine has resulted in an increase in *Moraxella catarrhalis* and *Staphylocccus aureus* as pathogens, in addition to strains of pneumococcus not seen in the vaccine.[20–22] As more vaccines are being developed to target pathogens in otitis media, one would expect a continuing shift in underlying microbiology of this disease.[23]

## EVALUATION

### History

Diagnosis of otitis media is based on history and physical exam. Children with acute otitis media often present with fever, irritability, otalgia, and hearing loss. Less commonly, children may also present with nausea, headache, and vomiting. Not infrequently, hearing loss or speech delay is the only presenting symptom in children with otitis media with effusion.

Otitis media is described as acute (less than three weeks duration), subacute (three to 12 weeks duration), or chronic (more than 12 weeks duration). Four or more episodes of acute otitis media within one year or three or more episodes within a six-month period is considered recurrent acute otitis media.[16] Otitis media with effusion refers to the presence of fluid behind the middle ear. Suppurative otitis media is characterized by the presence of purulent otorrhea typically in the presence of a tympanic membrane perforation or tympanostomy tube. Chronic suppurative otitis media (otorrhea present for more than three months) should raise concern for cholesteatoma.

### Physical Examination

Visualization of the tympanic membrane with pneumatic otoscopy often confirms the diagnosis of otitis media. The eardrum can appear red (in the setting of acute otitis media or crying) or opaque (consistent with an effusion) as shown in Fig. 4. Middle ear effusions can be purulent (opaque yellow or white), mucoid (clear or white), or serous (clear or translucent yellow). The tympanic membrane can be bulging in the setting of an acute otitis media (Fig. 4). Alternatively, the tympanic membrane may be retracted in the

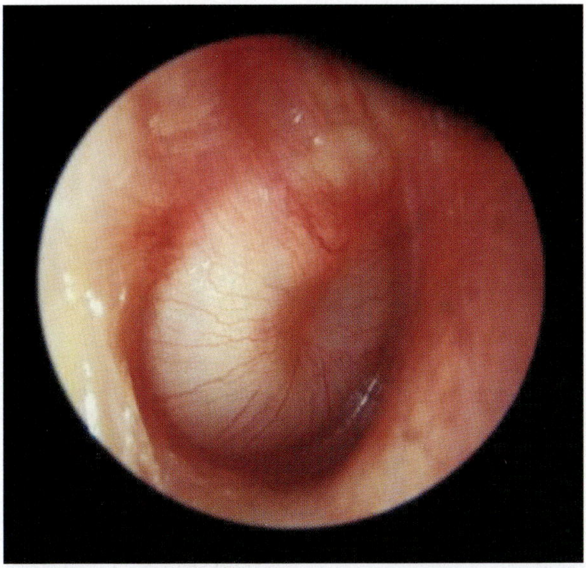

**Fig. 4.** Acute otitis media.

setting of negative middle ear pressure. Insufflation of air into the ear canal after forming a tight seal with the speculum can aid in the evaluation of the ear. In the presence of a middle ear effusion, pneumatic otoscopy will demonstrate an immobile or hypo-mobile tympanic membrane.

Patients with a tympanostomy tube, a tympanic membrane perforation, or cholesteatoma may have otorrhea. In congenital cholesteatoma, white opacification behind an intact tympanic membrane may be observed (Fig. 5). Additionally, changes of the tympanic membrane such as myringosclerosis (white thickened areas from scarring) or retraction pockets can be visualized. It is important to visualize the entire tympanic membrane, particularly the superior portion, or pars flaccida, in order to evaluate for cholesteatoma (Fig. 5) and retraction pockets, especially in a patient with chronic ear drainage.

Mastoid tenderness and an anteriorly rotated pinna may be suggestive of acute mastoiditis in the setting of otitis media. Lateral gaze

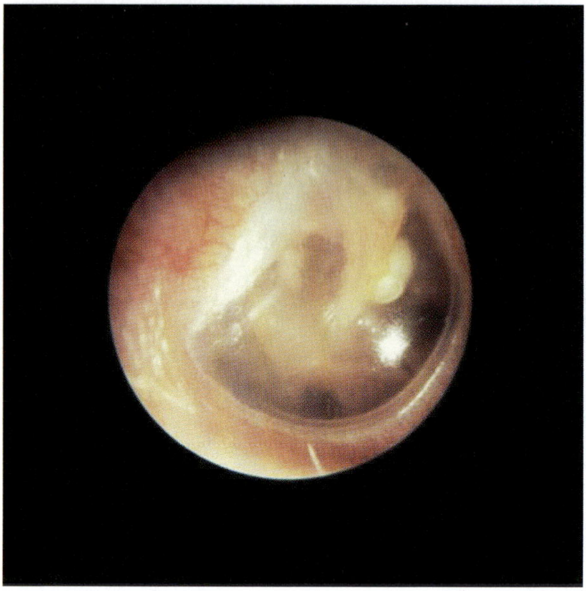

**Fig. 5.** A congenital cholesteatoma can be seen in the upper posterior quadrant just behind the tympanic membrane.

palsy or facial nerve paresis with nausea and vomiting are concerning signs for extra or intracranial complications of the disease. It is therefore important to perform a full cranial nerve exam on all patients.

## Audiologic Evaluation

All patients should undergo a formal hearing evaluation. This not only includes the audiometric examination of hearing thresholds, but also tympanometry, which evaluates the mobility of the tympanic membrane. A normal tympanogram (type A) has a peak transmission of sound at atmospheric pressure (0 daPa) (Fig. 6A). However, the presence of middle ear fluid will dampen the signal transmission, and typically result in a flattened curve across the entire pressure spectrum (type B) (Fig. 6B). Occasionally, children with eustachian tube dysfunction may have reduced middle ear pressure, resulting in

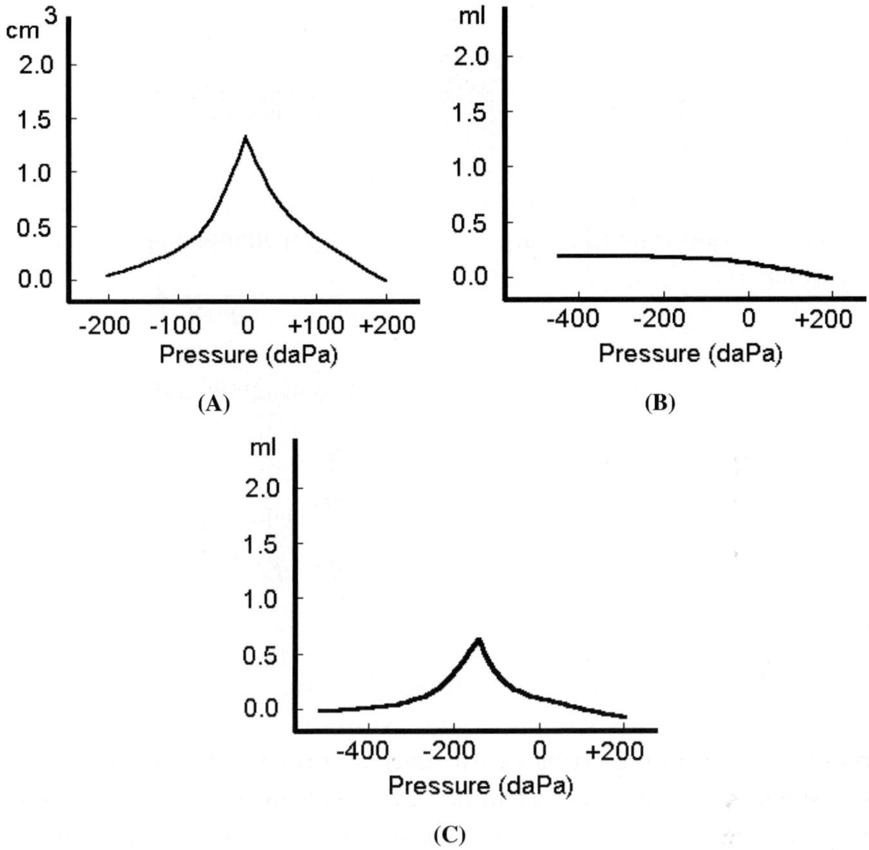


**Fig. 6.** **(A)** Type A tympanogram, **(B)** type B tympanogram and **(C)** type C tympanogram.

a retracted tympanic membrane. In these children, the pressure of maximum sound transmission is negative (type C) (Fig. 6C); however, the shape is similar to that of a type A tympanogram.

Audiometric testing varies according the children's age and can include behavior observational audiometry, visual reinforcement audiometry, play audiometry, conventional audiometry, otoacoustic emissions, and auditory brainstem response testing. Audiologic testing will usually distinguish a conductive hearing loss from a sensorineural hearing loss. Commonly, children with otitis media demonstrate mild to moderate conductive hearing loss in the affected ear(s) with a flat (type B) tympanogram(s).

## MANAGEMENT

The goal of treating otitis media is to avoid hearing loss that can impact speech and language as well to prevent the rarer otologic sequelae of tympanic retraction, ossicular erosion, cholesteatoma and extra- and intracranial complications. Clinical practice guidelines have been developed by the American Academy of Pediatrics (AAP), American Academy of Otolaryngology–Head and Neck Surgery (AAO–HNS), and American Academy of Family Physicians (AAFP) to treat both acute otitis media and otitis media with effusion in children between two months and 12 years of age.[24,25]

### Acute Otitis Media

According to the guidelines, the first step in management is confirming the diagnosis of otitis media which must include (1) a history of acute onset of signs and symptoms, (2) the presence of middle ear effusion, as demonstrated by bulging, decreased mobility, or the presence of an air-fluid level behind the tympanic membrane or otorrhea, and (3) signs and symptoms of middle ear inflammation, either as distinct erythema of the tympanic membrane or distinct otalgia.[24] Visualization of the tympanic membrane in small children can be difficult and tympanometry is a helpful tool to confirm the presence of middle ear effusion.

Not all patients require antibiotics. In fact, it is acceptable to wait 48 to 72 hours before instituting antibiotic treatment in a subset of patients.[26] Specifically, all patients greater than two years of age without a severe illness as defined by a temperature of greater than 39°C or severe otalgia can be observed. Likewise, in children between the ages of six months to two years without a severe illness and uncertain diagnosis, initial observation is also recommended. However, antibiotics should be given in all children less than six months regardless of diagnosis confirmation and in children under two years with a confirmed diagnosis.

Any child with severe symptoms should be given antimicrobial therapy immediately. Children should be re-examined if they have not improved after 48 to 72 hours. Those who underwent observation and have persistent symptoms should be treated with antibiotics and those who do not respond to initial antibiotics should be changed to a different antimicrobial. While there has been a general trend towards initial observation,[27,28] a recent meta-analysis of randomized controlled trials comparing antibiotic use versus placebo and antibiotic use versus watchful waiting showed that early antibiotic treatment resulted in an improved clinical course with decreased persistence of symptoms in children with acute otitis media, although there was no difference in cure rate.[29] Because of the persistence of symptoms such as fever and irritability, parents, on average, required an additional 0.3 to 4 quality-adjusted life-days for observing the child in lieu of antibiotic therapy.[30] There was no difference in the incidence of tympanic membrane perforations or development of middle ear effusions.[31] In addition, the early use of antibiotics resulted in increased side effects such as diarrhea.[29] Tympanocentesis (aspiration of fluid from the middle ear) does not appear to improve outcomes.

Although the early use of antibiotics has shown some benefit, their widespread use has resulted in increasing strains of resistant bacteria.[23] Since the 1990s, up to 70% of the *Streptococcus* isolated from children with acute otitis media are resistant to penicillin.[32] Therefore, in areas with high prevalence of *Streptococcus pneumoniae*, high-dose amoxicillin (80–90 mg/kg/day) for ten days is the recommended first-line therapy. Amoxicillin currently has little utility against *β-lactamase-positive Haemophilus influenza.* As a result, high dose amoxicillin-clauvulanate (90 mg/kg/day amoxicillin) is often used as the second-line therapy or first-line in patients with severe illness or recent prior history of antibiotic use for acute otitis media.[32] Macrolides have been used in the treatment of acute otitis media; however, they have high failure rates (>50%) in resistant bacteria.[33] An alternate second-line therapy to amoxicillin-clavulanate acid is intramuscular injection of ceftriaxone 50 mg/day for three days;[26] 97% eradication of *S. pneumoniae* could be achieved after three days as opposed to 52% after a one time dose of ceftriaxone.[34]

Recent evidence has demonstrated the clinical efficacy of childhood vaccinations against *Streptococcus pneumoniae* and *Haemophilus influenza* in preventing acute otitis media. In a study comparing children in New York and Tennessee, the use of the heptavalent pneumococcal conjugate vaccine has increased from <1% in 1998–1999 to 75% in 2000–2001 and correspondingly, the frequency of acute otitis media in these children by two years of age had decreased by 28% and 17%, respectively.[35] While a meta-analysis of vaccine prevention of acute otitis media shows a mild risk-reduction of 6%–7% in children vaccinated during infancy, trials involving vaccination of older children show no benefit in preventing further otitis media episodes.[36] It is therefore important to stress to parents the importance of timely vaccinations in their children. However, with the introduction of new vaccines other virulent strains not covered by existing vaccines are now emerging, and the microbial profile for otitis media is continuously changing.[23,37,38]

While many children are able to outgrow acute otitis media, it is currently recommended that children with three episodes in six months or four episodes over a 12-month span undergo surgical intervention with the placement of tympanostomy tubes.[14] However, recent studies have shown that children who develop acute otitis media during the first six months of life have an increased risk of recurrent acute otitis media[39] and some have proposed age-based risk stratification, with earlier tympanostomy tube placement in younger infants.[40]

## Chronic Otitis Media with Effusion

Children with chronic otitis media with effusion often present with fluid in the middle ear without any signs of acute ear infection. The diagnosis should be confirmed by pneumatic otoscopy and can be verified with tympanometry documenting Type B tympanograms. Documentation of laterality, duration of effusion and presence of associated symptoms is important to distinguish otitis media with effusion from acute otitis media. Children at risk for speech, language, or other forms of developmental delay should be identified and intervention should be expedited. Such children include those with speech delay, hearing loss independent of otitis media, associated syndromes (e.g. Down syndrome), craniofacial anomalies, autism or other pervasive developmental disorders, visual impairments or developmental delay.[16] These children may need more prompt intervention to avoid interference with their speech and language development.

Healthy children can be managed with watchful waiting for up to and possibly beyond three months. The natural course of otitis media with effusion is that 60% will have persistent effusion at one month, but 90% will have complete resolution by three months.[41] If after three months, the effusion persists, auditory testing is recommended. If there is documented hearing loss, surgical intervention may be warranted. Children who have normal hearing and speech development may be able to be observed for longer periods.[42] All children should be re-evaluated every three to six months to document resolution of effusion if pressure-equalization tubes have not been placed.

Medical intervention for otitis media with effusion is controversial. While some studies have shown short-term improvement in hearing loss with the use of steroids (oral or nasal) and antibiotics as compared to antibiotics alone, there was no difference in improvement over long term follow-up.[43] Additionally, there was no benefit in the use of antihistamines or decongestants in the resolution of the effusions. Rather, there was an 11% increased risk in side effects of these medicines.[44] As a result, the current evidence does not support use of decongestants, antihistamines, steroids or antibiotics for routine management of COME.[16]

Surgical intervention depends on multiple factors including duration of the effusion hearing status and associated speech and language delays, and other associated medical conditions that may place a child "at-risk."[25] Myringotomy with tympanostomy tube placement should be the first surgery performed for such children. A myringotomy alone to drain the effusion has no advantage over nonsurgical intervention.[45] Adenoidectomy, in addition to tympanostomy tube placement, may be considered in first-line treatment in children greater than four years and those with severe otitis media.[46] Myringotomy with tube placement resulted in a decreased number of patients with effusions (9%–16.4%) as compared to patients without intervention (56%) at one year follow-up.[47] However, 20%–50% of patients may continue to have recurrent or persistent effusions and may require repeat surgery after extrusion of their first set of tubes. Adenoidectomy at the time of repeat tympanostomy tube placement is strongly recommended as it has been shown to reduce the need for further surgery by 50%.[48]

## EMERGENCY EVALUATION AND TREATMENT

Acute otitis media rarely presents as an emergency. However, because of the potentially devastating effects of some complications, urgent evaluation with admission for high-dose intravenous antibiotic therapy may be indicated. A child with high fevers, altered mental status, headache, or cranial neuropathies should be seen immediately. Any child who continues to be symptomatic despite appropriate antibiotic therapy should be evaluated with an elevated level of suspicion for potential complications. A high-resolution temporal bone CT is often the first imaging modality of choice. However, in the setting of intracranial extension, an MRI may be also be indicated. If there is evidence of otitis media with possible intracranial extension, the child should be admitted immediately for high-dose intravenous antimicrobial therapy with potential surgical intervention.

## COMPLICATIONS AND THEIR MANAGEMENT

Although acute otitis media is usually a self-limiting disease, serious complications, though rare in the era of antibiotics, can arise in a subset of patients and can be associated with high mortality. The complications are often separated into two categories: extra-or intracranial and are listed in Table 1.

**Table 1. Complications of otitis media.**

| Extracranial | Intracranial |
|---|---|
| Hearing loss | Meningitis |
| Tympanic membrane perforation | Subdural empyema |
| Chronic suppurative otitis media | Brain abscess |
| Cholesteatoma | Extradural abscess |
| Tympanosclerosis | Lateral sinus thrombosis |
| Ossicular discontinuity/fixation | Otitic hydrocephalus |
| Mastoiditis | |
| Petrositis | |
| Labyrinthitis | |
| Facial paresis or paralysis | |
| Cholesterol granuloma | |

## Extracranial Complications

More minor extracranial complications such as hearing loss and/or tympanic membrane perforation, can be relatively common. Typically, hearing loss is due to acute suppurative otitis media or persistent perforation after a myringotomy. Hearing loss associated with a tympanic membrane perforation can range from 0 to 40 dB dependent on the size of the perforation and the status of the middle ear ossicles.[49] Chronic inflammation of the middle ear can lead to tympanosclerosis of the tympanic membrane and middle ear mucosa in 14% to 43% of the cases.[50,51] Tympanosclerosis limited to the tympanic membrane, also known as myringosclerosis, is usually not associated with hearing loss. However, with extension into the middle ear, the ossicular chain can become fixed, resulting in a conductive hearing loss.[52]

In the setting of persistent perforation, children can present with chronic suppurative otitis media. Otorrhea can be present due to chronic infection or inflammation of the middle ear, however this should always raise the suspicion for cholesteatoma. Cholesteatoma is an expanding mass of squamous debris within the middle ear. Because cholesteatoma can erode the ossicles, these children can have ossicular discontinuity resulting in conductive hearing loss.

The treatment for such cases is surgical and requires a referral to an otolaryngologist. If there is concern for a cholesteatoma, a high-resolution computed tomography imaging of the temporal bone is warranted. Rarely, cholesteatoma can lead to intracranial complications (see below).

Acute mastoiditis is a rare, but more serious complication in which the mastoid air cells are inflamed and filled with fluid. Children present with mastoid tenderness and erythema, fevers, otalgia, and anterolateral auricular protrusion (Fig. 7A). If left untreated, the infection can spread intracranially. A high-resolution CT should be obtained to diagnose coalescent mastoiditis, which is defined as erosion of the bony septations between mastoid air cells (Fig. 7B) Many cases of acute mastoiditis will resolve with

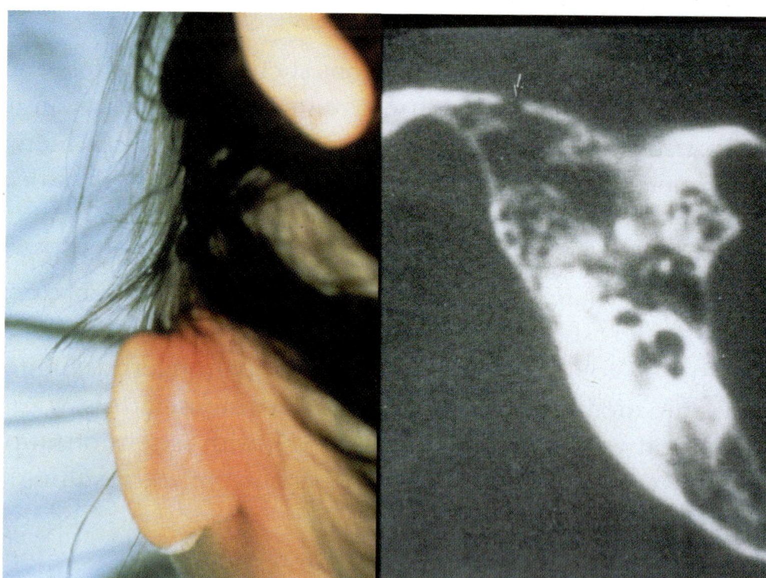

(A) (B)

**Fig. 7.** (**A**) The auricle of the ear is rotated forward and the mastoid tip is erythematous, common findings in a child presenting with acute mastoiditis. (**B**) CT scan of the mastoid in a child with mastoiditis. Notice the destruction of the bony septations of the mastoid air cells with destruction of bone at the most lateral aspect (arrow).

intravenous antimicrobial therapy, with the occasional requirement of a myringotomy with or without tube placement for culture and drainage of fluid. In patients with coalescent mastoiditis, or if conservative management fails for non-coalescent mastoiditis, a mastoidectomy should be performed.[49]

When severe, the suppurative process of mastoiditis can erode through the mastoid cortex and enter the superior neck space between the digastric and sternocleidomastoid muscles.[53] This laterocervical abscess is known as Bezold's abscess. The infection can then reach the deep compartments of the neck and even the mediastinum. Because Bezold's abscesses are associated with a well-pneumatized mastoid bone, which is rare in young children, this complication is uncommon in young children.[54,55]

The facial nerve courses through the temporal bone and before the antibiotic era, the incidence of facial nerve paresis (Fig. 8) due to otitis media was approximately 0.5%. Fortunately, it is now a rare occurrence.[56] Early development of facial paresis is thought to be due to acute edema of the nerve within the temporal bone. Later development is attributed to the bony erosion of the facial canal exposing the nerve to the disease itself.[57]

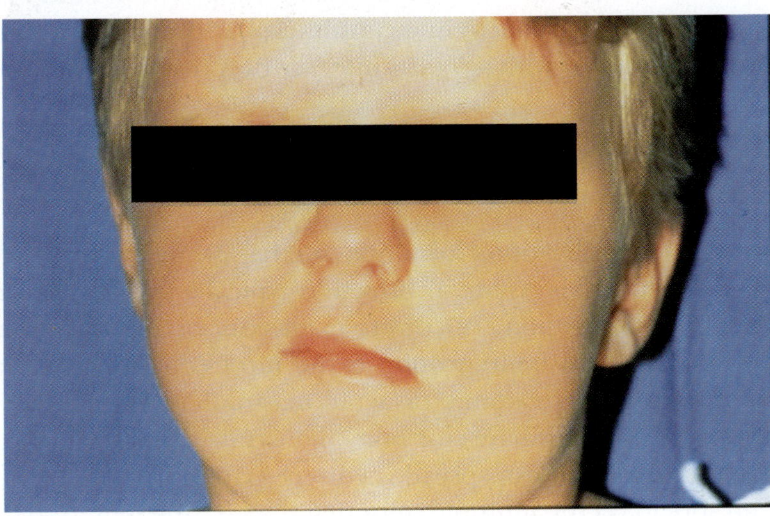

**Fig. 8.** Facial paralysis.

As in acute mastoiditis, intravenous antibiotics and myringotomy are employed as initial treatment. However, recent data also recommend the use of intravenous steroids.[56,58] In the event that the paralysis is refractory to conservative management, a high-resolution CT should be obtained and a mastoidectomy and possible facial nerve decompression should be considered.[49]

Labyrinthitis can occur as an isolated phenomenon or in conjunction with otitis media and typically presents with vertigo, nausea and vomiting. Patients often exhibit nystagmus. Treatment requires intravenous antibiotics to prevent intracranial spread and supportive therapy. If there is any concern for intracranial extension, a lumbar puncture is indicated and additional surgical intervention may be required.

Petrositis is a rare complication and classically presents with Gradenigo's triad of otorrhea, retro-orbital pain and abducens palsy; a constellation of symptoms that suggests infectious spread to the petrous apex. Because the petrous apex has poor drainage pathways and is adjacent to the central nervous system, it is more worrisome for intracranial extension.[49] While a high-resolution CT scan can detect bony erosion, an MRI scan assists in determining intracranial extension.[59] Like many of the other extracranial complications, high dose intravenous antibiotics and myringotomy are the first-line therapy with surgical intervention reserved for recalcitrant disease.

## Intracranial Complications

Intracranial complications of otitis media, while rare (0.13%–1.97%),[60,61] can be devastating. Infection typically spreads via three routes: (1) bone erosion, (2) direct extension, or (3) thrombophlebitis. Extension via bone erosion is the most common route and can be due to cholesteatoma, or acute mastoiditis. Alternatively, in the setting of a skull fracture or bony dehiscence, either congenital or acquired, infection can spread via direct extension. Finally, infection can spread via the multiple veins that traverse the temporal bone and lead to intracranial thrombosis of dural venous sinuses.[62]

Meningitis and brain abscesses are among the most common intracranial complications of otitis media.[60] Abscesses are typically located adjacent to the temporal bone and are most commonly due to spread via bony erosion. A transmastoid approach for drainage is typically adequate.[60] Lumbar puncture is indicated for the diagnosis of meningitis and should always be preceded by an imaging study (CT or MRI) to rule out risk factors for potential herniation.

The most common intracranial abscess is epidural and is most typically located between the temporal bone and the dura. This complication often precedes other intracranial complications and should be aggressively treated with transmastoid drainage and intravenous antibiotics.

Subdural empyemas are considerably rarer but have a high morbidity and mortality and consist of pus between the dura and arachanoid membrane. An MRI is the image of choice[63] and emergent surgical drainage with high dose intravenous antibiotics is indicated.[62] Lateral sinus thrombosis, also a rare entity, presents with fever, headache, nausea, vomiting and neck pain; 50% of the patients will present with papilledema. CT and MR imaging allow identification of thrombosis of the lateral (transverse) sinus. CSF cultures are typically low yield due to initiation of antibiotics prior to lumbar puncture.[64] Initial treatment includes high dose intravenous antibiotics, myringotomy with tympanostomy tube with possible mastoidectomy. Anticoagulation therapy and surgical drainage of sinus thromboses continues to be debated in the literature.[65]

Otitic hydrocephalus is a syndrome characterized by increased intracranial pressures without focal neurologic deficits except those due to hydrocephalus.[66] Children typically present with headache, drowsiness, blurry vision, nausea and vomiting, or diplopia weeks to years after the development of otitis media.[62,67] It often presents in the association with superior or lateral sinus thrombosis. Treatment should surgically address any middle ear or mastoid disease, as well as the elevated intracranial pressure, usually with steroids, mannitol or other diuretics.[68]

## OPERATIVE INTERVENTIONS

### Indications

Hearing loss is the primary reason for children with chronic otitis media with effusion to undergo surgical intervention. As stipulated previously, children at risk for developmental, speech and language delay are candidates for tympanostomy tubes. Additionally, children with bilateral hearing loss for greater than three months may be candidates as well. For children with acute otitis media, surgical intervention should be considered when children have frequent recurrent symptoms despite appropriate antibiotic and medical treatment.

### Myringotomy with Tube Placement

Children who have met criteria for tympanostomy tube insertion can undergo this procedure on an outpatient basis. The procedure includes a small incision, typically made in the anterior-inferior quadrant of the tympanic membrane, followed by insertion of a tympanostomy tube. Tympanostomy tubes remain in place for an average of 1.5 years and usually extrude spontaneously. Tubes that have remained in place for three or more years are sometimes removed. While a tympanostomy tube is in place and patent, children who develop otitis media can generally initially be treated with antibiotic otic drops targeting the middle ear directly, in lieu of systemic antibiotics. Complications from tympanostomy insertion are rare and can include otorrhea, hearing loss, tympanic perforation, tube obstruction, and early extrusion with need for repeat tympanostomy tube insertion. Therefore, children are typically followed every few months to evaluate for tube extrusion as well as for potential complications from surgery. After tube extrusion, audiograms with tympanometry should be obtained to document a child's hearing status and middle ear status.

### Adenoidectomy

Children who continue to have episodes of otitis media after the extrusion of the first set of tympanostomy tubes are candidates for adenoidectomy at the time of their second tympanostomy tube insertion. Randomized control trials have shown that children who undergo adenoidectomy at the time of their second tube placement suffered one-third fewer episodes of otitis media.[69] The procedure is typically done in an outpatient setting. The procedure requires general anesthesia and is done transorally. Prior to removal of the adenoids the palate should be examined for any submucosal clefts or uvular abnormalities that may suggest that the child will be at increased risk for velopharyngeal insufficiency. The nasopharynx can be viewed with a dental mirror. The adenoid pad sits midline between the eustachian tubes and can be removed via curettage, electrocautery or power-assisted instrumentation.[70,71] Complications from adenoidectomy include velopharyngeal insufficiency, adenoid regrowth, nasopharyngeal stenosis and injury to the eustachian tube.

## SUMMARY

Otitis media is a common disease in the pediatric population. Depending on the history and presenting symptoms, treatment may vary from watchful waiting to surgical intervention.

## REFERENCES


1. Vernacchio L, Vezina RM, Mitchell AA. Management of acute otitis media by primary care physicians: trends since the release of the 2004 American Academy of Pediatrics/American Academy of Family Physicians clinical practice guideline. *Pediatrics* 2007;120:281–287.
2. Auinger P, Lanphear BP, Kalkwarf HJ, *et al.* Trends in otitis media among children in the United States. *Pediatrics* 2003;112:514–520.
3. Tos M. Epidemiology and natural history of secretory otitis. *Am J Otol* 1984;5:459–462.
4. Kontiokari T, Koivunen P, Niemela M, *et al.* Symptoms of acute otitis media. *Pediatr Infect Dis J* 1998;17:676–679.
5. Casselbrant ML, Mandel EM. Epidemiology. In: Rosenfeld RM, Bluestone CD, eds. *Evidence-Based Otitis Media,* 2nd Ed. Hamilton, Ontario: BC Decker; 2003, pp. 147–162.

6. Couch ME. History, physical examination and the preoperative evaluation. In: Flint PW, *et al.*, eds. *Cummings Otolaryngology Head & Neck Surgery*, 5th Ed. Philadelphia, PA: Elsevier Mosby, 2010.
7. Corbeel L. What is new in otitis media? *Eur J Pediatr* 2007;166:511–519.
8. Bluestone CD. Anatomy and physiology of the eustachian tube system. In: Bailey BJ, Johnson JT, eds. *Head and Neck Surgery — Otolaryngology*. Philadelphia: Lippincott Williams & Wilkins; 2006, pp. 1253–1264.
9. Proctor B. Embryology and anatomy of the eustachian tube. *Arch Otolaryngol* 1967;86:503–514.
10. Ishijima K, Sando I, Balaban C, *et al.* Length of the eustachian tube and its postnatal development: computer-aided three-dimensional reconstruction and measurement study. *Ann Otol Rhinol Laryngol* 2000;109:542–548.
11. Holborow C. Eustachian tubal function: changes throughout childhood and neuro-muscular control. *J Laryngol Otol* 1975;89:47–55.
12. Seibert JW, Danner CJ. Eustachian tube function and the middle ear. *Otolaryngol Clin North Am* 2006;39:1221–1235.
13. Swarts JD, Rood SR. The morphometry and three-dimensional structure of the adult eustachian tube: implications for function. *Cleft Palate J* 1990;27:374–381.
14. Bluestone CD, Klein JO. Otitis media and eustachian tube dysfunction. In: Bluestone CD., *et al.*, eds. *Pediatric Otolaryngology*, 4th Ed. Philadelphia: Saunders 2003, pp. 474–685.
15. Tasker A, Dettmar PW, Panetti M, *et al.* Is gastric reflux a cause of otitis media with effusion in children? *Laryngoscope* 2002;112:1930–1934.
16. Kenna MA, Latz AD. Otitis media with effusion. Philadelphia: Lippincott Williams and Wilkins, 2006.
17. Shiao AS, Guo YC, Hsieh ST, *et al.* Bacteriology of medically refractory acute otitis media in children: a 9-year retrospective study. *Int J Pediatr Otorhinolaryngol* 2004;68:759–765.
18. Harrison CJ, Woods C, Stout G, *et al.* Susceptibilities of Haemophilus influenzae, Streptococcus pneumoniae, including serotype 19A, and Moraxella catarrhalis paediatric isolates from 2005 to 2007 to commonly used antibiotics. *J Antimicrob Chemother* 2009;63:511–519.
19. Black S, Shinefield H, Fireman B, *et al.* Efficacy, safety and immunogenicity of heptavalent pneumococcal conjugate vaccine in children. Northern California Kaiser Permanente Vaccine Study Center Group. *Pediatr Infect Dis J* 2000;19:187–195.

20. Benninger MS. Acute bacterial rhinosinusitis and otitis media: changes in pathogenicity following widespread use of pneumococcal conjugate vaccine. *Otolaryngol Head Neck Surg* 2008;138:274–278.
21. Casey JR, Pichichero ME. Changes in frequency and pathogens causing acute otitis media in 1995–2003. *Pediatr Infect Dis J* 2004;23:824–882.
22. Eskola J, Kilpi T, Palmu A, *et al.* Efficacy of a pneumococcal conjugate vaccine against acute otitis media. *N Engl J Med* 2001;344:403–409.
23. Vergison A. Microbiology of otitis media: a moving target. *Vaccine* 2008;26 Suppl 7:G5–10.
24. Neff MJ. AAP, AAFP release guideline on diagnosis and management of acute otitis media. *Am Fam Physician* 2004;69:2713–2715.
25. American Academy of Family Physicians, American Academy of Otolaryngology — Head and Neck Surgery, and American Academy of Pediatrics Subcommittee on Otitis Media with Effusion. Otitis media with effusion. *Pediatrics* 2004;113:1412–1429.
26. Subcommittee on Management of Acute Otitis Media. Diagnosis and management of acute otitis media. *Pediatrics* 2004;113:1451–1465.
27. Miller GE, Hudson J. Children and antibiotics: analysis of reduced use, 1996–2001. *Med Care* 2006;44:I36–44.
28. Arnold SR, Bush AJ. Decline in inappropriate antibiotic use over a decade by pediatricians in a Tennessee community. *Ambul Pediatr* 2006;6:225–229.
29. Vouloumanou EK, Karageorgopoulos DE, Kazantzi MS, *et al.* Antibiotics versus placebo or watchful waiting for acute otitis media: a meta-analysis of randomized controlled trials. *J Antimicrob Chemother* 2009;64:16–24.
30. Meropol SB. Valuing reduced antibiotic use for pediatric acute otitis media. *Pediatrics* 2008;121:669–673.
31. Falagas ME, Kotsantis IK, Vouloumanou EK, *et al.* Antibiotics versus placebo in the treatment of women with uncomplicated cystitis: a meta-analysis of randomized controlled trials. *J Infect* 2009;58:91–102.
32. Segal N, Leibovitz E, Dagan R, *et al.* Acute otitis media-diagnosis and treatment in the era of antibiotic resistant organisms: updated clinical practice guidelines. *Int J Pediatr Otorhinolaryngol* 2005;69:1311–1319.
33. Dagan R, Leibovitz E, Fliss DM, *et al.* Bacteriologic efficacies of oral azithromycin and oral cefaclor in treatment of acute otitis media in infants and young children. *Antimicrob Agents Chemother* 2000;44:43–50.

34. Leibovitz E, Piglansky L, Raiz S, *et al.* Bacteriologic efficacy of a three-day intramuscular ceftriaxone regimen in nonresponsive acute otitis media. *Pediatr Infect Dis J* 1998;17:1126–1131.
35. Poehling KA, Szilagyi PG, Grijalva CG, *et al.* Reduction of frequent otitis media and pressure-equalizing tube insertions in children after introduction of pneumococcal conjugate vaccine. *Pediatrics* 2007;119:707–715.
36. Jansen AG, Hak E, Veenhoven RH, *et al.* Pneumococcal conjugate vaccines for preventing otitis media. *Cochrane Database Syst Rev* 2009:CD001480.
37. Pichichero ME, Casey JR. Evolving microbiology and molecular epidemiology of acute otitis media in the pneumococcal conjugate vaccine era. *Pediatr Infect Dis J* 2007;26:S12–16.
38. McEllistrem MC, Adams JM, Patel K, *et al.* Acute otitis media due to penicillin-nonsusceptible *Streptococcus pneumoniae* before and after the introduction of the pneumococcal conjugate vaccine. *Clin Infect Dis* 2005;40:1738–1744.
39. Teele DW, Klein JO, Rosner B. Epidemiology of otitis media during the first seven years of life in children in greater Boston: a prospective, cohort study. *J Infect Dis* 1989;160:83–94.
40. Higgins TS, McCabe SJ, Bumpous JM, *et al.* Medical decision analysis: indications for tympanostomy tubes in RAOM by age at first episode. *Otolaryngol Head Neck Surg* 2008;138:50–56.
41. Teele DW, Klein JO, Rosner BA. Epidemiology of otitis media in children. *Ann Otol Rhinol Laryngol Suppl* 1980;89:5–6.
42. Paradise JL, Campbell TF, Dollaghan CA, *et al.* Developmental outcomes after early or delayed insertion of tympanostomy tubes. *N Engl J Med* 2005;353:576–586.
43. Thomas CL, Simpson S, Butler CC, *et al.* Oral or topical nasal steroids for hearing loss associated with otitis media with effusion in children. *Cochrane Database Syst Rev* 2006;3:CD001935.
44. Griffin GH, Flynn C, Bailey RE, *et al.* Antihistamines and/or decongestants for otitis media with effusion (OME) in children. *Cochrane Database Syst Rev* 2006:CD003423.
45. Mandel EM, Rockette HE, Bluestone CD, *et al.* Efficacy of myringotomy with and without tympanostomy tubes for chronic otitis media with effusion. *Pediatr Infect Dis J* 1992;11:270–277.

46. Gates GA, Avery CA, Prihoda TJ, *et al.* Effectiveness of adenoidectomy and tympanostomy tubes in the treatment of chronic otitis media with effusion. *N Engl J Med* 1987;317:1444–1451.
47. Mandel EM, Rockette HE, Bluestone CD, *et al.* Myringotomy with and without tympanostomy tubes for chronic otitis media with effusion. *Arch Otolaryngol Head Neck Surg* 1989;115:1217–1224.
48. Coyte PC, Croxford R, McIsaac W, *et al.* The role of adjuvant adenoidectomy and tonsillectomy in the outcome of the insertion of tympanostomy tubes. *N Engl J Med* 2001;344:1188–1195.
49. Gross ND, McMenomey SO. Aural complications of otitis media. In: Glasscock ME, Gulya AJ, eds. *Surgery of the Ear,* 5th Ed. Hamilton, Ontario: BC Decker, 2003.
50. Sheehy JL, House WF. Tympanosclerosis. *Arch Otolaryngol* 1962;76: 151–157.
51. Bhaya MH, Schachern PA, Morizono T, *et al.* Pathogenesis of tympanosclerosis. *Otolaryngol Head Neck Surg* 1993;109:413–420.
52. Kroon DF, Strasnick B. Diseases of the auricle, external auditory canal, and tympanic membrane. In: Glasscock ME, Gulya AJ, eds. *Surgery of the Ear,* 5th Ed. Hamilton, Ontario: BC Decker, 2003, pp. 345–367.
53. Gaffney RJ, O'Dwyer TP, Maguire AJ. Bezold's abscess. *J Laryngol Otol* 1991;105:765–766.
54. Marioni G, de Filippis C, Tregnaghi A, *et al.* Bezold's abscess in children: case report and review of the literature. *Int J Pediatr Otorhinolaryngol* 2001;61:173–177.
55. Hill FT. Bezold's abscess. *Ann Otol Rhinol Laryngol* 1968;77:984–985.
56. Popovtzer A, Raveh E, Bahar G, *et al.* Facial palsy associated with acute otitis media. *Otolaryngol Head Neck Surg* 2005;132:327–329.
57. Pollok RA, Brown LA. Facial paralysis in otitis media. In: Graham MD, House WF, eds. Disorders of the Facial Nerve. New York: Raven Press, 1982, pp. 221–224.
58. Joseph EM, Sperling NM. Facial nerve paralysis in acute otitis media: cause and management revisited. *Otolaryngol Head Neck Surg* 1998; 118:694–696.
59. Burston BJ, Pretorius PM, Ramsden JD. Gradenigo's syndrome: successful conservative treatment in adult and paediatric patients. *J Laryngol Otol* 2005;119:325–329.

60. Penido Nde O, Borin A, Iha LC, *et al.* Intracranial complications of otitis media: 15 years of experience in 33 patients. *Otolaryngol Head Neck Surg* 2005;132:37–42.
61. Osma U, Cureoglu S, Hosoglu S. The complications of chronic otitis media: report of 93 cases. *J Laryngol Otol* 2000;114:97–100.
62. Levine SC, De Souza C. Intracranial complications of otitis media. In: Glasscock ME, Gulya AJ, eds. *Surgery of the Ear,* 5th Ed. Hamilton, Ontario: BC Decker, 2003.
63. Weingarten K, Zimmerman RD, Becker RD, *et al.* Subdural and epidural empyemas: MR imaging. *AJR Am J Roentgenol* 1989;152:615–621.
64. Teichgraeber JF, Per-Lee JH, Turner JS, Jr. Lateral sinus thrombosis: a modern perspective. *Laryngoscope* 1982;92:744–751.
65. Christensen N, Wayman J, Spencer J. Lateral sinus thrombosis: a review of seven cases and proposal of a management algorithm. *Int J Pediatr Otorhinolaryngol* 2009;73:581–584.
66. Lenz RP, McDonald GA. Otitic hydrocephalus. *Laryngoscope* 1984; 94:1451–1454.
67. Tomkinson A, Mills RG, Cantrell PJ. The pathophysiology of otitic hydrocephalus. *J Laryngol Otol* 1997;111:757–759.
68. Sadoghi M, Dabirmoghaddam P. Otitic hydrocephalus: case report and literature review. *Am J Otolaryngol* 2007;28:187–190.
69. Paradise JL, Bluestone CD, Rogers KD, *et al.* Efficacy of adenoidectomy for recurrent otitis media in children previously treated with tympanostomy-tube placement. Results of parallel randomized and nonrandomized trials. *JAMA* 1990;263:2066–2073.
70. Rodriguez K, Murray N, Guarisco JL. Power-assisted partial adenoidectomy. *Laryngoscope* 2002;112:26–28.
71. Elluru RG, Johnson L, Myer CM, 3rd. Electrocautery adenoidectomy compared with curettage and power-assisted methods. *Laryngoscope* 2002;112:23–25.

# 2

# Otitis Externa

*Raymond C. Maguire and Joseph E. Dohar*

## INTRODUCTION

Otitis externa is an inflammatory condition of the external auditory canal (EAC) most commonly of infectious etiology. Approximately 10% of all individuals will experience otitis externa, and 90% of cases are unilateral.[1] The incidence of acute diffuse bacterial otitis externa (AOE) peaks between ages seven and 12 years, then declines after 50 years of age.[2] The spectrum of disease ranges from mild inflammation of the EAC skin to life threatening necrotizing osteomyelitis of the skull base.

## ANATOMY OF THE EAC

The external auditory canal is an epithelial lined 2.5-cm channel. The lateral one-third of the EAC is composed of a cartilaginous infrastructure lined with thick skin that contains hair, sebaceous and apocrine glands. Medially, the remaining two-thirds of the EAC is composed of a bony infrastructure lined with thin skin devoid of adnexal structures. The medial external auditory canal is richly supplied with nerve endings making it exquisitely sensitive to pain. If not offset by protective mechanisms, the warm temperature, humid environment and exfoliated skin combine to make the EAC a favorable environment for the growth of bacteria and fungi. Desquamation of skin in the external auditory canal proceeds in a medial to lateral direction and allows for natural egress of debris.

## PHYSIOLOGY OF THE EAC

Cerumen is produced in the lateral external auditory canal from the desquamation of the squamous epithelium and the secretion of lipids and peptides from pilosebaceous glands. Lipid rich cerumen is protective to the external auditory canal because of its hydrophobic nature, acidic pH, and lysozyme content all of which inhibit bacterial and fungal growth. The pH of cerumen ranges from 6.1–6.4 and its hydrophobic properties prevent water from penetrating and subsequently macerating the skin. Ideally, the external auditory canal should be self-cleansing, however, cerumen often impacts the EAC to the point where it compromises otologic health and function (i.e. conductive hearing). Cerumen impaction (see Fig. 1) may also obviate visualization of the tympanic membrane and middle ear, hence, interfering with the

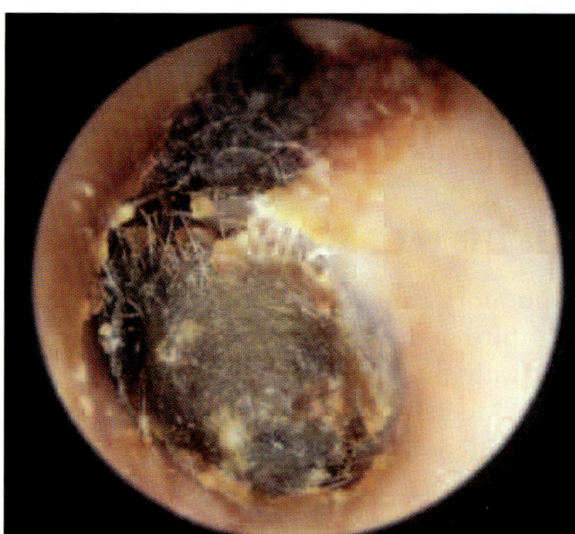

**Fig. 1.** Cotton swab abuse. Individuals who use cotton swabs may inadvertently push cerumen into the medial aspect of the external auditory canal. (Printed with permission from BC Decker Inc. from PDQ Otitis Externa, 2007.)

accurate diagnosis of pathological states. In such cases, cerumenectomy is indicated and most commonly performed with suction, irrigation, mechanical debridement or chemical cerumenolysis.

## PATHOPHYSIOLOGY OF AOE

AOE is most often precipitated by alteration of the EACs homeostatic acidity and humidity. Gray *et al.* have shown an elevated relative humidity of ear canals with a history of recurrent otitis externa compared to a control population. When the humidity exceeds 70%, an increased predisposition to recurrent AOE[3] occurs. Increased pH and inflammation support the growth of opportunistic bacteria and fungi that otherwise cannot thrive under normal physiologic EAC conditions. If water entry into the EAC removes the protective barrier of cerumen it, in turn, abruptly increases the EAC alkalinity thereby predisposing the external auditory canal to infection. Edema within the stratum corneum leads to occlusion of the apopilosebaceous units in the pre-inflammatory phase. This supports bacterial overgrowth, inflammation, pain, erythema, and otorrhea. Other predisposing factors in the development of acute otitis externa include dermatologic disorders (atopic dermatitis, psoriasis, and seborrheic dermatitis), immunocompromised states (HIV, diabetes), trauma, and prior temporal bone radiation exposure (see Table 1).

## DIAGNOSIS

Evaluation of patients with otitis externa begins with a complete medical history with care taken to identify possible comorbidities

**Table 1. Types of otitis externa.**

| |
|---|
| Furunculitis |
| Diffuse acute otitis externa |
| Chronic eczematoid otitis externa |
| Malignant otitis externa |
| Otomycosis |

**Table 2. Diagnosis of diffuse acute otitis externa.**[4]

1. Rapid onset (within 48 hours)
2. Symptoms
   - Otalgia, pruritis, aural fullness
   - +/– TMJ tenderness and hearing loss
3. Signs
   - Tenderness of the tragus and/or pinna
   - External auditory canal erythema and/or edema
   - +/– Otorrhea, lymphadenitis, tympanic membrane erythema, or cellulitis of the pinna or adjacent skin

such as diabetes, HIV, radiation exposure, dermatologic disorders, and any recent trauma. Pain is the most characteristic presenting symptom and is often out of proportion to physical findings (see Table 2). Diagnosis of AOE is heralded by the rapid onset of symptoms (usually within 48 hours) including otalgia, pruiritis, and aural fullness (see Fig. 2). Signs of AOE include tenderness to manipulation of the auricular cartilage, external auditory canal edema and erythema, with or without otorrhea, lymphadenitis or cellulitis of the pinnna (see Fig. 3). A complete physical exam including otoscopy, with pneumatic insufflation if tolerated, and removal of any debris that obscures adequate visualization is required for diagnosis.

Performing a thorough debridement of the external auditory canal is essential in arriving at the proper diagnosis and also maximizes treatment (see Table 3). Several techniques may be utilized when debriding the EAC including mechanical methods using "dry mopping," curette or suction. Advantages of suction include avoidance of trauma to the already inflamed epithelium, however, this instrumentation is rarely available in primary care settings and requires adequate training and experience. Dry mopping is best done with cotton twisted around a point to gently absorb serous secretions from the auditory canal. Sterile cotton-tip applicators may serve as a reasonable alternative. Commercially available Q-tips® should be avoided since their large size may traumatize the EAC and

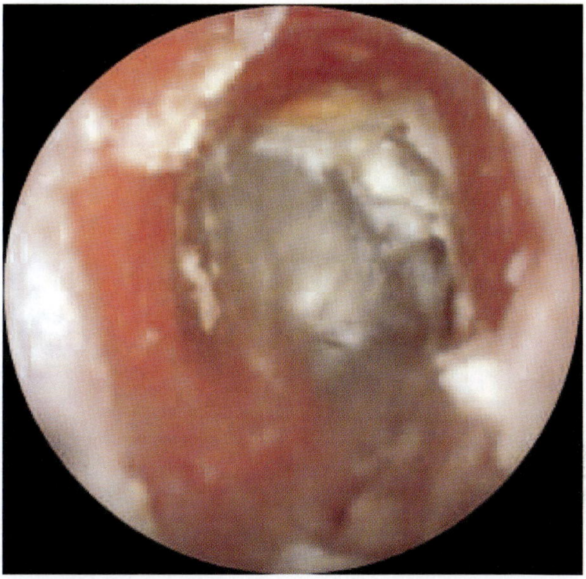

**Fig. 2.** Acute diffuse bacterial otitis externa. Characterized by a copious, creamy exudate that fills the medial canal with erythematous and edematous underlying skin. (Printed with permission from BC Decker Inc. from PDQ Otitis Externa, 2007.)

advance debris further medially. They are also too large to access debris in the bony EAC. Other methods of "aural toilet" include the placement and exchange of otowicks (see Fig. 4), and the use of antibiotic drops for thick crusted secretions. When the integrity of the tympanic membrane cannot be confirmed, avoid irrigation as the high pressure may disrupt the ossicles or potentially injure the cochlea and/or labyrinth. Also, irrigation may introduce infection into other compartments, such as the middle ear, not initially infected.

Acute diffuse otitis externa treatment guidelines have recently been published by the American Academy of Otolaryngology–Head and Neck Surgery (AAO–HNS) and are summarized in Table 4. The guidelines committee emphasized the importance of accurate diagnosis and careful attention to the treatment of pain associated with otitis externa. An evidence-based methodology was executed in order to arrive at the final recommendations (see Table 4).

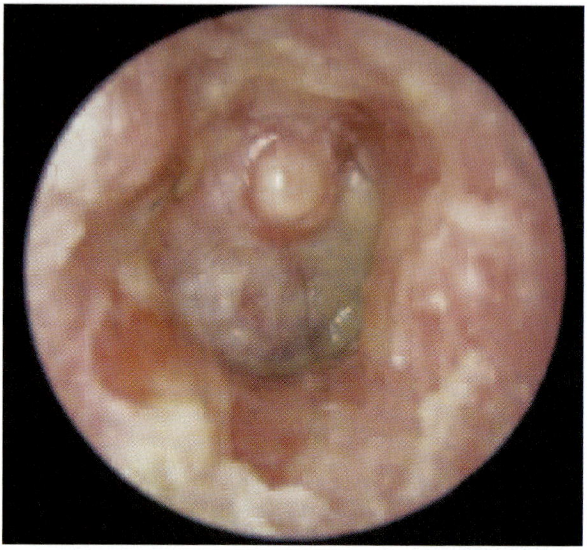

**Fig. 3.** Severe acute aspergillus otitis externa. The canal skin and tympanic membrane is often erythematous and ulcerated secondary to fungal invasion. Repeated aural toilet and application of antifungal agents is required. (Printed with permission from BC Decker Inc. from PDQ Otitis Externa, 2007.)

**Table 3. Clinical differential diagnosis.**

| Infectious | Non-infectious |
|---|---|
| Acute diffuse bacterial otitis externa | Allergic otitis externa (contact, atopic) |
| Chronic otitis externa | Irritant contact dermatitis |
| Necrotizing otitis externa | Psoriasis |
| Otomycosis | Seborrheic dermatitis |
| Viral otitis externa | Acne vulgaris |
| Furunculitis | Systemic lupus erythematosa |
| | Carcinoma |

Not unlike most medical conditions, arriving at the correct diagnosis is imperative. The primary challenge in making an accurate diagnosis lies in a facility with diagnostic pneumatic otoscopy. From the standpoint of history, other possible causes for otalgia and otorrhea should be eliminated. Some processes which mascarade as

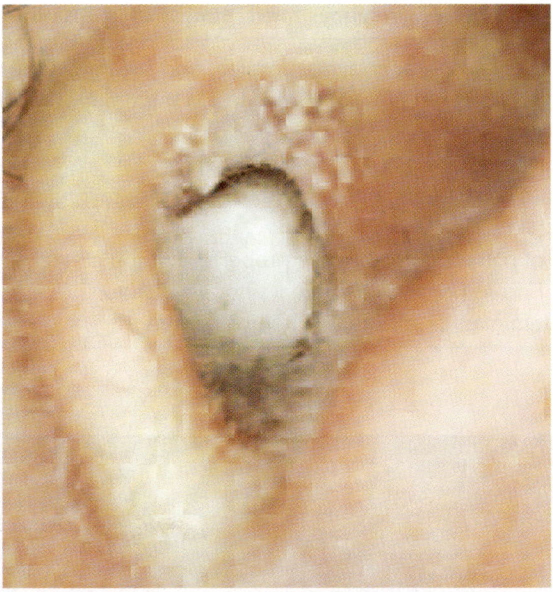

**Fig. 4.** Pope otowick. In severe cases of acute otitis externa, otowicks may need to be replaced daily to help debride the exudate from the canal. The wick is saturated with topical drops to increase the exposure of the antibiotic to the canal skin. Appropriate pain medication should be administered prior to otowick placement. (Printed with permission from BC Decker Inc. from PDQ Otitis Externa, 2007.)

acute diffuse bacterial otitis externa include other types of otitis externa such as furunculosis, eczema (i.e. dermatitic eczematoid otitis externa), sensitization to topical treatments (i.e. allergic otitis externa) and viral infections (i.e. herpes zoster oticus).

Furunculosis is differentiated from diffuse otitis externa in that in involves a focal segment of the external auditory canal, usually just one infected hair follicle in the lateral portion of the EAC. It presents with pain and otorrhea. Like acute diffuse otitis externa, it is of bacterial etiology most often caused by *S. aureus*. Treatment of furunculosis involves warm compresses, incision and drainage and antistaphyloccal topical possible systemic antibiotics.

Dermatologic conditions such as seborrhea (see Fig. 5), contact dermatitis, and eczema all result in inflammation of the ear canal skin, predisposing it to secondary infection. Contact dermatitis represents

**Table 4. AAO-HNS guidelines for treatment of acute otitis externa.**

| |
|---|
| Rule out other causes for otlagia, otorrhea, and inflammation |
| Identify factors that modify management: TM perforation, myringotomy tube, diabetes |
| Use of topical therapy as first line treatment |
| Use of non-ototoxic topical therapy in presence of myringotomy tube or perforation |
| Education of patents/caretakers on proper use of topical agents |
| Re-assess if no response to treatment after 48–72hours. |
| Use of systemic antibiotics only when warranted |

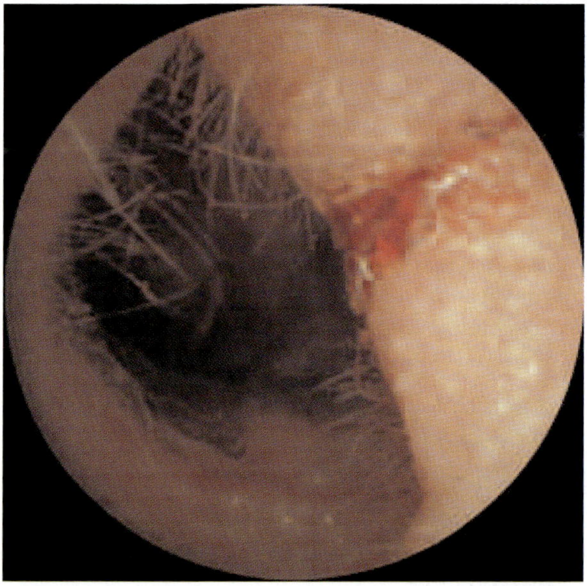

**Fig. 5.** External canal seborrheic dermatitis. Dry and scaly canal wall skin with excoriations indicate long standing seborrhea with puritis. (Printed with permission from BC Decker Inc. from PDQ Otitis Externa, 2007.)

allergic reactions to antigens such as metals, chemicals, drugs, and plastics. Neomycin is the most common otic preparation to cause sensitization and causes reactions in 5%–15% of individuals with chronic otitis externa[4] (see Fig. 6).

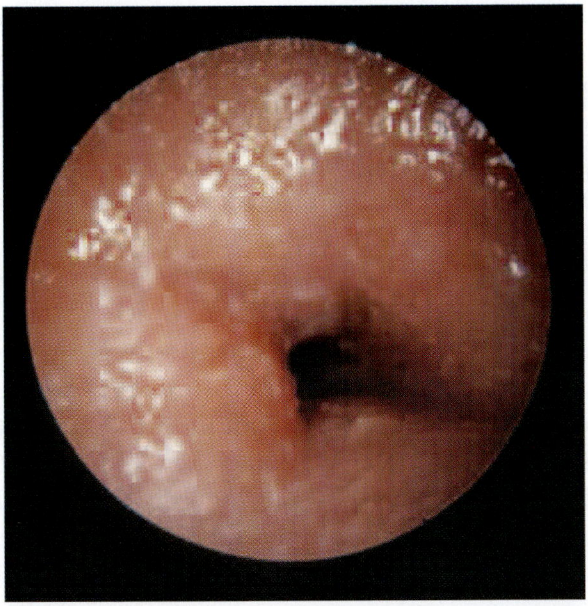

**Fig. 6.** Neomycin contact dermatitis. In long standing cases of external otitis the practitioner should consider underlying systemic disorders and allergic reactions. (Printed with permission from BC Decker Inc. from PDQ Otitis Externa, 2007.)

Comorbid factors must also be identified such as immunocompromise, past radiation exposure, trauma, and tympanic membrane perforation. These factors may alter the natural history of otitis externa and may warrant more advanced initial diagnostic investigations or more aggressive treatment.

Culture and sensitivity may be indicated when patients fail appropriate initial therapy (see Table 5). Indications for culture

**Table 5. When to culture in acute otitis externa.**

| | |
|---|---|
| 1. | Refractory cases |
| 2. | Recurrent cases |
| 3. | Disease extension beyond the EAC |
| 4. | Suppurative complications |
| 5. | Significant comorbidities (immunocompromise, diabetes) |
| 6. | Infection suspected to be atypical pathogen |

include refractory or recurrent cases, suppurative complications, significant comorbidities, and suspicion of atypical pathogens.

## ETIOLOGY

Acute diffuse otitis externa is most often bacterial, and infections tend to be polymicrobial with the most common pathogens including (Fig. 7) *Pseudomonas aeruginosa* and *Staphylococcus aureus*. Other less commonly isolated bacteria associated with acute diffuse otitis externa include *proteus* species, *Staphylococcus epidermidis*, *diptheriods*, and *E. coli*. Fungal pathogens isolated from the external auditory canal represent the next most common cause for otitis externa. Otomycosis is due to *Aspergillus niger* in 80% of patients, with *Candida albicans* and *Aspergillus fumigatus* is less commonly isolated.[5] Finally, otitis externa may also be caused by viral pathogens with the

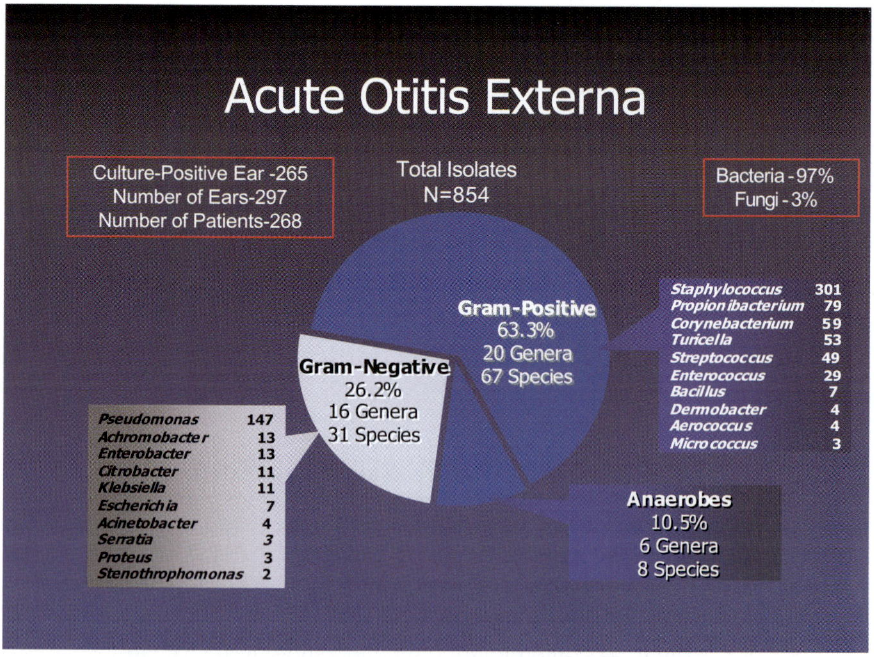


**Fig. 7.** Bacteriology of acute otitis externa. Oral communication from David Stroman.

most important cause being from the herpes virus. *Herpes zoster oticus* may be associated with significant morbidity which may include facial paralysis, hearing loss, and vertigo (Ramsey–Hunt syndrome). Vesicular eruptions delineate viral from bacterial or fungal causes of otitis externa. *Otitis externa hemmorrhagica* (*bullous myringitis*) is another viral type of acute otitis externa and is heralded by hemorrhagic bulla on the tympanic membrane.

## TREATMENT

The current recommendation for the initial treatment of diffuse acute otitis externa as set forth by the AAO–HNS employs ototopical preparations. Topical therapy should be used as first-line treatment in otherwise healthy individuals with diffuse acute otitis externa that is not complicated by osteitis, abscess formation, middle ear disease, or recurrent episodes of infection.[4] A list of FDA approved topical otic preparations is provided in Table 6. Advantages of topical therapy include direct delivery of medication to the target organs, less risk of treatment induced bacterial drug resistance, and fewer side effects. Also, courses of ototopical medications tend to be shorter in duration consisting of a week or less of treatment. Decreased treatment-induced resistance have been reported with topical medications most likely because topical agents are directly delivered to the site of infection at higher concentrations that far exceed the minimal inhibitory concentration for most bacterial pathogens. When canal edema is

**Table 6. Common topical otic preparations for treating acute otitis externa.**

| Active drug(s) | Trade name |
|---|---|
| • Acetic acid, aluminum acetate | • Otic Domeboro |
| • Acetic acid, hydrocortisone | • VoSol HC |
| • Neomycin, polymyxin B, hydrocortisone | • Cortisporin Otic |
| • Ciprofloxacin, hydrocortisone | • Cipro HC |
| • Ciprfloxacin, dexamethasone | • Ciprodex |
| • Ofloxacin | • Floxin Otic |

severe, it may be necessary to place a wick in the external auditory canal to enhance topical drug delivery. Wicks should be made of cellulose that expand as it is saturated with an aqeous solution and also allow for easy removal. One should avoid the use of cotton as this may fragment and become lodged in the ear canal.

There are currently many preparations available for the topical treatment of acute otitis externa. Various agents such as Cortisporin® Otic, combine multiple antibiotics in a single formulation. Historically, multiple antibiotics were combined to cover for *P. aeruginosa* and *S. aureus,* because no single agent was effective against both bacteria. Currently, newer agents in the fluoroquinolone family (Ciprodex®, Floxin® Otic, Cipro-HC®) have solved this dilemma with antimicrobial activity that covers both pathogens as monotherapy.[6,7] Furthermore, ototopical fluroquinolones as monotherapy have been shown to be as efficacious as the combination of topical and oral antibiotic treatment in otitis externa, with less propensity for resistance and adverse medication reactions.[8] Of note, cost is often less with ototopical monotherapy.

## COMBINATION OTOTOPICAL THERAPY

The use of steroids in ototopical preparations has also been extensively studied. Topical steroids in combination with aural antibiotics have resulted in a more rapid resolution of otalgia related to otitis externa (19 hours sooner in one study). It also appears that more potent steroids such as dexamethasone (compared to hydrocortisone) provide a greater anti-inflammatory response, especially in more severe cases. Furthermore, combination ototopical therapy has been shown to be superior to ototopical antibiotics without steroids and oral antibiotics, as well as reducing the incidence of antibiotic resistant organisms.[9]

## ROLE OF SYSTEMIC ANTIBIOTICS

Systemic antibiotics are rarely indicated in the treatment of acute otitis externa (see Table 7). For cases of persistent otitis externa,

**Table 7. Indication for using systemic antibiotics.**

| |
|---|
| Persistent otitis externa |
| Associated otitis media |
| Infection progression beyond the external auditory canal |
| High-risk patients |
| Signs of necrotizing otitis externa |
| Toxic appearance |

**Table 8. Treatment of otitis externa.**

| |
|---|
| Aural toilet |
| Topical antibiotics |
| Systemic antibiotics |

culture directed adjunctive systemic antibiotics may be considered, especially when compliance or inadequate delivery of a topical agent is suspected. One must also consider whether the organism is a true pathogen or merely a colonizing saprophyte. Such a distinction is not always trivial to make and is especially relevant in fungal otitis externa. Although a chapter unto itself, isolating a fungal organism from a draining ear suggests any one of six potential roles that the fungus may be playing. When infection is present in the middle ear or has progressed beyond the external auditory canal systemic antibiotics are also indicated. Finally, high risk patients or those with severe disease such as necrotizing otitis externa, require systemic antibiotic therapy. In the latter case, the mode of administration of the systemic antibiotic may also need to be considered. Although once a standard, intravenous or intramuscular systemic antibiotics are not always needed in such cases (see Table 8).

## RECURRENT OTITIS EXTERNA

Preventing the occurrence or recurrence of otitis externa relies on avoiding predisposing factors and appropriately treating underlying dermatologic conditions. Individuals with acute otitis externa should avoid swimming and any other activity that allows moisture to enter the external ear until the infection has resolved. A good measure of resolution is when cerumen production returns to normal. Avoiding swimming may be impractical. Considering alternatives such as ear plugs, drying agents, and prophylactic ototopicals is reasonable in such cases. Avoidance of trauma (e.g. Q®-tips, bobby-pins, pen caps) to the external auditory is paramont and dermatologic disorders should be aggressively treated as indicated with topical and/or systemic steroid medications. The use of acidifying and astringent solutions may also aid in prevention of otitis externa by restoring physiologic acidic pH of the external auditory canal and effectively drawing excess water from epithelial cells, respectively. Examples of such solutions include Otic Domeboro® which contains acetic acid (acidifying) and aluminum acetate (astringent). These precautions are especially valid for those individuals who suffer from recurrent otitis external and have repeated exposure to water.

## Necrotizing Otitis Externa

In the spectrum of otitis externa certain disease processes warrant further discussion not the least of which is necrotizing otitis externa. An older term no longer used, "malignant," emphasized the seriousness of this infection. Because of confusion that the term implied a neoplastic process, it has fallen out of favor. Other names for this disease include progessive, fulminant, and invasive otitis externa. Necrotizing otitis externa, by definition, is osteomyelitis of the skull base involving the cancellous bone of the skull, periosteum, dura, major blood vessels, and cranial nerves. These infections typically arise in hosts with compromised immunity such as in diabetics and patients undergoing chemotherapy. Signs and symptoms of necrotizing otitis externa include granulation tissue of the external auditory canal at the bony cartilaginous junction (see Fig. 8) and disproportionate otalgia and headache despite adequate topical treatment. Osteomyelitis of the skull base follows a particular pattern of spread from the epithelium of the external auditory canal into the retromandibular fossa through the fissures of Santorini into

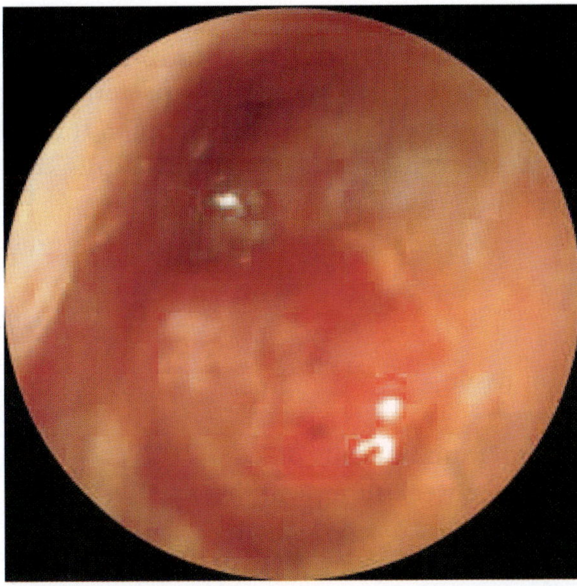

**Fig. 8.** Necrotizing otitis externa. Inflamed, erythematous canal skin with granulation tissue present at the bony/cartilaginous junction. (Printed with permission from BC Decker Inc. from PDQ Otitis Externa, 2007.)

the parotid space or through the tympanomastoid suture. Facial nerve palsy may result from infection around the stylomastoid foramen, with nerves of the jugular foramen representing the next most commonly affected structures.[10] Infection then progresses to involve the mastoid tip and jugular foramen with the potential to thrombose the sigmoid sinus. Dissemination of septic emboli and cranial nerve palsies may ensue along with progression of the osteomyelitis to involve the petrous apex, posterior and middle cranial fossa, base of the sphenoid sinus and clivus.

Necrotizing otitis externa is thought to result from either progression of acute disease, hematogenous seeding, or microvascular disease. Diminished blood supply in microvascular disease limits effective host immunologic response and, in turn, host defense against infection. Diabetes is the most common comorbidity and is present in 65%–90% of effected patients. Necrotizing otitis externa may result from bacterial or fungal infections and may also present with out any identifiable pathogen (culture-negative specimen). *Pseudomonas aeruginosa* represents the most common bacterial pathogen with *Aspergillus fumigatus* being then the most common fungal pathogen.[10]

Major diagnostic criteria for necrotizing otitis externa as outlined by Cohen and Friedman[11] include:

- Pain
- Exudate
- Edema
- Granulation tissue
- Microabscesses
- Positive technetium-99 scan
- Failure after one week of topical therapy
- Presence of *Pseudomonas aeruginosa*

The minor criteria include a positive CT scan, age greater 50 years, cranial nerve palsy, and diabetes mellitus. Skull base osteomyelitis may present from one month to one year after clinical resolution of more contained episodes of necrotizing otitis externa. The presence of low-grade fever, malaise and a unilateral unremitting headache requiring narcotic analgesia should alert the clinician to the potential for necrotizing otitis externa.

Staging of malignant otitis externa is facilitated with the use of radionucleotide imaging. Gallium-67 scanning identifies inflammation in the presence of functioning white blood cells, whereas, technetium-99 bone scanning reflects increased osteoblastic activity. A three-level staging system proposed by Benecke includes:

- Deep invasion into the soft tissue without bone involvement
- Extent of disease into the mastoid with early osteomyelitis and positive gallium and technetium scans
- Extensive skull base osteomyelitis with markedly positive gallium and technetium scans

Multiple studies have evaluated the relationship of comorbidities as they relate to the prognosis of necrotizing otitis externa.[12,13] The association of facial paralysis alone is not an adverse prognostic factor. Nasopharyngeal involvement was found to carry a grave prognosis. These studies indicate that patients with vascular pathology (elderly diabetics), exhibit worse outcomes most likely due to the impaired immunologic capacity of the ischemic tissues.

Treatment includes prolonged systemic antibiotic therapy with intravenous third generation cephalosporins or oral fluroquinolones and appropriate control of any metabolic derangements (tight blood sugar control). The excellent absorption of fluroquinolone antibiotics from the gastrointestinal tract allow for the oral administration of these medications for durations ranging from six weeks to six months with good rates of cure. For treatment of fungal necrotizing otitis externa intravenous amphotericin B has traditionally been the medication of choice, although recently the use of voriconazole has become the first line treatment of aspergillus necrotizing otitis externa secondary to its more favorable side effect profile.[14] Other adjunctive medical therapies for necrotizing otitis externa include hyperbaric oxygen treatments. Hyperbaric oxygen effectively increases wound $PO_2$ levels, enhances phagocytic oxidative killing of aerobic organisms and promotes angiogenesis and osteoneogenesis. Typical treatment courses involve administration of 100% oxygen for 90 minutes at 2.5 atmospheres of pressure five days per week for four weeks.

Surgical intervention is rarely indicated in necrotizing otitis externa, however, in situations where necrotic tissue or sequestrations of devitalized bone are present, debridement may be necessary. One should take caution in performing surgery because of the possibility of exposing facial planes not previously infected and surgery should be individualized to specific cases.

Disease progression can be followed with gallium-67 scanning and sedimentation rates. Multiple cranial neuropathies are poor prognostic signs. If present despite adequate antimicrobial and adjunctive therapies, multiple cranial neuropathies result in high mortality rates. Overall, when appropriate and timely treatment is implemented, recent cure rates in the range of 80%–100% have been reported.

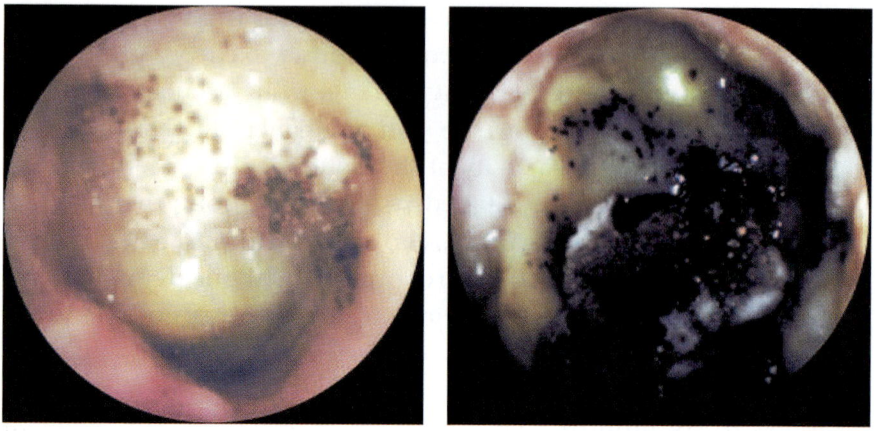

(a) (b)

**Fig. 9.** Otomycosis. **(a)** Small black tufts and white exudate may be visualized on otoscopy. **(b)** *Aspergillus niger* is characterized by black mycelia. (Printed with permission from BC Decker Inc. from PDQ Otitis Externa, 2007.)

## Otomycosis

Otomycosis is a superficial, fungal infection of the external auditory canal with symptoms of pruritis, scaling, otalgia, and otorrhea. The discharge may be fluffy and white but may also be black, gray, bluish-green, or yellow depending on the organism (see Fig. 9). Commonly, black or white conidiophores on white hyphae are visualized and associated with *aspergillus* infections. *Apergillus* species represent the most common pathogens associated with otomycosis with 80%–90% of infections resulting from *A. niger, A. flavus,* or *A. fumigatus.* Other common pathogens include *Candida albicans* and rarely *Phycomycetes, Rhizopus, Actinomyces,* and *Penicillium.* Typically, otomycosis occurs after prolonged bacterial otitis externa although may result from overzealous use of topical steroid preparations which render the external auditory canal vulnerable to such opportunistic infections.

An understanding of the normal physiology of the external auditory canal is critical in appropriate management of otomycosis. Uncomplicated presentations of otomycosis may be treated with topical antifungal drops such as clotrimazole. Other authors have advocated the use of mechanical debridement, topical ketoconazole or cresylate otic drops, in patients with intact tympanic membranes.[15] Restoration of external auditory canal pH, adequate debridement, and moisture reduction are essential and sometimes the only intervention required for resolution of infection. Rarely is systemic antifungal medication such as fluconazole, or surgical debridement indicated. Patients may present with fungal id reactions manifesting in the external auditory canal. These infections occasionally require systemic antifungal therapy as certain diseases, such as onychomycosis, may not be treated adequately with topical therapy alone. In addition, allergic fungal otitis may warrant specific skin testing and desensitization immunotherapy for effective treatment. Finally, invasive fulminant infection may be seen in profoundly immunocompromised hosts. In such cases, the prognosis depends largely on the extent to which the immunocompromised state can be treated and reversed. Most of these patients require surgical excision of the infected area. The most common procedure in such cases is a lateral temporal bone resection. In no other circumstance is it more important to employ an interdisciplinary approach to both diagnosis and management. Radiologists, infectious disease experts, intensivists, oncologists, endocrinologists, and otolaryngologists are often integral to such a team.

## Herpes Zoster Oticus

*Herpes zoster oticus* is a viral infection caused by varicella zoster. Latent viral infection within the geniculate ganglion and cell bodies of sensory nerves innervating the ear are the source of this infection. The typical presentation involves a two- to three-day prodrome of pain and burning which then manifests as a vesicular rash. Ramsey Hunt syndrome is a *herpes zoster* infection involving the seventh cranial nerve and is characterized by intense otalgia, a rash around the ear, mouth, face, neck, and scalp, and paralysis of facial nerves (see Fig. 10). Occasionally hearing loss, tinnitus, and veritigo may also be present in Ramsey–Hunt syndrome. Dysgeusia, xerostomia, and

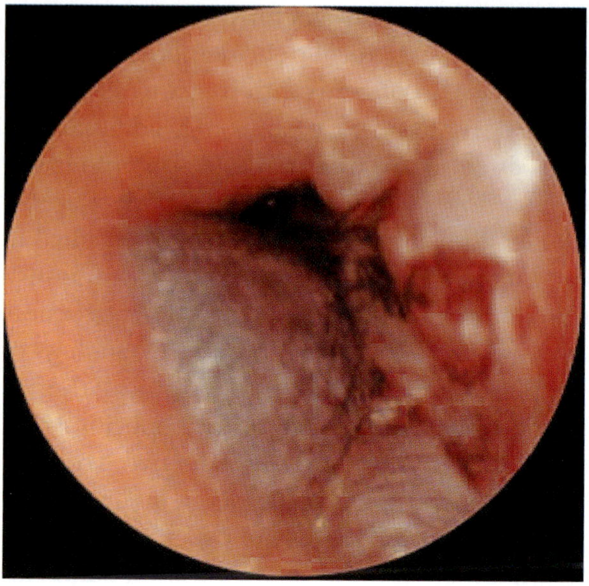

**Fig. 10.** Herpes zoster oticus (Ramsey–Hunt syndrome). Vesicles involving the canal skin and tympanic membrane may result from a herpes zoster infection of the seventh cranial nerve. (Printed with permission from BC Decker Inc. from PDQ Otitis Externa, 2007.)

lagophthalmos are also expected findings as the meatal foramen is the most narrow segment of the intra-temporal facial nerve and the nerves of taste, salivation and facial expression are all transmitted through this foramen.

Patients 60 years of age and older are most likely to develop *herpes zoster oticus,* which requires a previous varicella-zoster infection. Ramsey–Hunt syndrome represents approximately 12% of all cases of facial paralysis in the United States.

Treatment of *herpes zoster oticus* is mainly symptom related with the use of NSAIDS, wet dressings and lotions for relief of discomfort. Various antiviral medications, steroids, and ocular protection are indicated in cases of Ramsey–Hunt syndrome. Post-herpeic neuralgia is a common long-term complication of *herpes zoster oticus* and is characterized by pain that persists one month after resolution of the vesicular rash. The incidence of post-herpetic neuralgia increases with age and usually resolves within six months.

Methods for prevention of *herpes zoster oticus* are currently available in the form of the vaccine Zostavax®. Zostavax® is indicated for persons 60 years of age and older with a history of varicella-zoster and immunocompromise due to cancer, HIV, active tuberculosis, or chronic immunosuppressive medication use. The vaccination is administered as one injection and reduces the chances of developing shingles by 51%.

## REFERENCES


1. Lee KJ. *Essential Otolaryngology*. New York: McGraw Hill, 2003, Chap. 23, p. 466.
2. Osguthorpe JD, Nielson DR. Otitis externa: review and clinical update. *Am Fam Physician* 2006;74(9):1510–1516.
3. Gray RF, Sharma A, Vowler SL. Relative humidity of the external auditory canal in normal and abnormal ears, and its pathogenic effect. *Clin Otolaryngol* 2005;30:105–111.
4. Rosenfeld RM, Brown L, Cannon CR, Dolor RJ, Ganiats TG, Hannley M, Kokemueller P, Marcy M, Roland PS, Shiffman RN, Stinnett SS, Witsell DL. Clinical practice guideline: acute otitis externa. *Otolaryngol Head Neck Surg* 2006;134:S4–23.
5. Santos F, Selesnick SH, Grunstein E, Lalwani AK (ed.). *External Ear: Current Diagnosis and Treatment in Otolaryngology-Head and Neck Surgery*. McGraw-Hill, 2004, Chap. 46, pp. 660–661.
6. Drehobi M, Guerrero JL, Lacarte PR, Goldstein G, Mata FS, Luber S. Comparison of efficacy and safety of ciprofloxacin otic solution 0.2% versus polymyxin B-neomycin-hydrocortisone in the treatment of acute diffuse otitis externa. *Curr Med Res Opin* 2008;24(12):3531–3542.
7. Dohar J. Evolution of management approaches for otitis externa. *Pediatr Infect Dis J* 2003;22:299–308.
8. Roland PS, Belcher BP, Bettis R, Makabale RL, Conroy PJ, Wall GM, Dupre S, Potts S, Hogg G, Weber K. A single topical agent is clinically equivalent to the combination of topical and oral antibiotic treatment for otitis externa. *Am J Otolaryngol Head Neck Med Surg* 2008;29:255–261.
9. Wall GM, Stroman DW, Roland PS, Dohar J. Ciprofloxacin 0.3%/Dexamethasone 0.1% sterile otic suspension for the topical treatment of ear infections. *Pediatr Infect Dis J* 2009;28:141–144.

10. Carfrae MJ, Kesser BW. Malignant otitis externa. *Otolaryngol Clin North Am* 2008;41:537–549.
11. Cohen D, Friedman P. The diagnostic criteria of malignant external otitis. *J Laryngol Otol* 1987;101:216–221.
12. Soudry E, Joshua BZ, Sulkes J, Nageris BI. Characteristics and prognosis of malignant external otitis with facial paralysis. *Arch Otolaryngol Head Neck Surg* 2007;133(10):1002–1004.
13. Joshua BZ, Sulkes J, Raveh E, Bishara J, Nageris B. Predicting outcome of malignant external otitis. *Otol Neurotol* 2008;29:339–343.
14. Parize P, Chandesris MO, Lanternier F, Poirée S, Viard JP, Bienvenu B, Mimoun M, Méchai F, Mamzer MF, Herman P, Bougnoux ME, Lecuit M, Lortholary O. Antifungal therapy of *aspergillus* invasive otitis externa: efficacy of voriconazole and review. *Antimicrob Agents Chemother* 2009; Mar:1048–1053.
15. Ho T, Vrabec JT, Yoo D, Coker NJ. Otomycosis: clinical features and treatment implications. *Otolaryngol Head and Neck Surg* 2006;135: 787–791.

3

# Hearing Loss and Balance Disorders

*Jodi L. P. Jones and Deborah S. F. Kacmarynski*

## ANATOMY AND PHYSIOLOGY

### Conductive System

The conductive system is composed of the tympanic membrane and three ossicles, the malleus, incus and stapes, and the connection of the stapes footplate to the oval window. This system transfers the energy of sound from vibration of air to waves in liquid. The amplification gains of the system are from the size decrease of the tympanic membrane to the oval window and the lever ratio of the malleus to the incus. Anything that hinders the free motion of the system or changes the physics of the motion can potentially create a conductive hearing loss (see Fig. 1).

### Sensorineural System

The sensorineural system takes the vibration of the fluid at the oval window and transmits it through the membranous cochlea to the Reissner's membrane in a tonotopic fashion. The highest pitches are transduced at the base of the cochlea and the lowest frequencies travel in longer fluid waves to the apex of the cochlea. The vibration at the Reissner's membrane is transduced to electrical energy

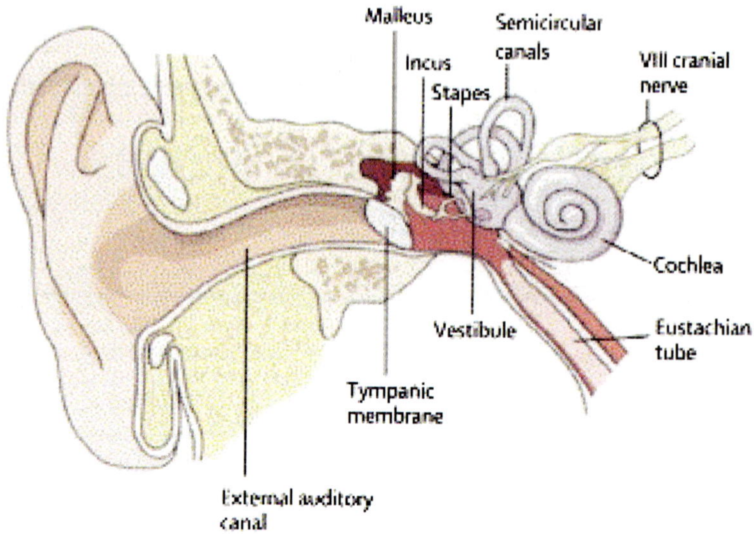


**Fig. 1.** Outer, middle and inner ear cross-section. Used with permission from Ref. 36.

through the inner hair cells, which change their signal frequency to the auditory nerve when stimulated with sound (see Fig. 2). The hair cell function is dependent on a voltage difference between the two fluids of the labyrinth, the endolymph and the perilymph. Insults to the hair cells or the fluid composition are two ways to create cochlear hearing loss. The inner hair cells send neural signals into the cochlear nerve fibers which proceed through the spiral ganglion to coalesce into the auditory nerve and pass into the cochlear ganglion. Insults to the nerve or pathways beyond create hearing loss through auditory neuropathy.

The peripheral vestibular system is composed of a bony outer labyrinth and a membranous inner labyrinth. It contains two otolith organs and three semicircular canals (SCC). The otolith organs (utricle and saccule) are responsible for the sensation of linear acceleration. The SCCs (lateral, posterior and superior) sense angular acceleration. The SCCs are paired and lie in orthogonal planes — the two lateral canals, the right superior and left posterior, and the right posterior and left superior. The nerve supply to the

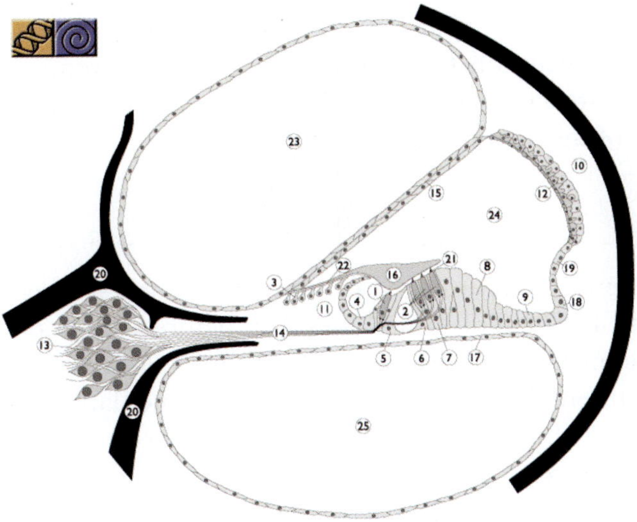


**Fig. 2.** Inner ear cells. Used with permission from Ref. 10.

vestibular system arises from the inferior and superior divisions of the vestibular nerve (CN VIII).

The primary sensory organ of the SCC is the organ of Corti (see Fig. 2) which lies within the ampullated end of the SCC. It is divided into the scala vestibuli, the scala media and the scala tympani. The scala vestibuli and the scala tympani contain perilymph, a fluid with similar composition to cerebrospinal fluid. The scala media is filled with endolymph, a fluid high in potassium. Inner and outer hair cells are topped by the tectorial membrane. When head movements occur, fluid shifts within the scala media stimulate or inhibit neural firing by bending the hair cells, triggering an action potential. In the horizontal SCC, stimulation occurs with ampullopetal movement of fluid while in the remaining SCC, it occurs with ampullofugal movement. The otolith sensory organ is in the macular area, in which hair cells project into a gelatinous matrix of calcium carbonate crystals.

Electrical signals from the otolith organs and the SCC then travel to the vestibular nuclei in the brainstem, forming second-order neural pathways — vestibulo-ocular reflex (VOR), vestibulospinal reflex and the vestibulocerebellar reflex. The VOR is critical to maintaining a stable image on the retina during head movement. Insult to any of these structures in the vestibular system results in the aberrant sensation of movement, known as vertigo.

## HEARING LOSS

Hearing loss is present in one to three per 1000 newborn children; an additional one in 1000 children becomes deaf before adulthood. This represents the most common sensory deficit in children. Early diagnosis and treatment lead to optimized speech and language development in young children and continued optimal educational outcomes in older children.

Many patients with congenital hearing loss are now diagnosed initially with the newborn hearing screening. Universal newborn hearing screening is rapidly becoming a worldwide practice. By 2005, 95% of newborn infants in the United States were screened for hearing loss prior to hospital discharge and every state had implemented a newborn hearing-screening program.[1] When screening is performed with otoacoustic emissions (OAE), conductive or sensory hearing loss of 40 dB or greater will be detected. When automated auditory brainstem response (ABR) is used as a single screening, neural auditory disorder will also be detected. When automated ABR is used as initial screening, OAE should not be used subsequently to "pass" the child's rescreening as this would miss auditory neuropathy/dyssynchrony.[1] When a neonate fails her initial screen, she needs a repeat screening performed in a short timeframe. All infants should be screened by one month of age.[1] If this fails, a referral to an audiologist is made for a comprehensive audiological evaluation. This should occur no later than three months of age.[1] An ABR is needed if the OAE refers again. An ABR should be performed after an otoscopic exam to determine if cerumen, canal obstruction or middle ear effusion is contributing to the failed hearing screens. If there is a treatable problem on otoscopy, this should be addressed. Treat acute otitis media with antibiotics and repeat exam, obstruction with a canal cleaning, or chronic otitis media with effusion with myringotomies if bilateral hearing loss and effusions have persisted three months. An ABR can be performed during the same anesthetic with myringotomy and tubes or subsequently after the remaining effusion has cleared at a separate setting.

Potential false negatives to the congenital hearing screening can occur. Auditory neuropathy and dyssynchrony will be missed by OAEs. Mild hearing loss will be missed, and losses outside of the range of screening will be missed. The most common reason that the congenital hearing loss patient is not appropriately treated is a failure to follow up with additional diagnostic and therapeutic visits. This is an important area of progress in public health, and improving communication and reducing barriers to further care helps, but does not completely eliminate this problem.

Parents may suspect progressive hearing loss due to inappropriate responses to noises at home. Medical caregivers may participate in the quick diagnosis of progressive hearing loss by appropriate questioning of parents, interactions during examinations and routine hearing screens. School screens also assist in monitoring hearing and capturing children with progressive hearing loss.

For a complete discussion of hearing tests, please refer to Chapter 4 "Audiologic Assessment in Children". In brief, audiologic tests may measure hearing threshold, speech recognition, middle ear function, cochlear function, neural synchrony and vestibular function. The tests that measure these functions are pure-tone audiometry, speech recognition, immittance battery, otoacoustic emissions, electrophysiology and electronystagmography. Electrophysiology includes auditory brainstem, middle latency responses, auditory steady state response, electrocochleography and evoked cortical potentials.[2]

For the youngest babies, tympanometry, otoacoustic emissions and auditory brainstem response form the toolset allowing early diagnosis of hearing loss. Babies with severe hearing loss or worse need hearing aids in place by six months in order to follow progress in auditory development over some months, and allow cochlear implantation by 12 months of age in those children not progressing with hearing aids.

Increasing age allows increasing interaction and purposeful response, which improves the efficiency of the audiologic assessment. Visual reinforcement audiometry, conditioned play audiometry and conventional audiometry are methods used for children of increasing age and cooperation.[3] Tympanograms are an important tool in the diagnosis of hearing loss. A flat tympanogram can be consistent with a middle ear effusion if the canal volume is normal. It can be consistent with a perforation or patent tympanostomy tube if the canal volume is large. A negative peak value can be consistent with eustachian tube dysfunction.

Otoscopy is an important part of the diagnostic evaluation, and pneumatic otoscopy is helpful to determine if the tympanic membrane is moving normally. A microscopic ear exam allows much improved depth perception and also allows for increased magnification. Removing obstructing cerumen from the external auditory canal is a frequent part of the ear examination in children. Ear drops and irrigations should be used with caution if the integrity of the tympanic membrane is in question to protect the ear from any traumatic or ototoxic damage to hearing.

Children with hearing loss have often had their radiographic evaluation delayed until a later date to minimize the difficulties with sedation and early radiation. The most commonly used modality has been a high resolution computed tomography (HRCT) scan. A second option is the magnetic resonance imaging (MRI) modality with gadolinium contrast and a protocol with high resolution of the auditory system. Proponents of the HRCT note that it is rapid, readily accessible, relatively less expensive, that it gives fine, bony detail of the temporal bone, clearly shows the facial nerve course and typically requires less sedation.[4] Advocates of the MRI promote its lack of radiation exposure with attendant risk of malignancy and excellent visualization of the soft tissue structures of the membranous labyrinth.[5] They also note that a number of important diagnoses are visible on MRI that can be missed on HRCT. These include auditory nerve agenesis or abnormality, modiolar deficiencies, cochlear obstruction by soft tissue or bone, endolymphatic sac enlargement and brainstem or temporal lobe abnormalities.[4] Some of these abnormalities visualized only on MRI may help guide treatment, such as which cochlea to implant, or clarify prognosis for future speech and language development.

## DIFFERENTIAL DIAGNOSIS OF HEARING LOSS

### Non-Organic Hearing Loss

Non-organic hearing loss is a pediatric form of functional hearing loss with poorly understood or identified motives, but very high prevalence. Non-organic hearing loss in children has been reported to be between 1.5% and 8% in prevalence. This is a difficult diagnosis to obtain, but is greatly aided by adding speech audiometry and OAEs or ABR to pure-tone audiometry. Non-organic hearing loss does not respond well to direct confrontation or accusation of the pediatric patient, but has good prognosis with reassurance. The various forms are nicely described by Austen and Lynch, but do respond well to early diagnosis, reassurance, encouragement and occasional psychologic intervention.[6,7]

### Conductive Hearing Loss

External auditory canal (EAC) abnormalities are not typically difficult to diagnose as they are most often readily visible on examinations with the naked eye and simple otoscopy. Some milder abnormalities will be clarified with otomicroscopy; radiographic imaging can clarify the middle and inner ear abnormalities that are commonly associated.

Tympanic membrane (TM) abnormalities can cause variable levels of conductive hearing loss. The location and size of perforation can have a very large impact on hearing, depending on the impact of sound waves on the round and oval windows. Tympanosclerosis may have variable contributions to hearing loss, but is often present without causing the loss. Retractions and atalectasis may have directly caused hearing loss or may be associated with the inflammation and scarring that also affect the hearing more directly through partial ossicular fixation.

The middle ear space is usually partially visible through the translucent TM. It may be difficult to clearly diagnose in the office examination with an otoscope when significant abnormalities are present. The examination is greatly enhanced with a close inspection through an otomicroscope. Restraint may be necessary to obtain a proper diagnosis in younger children. Otitis media with effusion will often decrease the translucency of the TM, cast a yellowish hue, or reveal itself with bubbles, retraction and decreased movement with pneumotoscopy. Cholesteatoma will often be visible as a pearly white mass and may be visible through a perforation or deep in a retraction pocket. Glomus or dehiscent or misplaced vessels will often cast a blue or red hue through the TM. A high-riding jugular bulb may give conductive hearing loss with venous hum or tinnitus with bluish hue behind intact tympanic membrane.[8] Pulsatile tinnitus may accompany a dehiscent carotid artery. Congenital perilymphatic fistula may occur in oval window, fundus of the modiolus, fissulae ante fenestram or round window with increased risk of meningitis.[8]

Ossicular abnormalities are numerous and are a common cause of conductive hearing loss. Many abnormalities have been reported and a complete list may be found in many otolaryngology textbooks or review articles.[8,9] Malleus head fixation is likely the most common abnormality and is associated with incomplete pneumatization of the epitympanum. The most common discontinuity is congenital absence of long process of the incus. The stapes may be displaced or abnormal; examples include isolated congenital stapes ankylosis or stapes fixation with perilymphatic gusher and profound or mixed hearing loss. Other anomalies include atresia of the oval window or persistent stapedial artery.[8]

## Sensorineural Hearing Loss

Although categorizations such as genetic vs. acquired organize our differential, there are complex causes such as the genetic disposition toward hearing loss sensitivity from aminoglycosides caused by mutations in mitochondrial gene 12SrRNA.[10] Nonetheless, we will organize our discussion around these categories.

Genetic causes of hearing loss can be divided into syndromic vs. non-syndromic. Secondary findings directing us towards syndromic can be obvious or subtle. An ophthalmology consult can assist in diagnosing the many syndromes with ocular involvement. An abdominal ultrasound and urinary analysis will assist in diagnosing many of the renal abnormalities. An EKG is simple and inexpensive to evaluate the QT interval for Jervell-Lange-Nielsen syndrome. The subtleties of the many syndromes associated with hearing loss justify offering a consultation with a geneticist for a child with hearing loss.

Classic clinical findings for the main syndromes including hearing loss are discussed briefly here. More complete discussions including current knowledge of genetic research are referenced and updated on the Hereditary Hearing Loss Homepage.[10] Alport syndrome is associated with renal and ocular abnormalities including hematuria with progressive renal failure and lenticonus and retinal flecks. Branchio-Oto-Renal syndrome has branchial clefts, cysts or fistulas and renal malformations. Jervell-Lange-Nielsen has prolonged QT interval with syncopal attacks, torsade de pointe arrhythmias and risk of sudden death. Neurofibromatosis II has bilateral vestibular schwannomas, meningiomas, schwannomas, gliomas, scalp neurofibromas and juvenile subcapsular cataract. Norrie disease classically has ocular abnormalities including retinal hyperplasia, cataracts and pseudotumor of the retina, as well as mental retardation and hearing loss. Pendred syndrome has goiter. Stickler syndrome has ocular abnormalities including progressive myopia and cataract, arthropathy (spondyloepiphyseal dysplasia), midface hypoplasia, vertebral body irregularities and cleft palate. Treacher Collins syndrome has malformations in both the middle and inner ear and distinct craniofacial abnormalities including lower eyelid coloboma, micrognathia, microtia, zygomatic arch hypoplasia, macrostomia and inferior placement of the lateral canthi relative to the medial canthi. Usher syndrome has retinitis pigmentosa. Waardenburg syndrome has dystopia canthorum (lateral displacement of the inner canthum of the eye) and abnormalities of the pigment of skin, hair and iris (heterochromia iris).[10]

Non-syndromic disorders are divided into groups based on inheritance patterns, including autosomal recessive, autosomal dominant or X-linked. The most important X-linked genetic cause of hearing loss is from mutations to gene POU3F4 and can be associated with stapes fixation and perilymphatic gusher and conductive, mixed or sensorineural hearing loss.[10]

Autosomal recessive genes are identified by locus (DFNB1), by gene (GJB2) and by protein (Connexin 26 or Cx26). As of 2011, forty-two genes are listed on the Hereditary Hearing Loss Homepage[10] as causes of autosomal recessive non-syndromic hearing loss. Up to 50% of patients with autosomal recessive non-syndromic prelingual deafness have mutations affecting Connexin 26 via the gap junction protein, beta 1 (GJB2) gene located at locus DFNB1 on chromosome 13q12.[11] The second most common non-syndromic cause is Connexin 30 protein from the gene GJB6 also at the locus DFNB1. These genes can combine as digenic abnormalities and cause hearing loss with heterozygous abnormalities in both GJB2 and GJB6. The gap junction proteins are subunits of gap junction channels that mediate ion and metabolite diffusion between adjacent cells.[10]

As of 2011, twenty-four genes are identified as causes of autosomal dominant non-syndromic hearing loss.[10] Some of the same genes can cause either autosomal dominant or recessive hearing loss depending on the mutation. The loci are named DFNA with an integer following. Proteins affected include gap junction proteins, myosins and tectorial membrane proteins.

Mitochondrial hearing impairment is maternally inherited; multiple mutations have been identified that cause syndromic and non-syndromic hearing loss. Causes include large rearrangements involving several genes and point mutations in transfer RNA (tRNA) genes in addition to mutations in ribosomal RNA (12S rRNA) which are associated with aminoglycoside induced hearing loss. Syndromes include Kearns-Sayre syndrome (KSS), myoclonic epilepsy and ragged red fibers (MERRF), mitochondrial encephalopathy, lactic acidosis and stroke-like episodes (MELAS) and maternally inherited diabetes and deafness (MIDD). KSS involves progressive external ophthalmoplegia and retinopathy presenting in the second decade. Ataxia, heart block or cerebrospinal fluid protein elevation can develop. MERRF includes myoclonus, epilepsy and ataxia with frequent addition of dementia, optic atrophy and variable degree of hearing loss. MELAS occurs in childhood with recurrent cerebral insults resembling strokes and causing hemiparesis and cortical blindness. Proximal limb weakness and intermittent vomiting are characteristic and short stature occurs frequently. Hearing loss occurs in a third of patients. MIDD occurs with diabetes mellitus and sensorineural hearing loss in a maternally inherited pattern. A given mutation may cause one or another of the syndromes in given families and individuals.[10]

Ototoxic medications and intrauterine teratogenic exposure have become less frequent causes of hearing loss due to improved knowledge and awareness. One of the most useful classes of antibiotics, aminoglycosides, still does have the risk of ototoxicity. Gentamicin is still routinely used for treating infections in neonates. Increasing ease of genetic testing may soon provide a means to determine genetic susceptibility to hearing loss from gentamicin due to 12S rRNA mutations. When treating cancer, the risk of ototoxicity should be discussed and balanced with the need for treating the malignancy effectively. An important part of treating children with ototoxic antineoplastic agents such as cisplatin or carboplatin is monitoring hearing function. The onset of hearing loss may be during treatment or may be years after treatment is completed.[12]

Overall, infectious causes of hearing loss such as otitis media, maternal rubella infections and bacterial meningitis have decreased as antibiotics, vaccines and awareness have increased. Some shifts in the relative frequency of various causes have occurred as more infectious diseases are being prevented or quickly treated. Human immunodeficiency virus (HIV) causes sensorineural hearing loss by both peripheral and central auditory pathologies. Cytomegalovirus (CMV) continues to be a significant cause of hearing loss and can be difficult to differentiate from a common upper respiratory infection during pregnancy.

Noise is increasing as a cause of hearing loss in older children due to the regular use of headphones and earplugs in addition to loud concerts. Counsel regarding proper hearing protection and volume settings should be given to minimize further hearing loss.[13]

Membranous portion of labyrinth only or bony and membranous components can cause hearing loss, but the bony changes are more discernable by current imaging methods. Imaging abnormalities discernable on CT that cause mixed hearing loss include large vestibular aqueduct, lateral semicircular canal dysplasia and enlarged internal auditory canal. Bony abnormalities that cause sensorineural hearing loss are thought to be caused by failures of development. Jackler published a classification of inner ear anomalies based on embryogenesis in 1987; this is most commonly used.[8] Michel aplasia (complete labyrinthine aplasia) can be differentiated from labyrinthitis obliterans on CT by the lack of promontory bulge in the first and its presence in second, or by MRI.[8]

Premature infants have numerous causes of increased risk of hearing loss, thus they need close monitoring of hearing and language development during childhood.[14] Bronchopulmonary dysplasia is associated with auditory dysfunction in premature infants.[15] Hyperbilirubinemia has been shown to cause hearing loss in neonates, both sensorineural hearing loss and auditory neuropathy. However, hyperbilirubinemia has not been proven to cause speech delay at age 3 in NICU graduates,[16] nor was it proven to cause speech delay at severe levels in term infants.[17] Reversible auditory dysfunction has also been reported due to indirect hyperbilirubinemia, with effects at both the peripheral and brainstem level.[16] Please see Table 1 for a more complete list of possible causes of hearing loss.

## OUTPATIENT VS. INPATIENT MANAGEMENT OF HEARING LOSS

Most of the management of hearing loss is performed on an outpatient basis with the exception of the universal newborn hearing screening process, which is performed in the hospital after birth, prior to discharge.

**Table 1. Differential diagnosis of hearing loss.**

| Non-Organic Hearing Loss | Sensorineural Hearing Loss | Sensorineural Hearing Loss | Conductive Hearing Loss |
|---|---|---|---|
| | ***Genetic*** | ***Acquired*** | |
| | *Syndromic* | *Toxins* | *External auditory canal* |
| | Alport | Aminoglycosides | Cerumen impaction |
| | Branchio-oto-renal | Platins | Atresia |
| | Jervell and Lange Nielsen | Erythromycin | Stenosis |
| | Neurofibromatosis II | Loop diuretics | |
| | Norrie disease | Quinines | *Tympanic Membrane (TM)* |
| | Pendred | Salicylates | TM retraction |
| | Stickler | | Tympanosclerosis |
| | Treacher-Collins | *Infectious* | TM perforation |
| | Usher | CMV | TM atalectasis |
| | Waardenburg | EBV | |
| | | Herpes simplex virus | *Middle Ear Space* |
| | *Non-syndromic* | HIV | Otitis media with effusion |
| | Autosomal-recessive | Meningitis | Cholesteatoma |
| | Loci DFNB 1-30 | Mumps | Glomus |
| | Autosomal dominant | Rubella | High-riding jugular bulb |
| | Loci DFNA 1-39 | Syphilis | Dehiscent carotid artery |
| | X-Linked Loci DFN 1-6 | | Perilymphatic fistula |
| | Mitochondrial | *Other* | Other masses |
| | | Noise Trauma | |
| | | Perilymph fistula | *Ossicles* |
| | | Hyperbilirubinemia | Discontinuity |
| | | Multiple sclerosis | Atresia of the oval window |
| | | Endolymphatic hydrops | Displaced |
| | | Michel aplasia | Persistent stapedial artery |
| | | Labyrinthitis obliterans | Agenesis |

A full audiologic evaluation with appropriate pediatric expertise is necessary to understand the type and extent of hearing loss. Please see Chapter 4 for a full discussion of hearing evaluations in children. Imaging studies may be performed on outpatients with possible sedation depending on age and ability to cooperate with the examinations. This may be coordinated with ABR if sedation is needed for both evaluations.

Hearing aid evaluations are performed outpatient and typically involve a series of visits to create molds, order and fit hearing aids and monitor progress with language development and use of hearing aids.

## EMERGENCY EVALUATION AND TREATMENT OF HEARING LOSS

The most common reason for sudden hearing loss in children is non-organic hearing loss, over 50% in one study. Non-organic hearing loss prevalence is estimated at 7% in children aged six to 17.[6] The second most common reason was idiopathic; other rare causes include enlarged vestibular aqueduct syndrome, acoustic trauma, multiple sclerosis, herpes virus infection, acoustic neuroma, and sudden intracranial hypotension.[18–20] Patients with sudden hearing loss need an immediate audiogram with an experienced audiologist to evaluate for non-organic or conductive causes. If sudden sensorineural hearing loss is diagnosed, an urgent workup is in order including imaging and consideration of possible treatment with oral antiviral and steroid medical management.

Please refer to Chapter 1 on otitis media and complications.

## OPERATIVE INTERVENTIONS OF HEARING LOSS

Surgery for hearing loss may be as simple as myringotomy with tympanostomy tube for middle ear effusions or retraction. An exploratory tympanoplasty can be performed for other conductive losses with possible ossiculoplasty or repair of perilymph fistula. Canaloplasty may be performed for external auditory canal atresia or stenosis as early as six years of age, but a preoperative CT scan should reveal sufficiently developed middle ear structures by Jahrsdoerfer's criteria to give good hearing prognosis for this procedure.[21] A bone-anchored hearing aid may be recommended for patients with significant conductive hearing loss or unilateral profound hearing loss in patients desiring sound awareness on the non-hearing side. A study of the findings of 67 patients from middle ear explorations showed no improvement in air-bone gaps postoperatively in half the patients. Two-thirds of patients with a mobile stapes had a postoperative air-bone gap of less than 30 dB.[9]

Profound and some severe bilateral hearing losses can be treated with cochlear implantation in the proper candidates. Currently, candidacy includes lack of auditory skills development and minimal hearing aid benefit as documented by parent questionnaire in 12–24-to month-old children and word recognition scores <30% in older children. Current FDA guidelines recommend implantation at 12 months of age or older. Earlier implantation in congenitally deaf children provides significant advantages in language development.[22,23] Recent literature is beginning to document the benefits of bilateral cochlear implantation and increasing numbers of children are undergoing their second cochlear implantation on the contralateral side.[24] Others are receiving bilateral implants at their initial operative setting.[25]

## BALANCE DISORDERS

As with any adult patient who presents with a complaint of vertigo or balance disturbance, a thorough and detailed history is critical in determining the etiology of pediatric balance disorders. Unfortunately, children are often too young to be able to provide an accurate history and therefore it is only available from the parents or caregivers. This makes the diagnosis of balance disorders in children more challenging. Healthcare professionals are often anxious in managing and investigating vestibular disorders in children for fear of missing a potentially devastating diagnosis, such as a posterior fossa tumor. The reality is that such tumors are rare, therefore the use of expensive radiologic investigations is usually not indicated.

A detailed description of the symptoms is important in directing further investigations. Important features include type of "vertigo" (spinning, turning, imbalance, lightheadedness), duration, timing, associated symptoms, aggravating and relieving factors, progression or variation, and other neurologic symptoms or signs. One also needs to elicit a complete otologic history including acute otitis media, otitis media with effusion, otorrhea, tinnitus, fullness, hearing loss, and a history of otologic surgery. Additional contributory information includes a history of motion sickness, a positive family history for migraine and/or vestibular disorders, history of head trauma and any exposure to ototoxic medications.

Physical exam findings may often be absent in children with balance disorders, however a complete otologic/neurotologic evaluation is essential. Presence of middle ear effusions or other ear anomalies should be documented. The presence and character of nystagmus is also important as it may help distinguish peripheral from central disorders. Dix-Hallpike maneuvers should be performed where possible as well as a fistula test. A complete neurologic exam must also be done to rule out central lesions. Given that vision is so critical in the maintenance of balance, an ophthalmologic assessment should be performed. Additional testing will be discussed later in this chapter.

## DIFFERENTIAL DIAGNOSIS OF BALANCE DISORDERS

Vestibular disorders in children and adolescents are typically grouped into two categories — peripheral and central disorders. The most common etiologies in each of these broad groups will be discussed. Please see Table 2 for a differential diagnosis of balance disorders.

**Table 2. Differential diagnosis of balance disorders.**

| Peripheral causes | Central causes |
|---|---|
| Otitis media | Migraine |
| Congenital inner ear anomalies | BPV |
| Vestibular neuronitis | Posterior fossa tumors |
| BPPV | Seizure disorder |
| Endolymphatic hydrops | Psychiatric origin |
| Perilymphatic fistula | |
| Post-traumatic | |
| Ototoxicity | |

## Peripheral Vestibular Disorders

### *Otitis media*

Acute otitis media is one of the most common diagnoses in pediatric patients and perhaps the most common reason to seek medical attention. Complications from acute otitis media are many and include otitis media with effusion which can lead to hearing loss. However, Casselbrant *et al.* recently reviewed the literature on balance disorders resulting from otitis media with effusion and found that many children suffer motor and balance difficulties during acute otitis media and/or in the presence of chronic middle ear effusions.[26] Their performance on tests to measure balance was diminished when compared to children who did not have fluid at the time of testing. Reviews by Balatsouras *et al.* and Bower *et al.* revealed otitis media to be one of the three most common diagnoses in pediatric vestibulopathy.[27,28]

### *Congenital inner ear anomalies*

Congenital malformations of the temporal bone may be associated with balance disorders in children. The most common inner ear malformation is that of a dilated vestibular aqueduct. Such an anomaly can result in progressive sensorineural hearing loss in affected individuals, particularly following trauma. In addition to hearing loss, children may also experience vestibular symptoms, most commonly episodic vertigo.[29]

*Vestibular neuronitis*

Usually caused by a viral illness, vestibular neuronitis can occur in children. The vertigo is typically of a longer duration (days) and is related to a viral illness. Neuronitis should be distinguished from bacterial labyrinthitis by the associated hearing loss and typical presence of otitis media in the latter. Once the acute illness has resolved, children may be prone to developing a delayed endolymphatic hydrops, producing symptoms resembling Meniere's disease (see below).

*Other peripheral causes*

While benign paroxysmal positional vertigo is the most common peripheral cause of vertigo in adults, it is uncommon in children. It is characterized by brief episodes of spinning vertigo typically brought on by changes in head position. Torsional nystagmus is present on Dix-Hallpike testing, is delayed in onset and is fatiguable with repeated maneuvers. It is thought to be the result of canalithiasis, making canalith repositioning maneuvers (e.g. Epley) a useful treatment.

Endolymphatic hydrops (also known as Meniere's disease), is also uncommon in children. A study by Choung *et al.* reported that 2.6% of patients with endolymphatic hydrops are pediatric.[29] Additionally, only 2% of children with vestibular complaints are found to have this condition characterized by episodes of vertigo, aural fullness, tinnitus and hearing loss.

Children with profound sensorineural hearing loss may also have vestibular dysfunction. Wiener-Vacher reported that 20% will have complete bilateral vestibular loss, 40% will have normal vestibular function, and the remaining 40% will have incomplete or asymmetric loss.[30] These children will often exhibit delays in psycho-motor development, therefore the diagnosis should be made early in order to introduce rehabilitation to facilitate normal development.

Children may experience vestibular symptoms following head injuries. A review by Wiener-Vacher of 2000 children referred for vestibular evaluation showed that 10% of cases were related to head trauma.[30] This may be related to temporal bone fractures, the presence of a perilymphatic fistula, or a labyrinthine concussion.[31] A history of prior head injury should be elicited in the evaluation of all children with vestibular disorders. Patients will experience vertigo, gait unsteadiness, nausea and vomiting, all of which may last from four to six weeks. Fortunately, due to the plasticity and adaptability of the pediatric vestibular system, children will habituate to the vestibular dysfunction.

Children may also suffer insults to the vestibular system resulting from administration of ototoxic medications. Injury is typically bilateral in nature and therefore patients often present with symptoms of imbalance and dysequilibrium as opposed to spinning vertigo which is more typical of unilateral lesions.

## Central Vestibular Disorders

### *Migraine*

Migraine is the most common etiology of vestibular disorders in children and adolescents.[27,32] It presents with headache, nausea and vomiting, and may last for several hours. The headache is usually frontal or periorbital.[33] It may be triggered by psychosocial stressors or sleep deprivation.[30] The typical profile of the patient with vestibular migraine is an adolescent female with headache, dizziness, past history of motion sickness, family history of migraine and a normal neurologic exam.[33] A trial of prophylactic therapy is indicated in such patients as described below.

### *Benign paroxysmal vertigo of childhood*

Benign paroxysmal vertigo (BPV) was first described by Basser in 1964 and is one of the most common causes of pediatric vertigo.[27,28,32,34] It most commonly affects children aged two to four years. The onset of this condition is sudden with children exhibiting anxiety and fear, clinging to their parents, remaining immobile.[35] When able, children may describe a sensation of movement or falling. The duration of each episode is brief, lasting seconds to minutes. They may occasionally be associated with other symptoms such as pallor, nausea and unusual head positions. The episodes will occur anywhere from daily to once every few months, with a decreasing frequency over time. The condition will resolve spontaneously in essentially all cases. The diagnosis is confirmed by the recurring nature of the vestibular attacks in young children in the presence of a normal neurologic exam. In a study by Drigo *et al.*, the mean duration of symptoms was 22 months.[35] Wiener-Vacher found BPV to be present in 20% of children referred for vestibular evaluation.[30] The etiology of BPV is unknown, however it is thought to be related to migraine as many children who have BPV have a strong family history of migraine and/or have gone on to develop migraines themselves.[33] BPV does not require any treatment and parents should be reassured of the benign nature of the condition as well as its propensity for spontaneous resolution.

*Posterior fossa tumors*

While posterior fossa tumors are the most feared diagnosis in a child with vestibular symptoms, they are very uncommon, presenting in less than 1% of cases referred for vestibular evaluation.[30] Posterior fossa tumors are accompanied by other neurologic symptoms and signs. Any neurologic features present in a child who presents with vestibular dysfunction should alert the otolaryngologist to the possibility of an intracranial mass. These may include, but are not limited to, lateralizing weakness or cranial nerve dysfunction, hypotonia, sensory deficits and abnormal reflexes.

*Other central disorders*

Seizure disorders can present with vertiginous symptoms. They would be distinguishable from migraines by a loss of consciousness, visual or auditory hallucinations, and neurologic signs.

Children may also present with vertigo of psychiatric origin. These children are slightly older, eight to ten years of age, and have exaggerated symptoms. They may present with atypical findings that fail to correlate with a distinct clinical picture. They are also able to perform autonomic tasks without any impairment. A careful history should elicit the underlying cause for the child's symptoms.

## OUTPATIENT MANAGEMENT OF BALANCE DISORDERS

As previously stated, the most useful components in the evaluation of pediatric balance disorders are a careful history and physical exam. This will, in many cases, reveal the likely diagnosis and eliminate the need for unnecessary tests. Bower *et al.* in 1995 published a review of vertigo in children in their institution and evaluated the use of ancillary tests.[28] They concluded that audiometry and tympanometry were the most useful tests in such cases and should generally be ordered on all children. With the exception of otitis media, most children should also undergo electronystagmography and caloric testing in order to assess vestibular function.

Computed tomography and magnetic resonance imaging are very costly investigations and are usually normal in this population. Posterior fossa tumors are present in less than 1% of cases of vertigo in children and therefore imaging should only be reserved for children with other neurologic features suggestive of an intracranial process. When seizure disorders are suspected, electroencephalography should be performed.

Visual disturbances may be the cause or the aggravating factor in children with presumed balance disorders. A complete ophthalmologic evaluation should be performed in children with an unclear diagnosis, particularly those with migraine, as visual impairment may act as a trigger.

Children diagnosed with a balance disorder related to otitis media should be treated with a standard course of antimicrobial therapy. Vestibular symptoms should resolve after the infection has resolved. Children who suffer from migraines should initially be instructed on avoidance of triggers. If this fails, medical therapy should be instituted. Ibuprofen is often very effective at managing migraine-related pain once it occurs. For children who have frequent, severe attacks, prophylactic therapy should be considered, such as beta blockers. Ergot derivatives are not recommended for long-term use in children.[30] Serotoninergic derivatives are not approved for use in children under age 12, though these have been used in refractory cases. As previously mentioned, ophthalmologic evaluation of children with migraines should be performed as this can be an aggravating factor. Children with symptomatic endolymphatic hydrops can be started on a prolonged course of betahistine.

## INPATIENT MANAGEMENT OF BALANCE DISORDERS

In general, balance disorders in children and adolescents can be managed in an outpatient environment. Admission would be reserved for children with refractory nausea and vomiting or those requiring invasive procedures for intracranial lesions. Children with other complications from otitis media (e.g. meningitis, mastoiditis) should be admitted for appropriate intravenous antimicrobial therapy as well as myringotomy, culture and placement of pressure equalization tubes.

## OPERATIVE INTERVENTION OF BALANCE DISORDERS

Given that the most common causes of pediatric balance disorders are migraines, otitis media and benign paroxysmal vertigo of childhood, surgical management is often not required. Pressure equalization tubes should be placed according to standard criteria relating to frequency of otitis media and duration of middle ear effusions. A neurosurgical consultation would be required for those rare cases where vertigo is caused by a posterior fossa tumor.

## ACKNOWLEDGMENTS

We would like to express our deepest appreciation for inspiration, guidance and assistance to Richard J. H. Smith, MD, our mentor and fellowship director during pediatric otolaryngology fellowship at the University of Iowa.

## REFERENCES

1. American Academy of Pediatrics, Joint Committee on Infant Hearing. Year 2007 position statement: principles and guidelines for early hearing detection and intervention programs. *Pediatrics* 2007 Oct;120(4): 898–921.
2. Sweetow RW, Sabes JH. Audiologic testing. In: Lalwani AK, ed. *Current Diagnosis and Treatment in Otolaryngology Head and Neck Surgery*, 2nd Ed. New York: McGraw-Hill Medical, 2008, pp. 596–606.
3. Nozza RJ. The assessment of hearing and middle-ear function in children. In: Bluestone CD, Stool SE, Alper CM, Arjmand EM, Casselbrant ML, Dohar JE, *et al.*, eds. *Pediatric Otolaryngology*, 4th Ed. Philadelphia: Saunders 2003, pp. 187–229.
4. Parry DA, Booth T, Roland PS. Advantages of magnetic resonance imaging over computed tomography in preoperative evaluation of pediatric cochlear implant candidates. *Otol Neurotol* 2005 Sep;26(5):976–982.
5. Silver RD, Djalilian HR, Levine SC, Rimell FL. High-resolution magnetic resonance imaging of human cochlea. *Laryngoscope* 2002 Oct;112(10):1737–1741.
6. Austen S, Lynch C. Non-organic hearing loss redefined: understanding, categorizing and managing non-organic behaviour. *Int J Audiol* 2004 Sep;43(8):449–457.
7. Saravanappa N, Mepham GA, Bowdler DA. Diagnostic tools in pseudohypacusis in children. *Int J Pediatr Otorhinolaryngol* 2005 Sep;69(9): 1235–1238.
8. Rodriguez K, Shah RK, Kenna M. Anomalies of the middle and inner ear. *Otolaryngol Clin North Am* 2007 Feb;40(1):81, 96, vi.
9. Raveh E, Hu W, Papsin BC, Forte V. Congenital conductive hearing loss. *J Laryngol Otol* 2002 Feb;116(2):92–96.
10. Hereditary Hearing Loss homepage [homepage on the Internet]. Available from: http://hereditaryhearingloss.org/.
11. Green GE, Scott DA, McDonald JM, Woodworth GG, Sheffield VC, Smith RJ. Carrier rates in the midwestern united states for GJB2 mutations causing inherited deafness. *JAMA* 1999 Jun 16;281(23):2211–2216.

12. Jehanne M, Lumbroso-Le Rouic L, Savignoni A, Aerts I, Mercier G, Bours D, *et al.* Analysis of ototoxicity in young children receiving carboplatin in the context of conservative management of unilateral or bilateral retinoblastoma. *Pediatr Blood Cancer* 2009 May;52(5):637–643.
13. Biassoni EC, Serra MR, Richtert U, Joekes S, Yacci MR, Carignani JA *et al.* Recreational noise exposure and its effects on the hearing of adolescents. part II: development of hearing disorders. *Int J Audiol* 2005 Feb;44(2):74–85.
14. Robertson CM, Watt MJ, Dinu IA. Outcomes for the extremely premature infant: what is new? And where are we going? *Pediatr Neurol* 2009 Mar;40(3):189–196.
15. Wilkinson AR, Brosi DM, Jiang ZD. Functional impairment of the brainstem in infants with bronchopulmonary dysplasia. *Pediatrics* 2007 Aug;120(2):362–371.
16. Amin SB, Prinzing D, Myers G. Hyperbilirubinemia and language delay in premature infants. *Pediatrics* 2009 Jan;123(1):327–331.
17. Ogun B, Serbetcioglu B, Duman N, Ozkan H, Kirkim G. Long-term outcome of neonatal hyperbilirubinaemia: subjective and objective audiological measures. *Clin Otolaryngol Allied Sci* 2003 Dec;28(6):507–513.
18. Ioannis P, Georgios K, Alexandra K, Dimitrios D, Michael T. Pseudohypacusis: the most frequent etiology of sudden hearing loss in children. *Eur Arch Otorhinolaryngol* 2009 Dec;226(12):1857–1861.
19. Uysal S, Albayram S, Ercan TE. Spontaneous intracranial hypotension: a case report. *J Child Neurol* 2008 Nov;23(11):1312–1315.
20. Mazzoni A, Dubey SP, Poletti AM, Colombo G. Sporadic acoustic neuroma in pediatric patients. *Int J Pediatr Otorhinolaryngol* 2007 Oct;71(10):1569–1572.
21. Jahrsdoerfer RA, Yeakley JW, Aguilar EA, Cole RR, Gray LC. Grading system for the selection of patients with congenital aural atresia. *Am J Otol* 1992 Jan;13(1):6–12.
22. Fitzpatrick E, Olds J, Durieux-Smith A, McCrae R, Schramm D, Gaboury I. Pediatric cochlear implantation: how much hearing is too much? *Int J Audiol* 2009 Feb;48(2):91–97.
23. Johnston JC, Durieux-Smith A, Angus D, O'Connor A, Fitzpatrick E. Bilateral paediatric cochlear implants: a critical review. *Int J Audiol* 2009;48(9):601–617.

24. Zeitler DM, Kessler MA, Terushkin V, Roland TJ Jr, Svirsky MA, Lalwani AK, *et al.* Speech perception benefits of sequential bilateral cochlear implantation in children and adults: a retrospective analysis. *Otol Neurotol* 2008 Apr;29(3):314–325.
25. Ramsden JD, Papaioannou V, Gordon KA, James AL, Papsin BC. Parental and program's decision making in paediatric simultaneous bilateral cochlear implantation: who says no and why? *Int J Pediatr Otorhinolaryngol* 2009 Jul 16 [Epub ahead of print].
26. Casselbrant ML, Villardo RJ, Mandel EM. Balance and otitis media with effusion. *Int J Audiol* 2008 Sep;47(9):584–589.
27. Balatsouras DG, Kaberos A, Assimakopoulos D, Katotomichelakis M, Economou NC, Korres SG. Etiology of vertigo in children. *Int J Pediatr Otorhinolaryngol* 2007 Mar;71(3):487–494.
28. Bower CM, Cotton RT. The spectrum of vertigo in children. *Arch Otolaryngol Head Neck Surg* 1995 Aug;121(8):911–915.
29. Choung YH, Park K, Moon SK, Kim CH, Ryu SJ. Various causes and clinical characteristics in vertigo in children with normal eardrums. *Int J Pediatr Otorhinolaryngol* 2003 Aug;67(8):889–894.
30. Wiener-Vacher SR. Vestibular disorders in children. *Int J Audiol* 2008 Sep;47(9):578–583.
31. Eviatar L, Bergtraum M, Randel RM. Post-traumatic vertigo in children: a diagnostic approach. *Pediatr Neurol* 1986 Mar-Apr;2(2):61–66.
32. Erbek SH, Erbek SS, Yilmaz I, Topal O, Ozgirgin N, Ozluoglu LN, *et al.* Vertigo in childhood: A clinical experience. *Int J Pediatr Otorhinolaryngol* 2006 Sep;70(9):1547–1554.
33. Weisleder P, Fife TD. Dizziness and headache: a common association in children and adolescents. *J Child Neurol* 2001 Oct;16(10):727–730.
34. Worden BF, Blevins NH. Pediatric vestibulopathy and pseudovestibulopathy: differential diagnosis and management. *Curr Opin Otolaryngol Head Neck Surg* 2007 Oct;15(5):304–309.
35. Drigo P, Carli G, Laverda AM. Benign paroxysmal vertigo of childhood. *Brain Dev* 2001 Mar;23(1):38–41.
36. Smith RJ, Bale J, James F, White KR. Sensorineural hearing loss in children. *Lancet* 2005 Mar;365(9462):879–890.

# 4

# Basic Audiometric Assessment of Children

*Yvonne S. Sininger*

## INTRODUCTION

This chapter will discuss the basic philosophy and techniques of audiologic assessment of children. There are multiple purposes for evaluating auditory system function in children including determination of hearing handicap, monitoring of hearing/ear functions including middle ear status and sensorineural hearing levels or determination of higher-order auditory functions and central auditory system disorders. Assessment of the auditory system must include test batteries and generally cannot be based on a single test. Assessments must be developmentally appropriate and can change dramatically with the age and ability of the child.

Close communication between the Pediatric Otolaryngologist and the Audiologist is important to assure appropriate assessment and management of children with auditory system dysfunction. Especially with infants and toddlers, test time is significantly limited by factors such as attention span. To assure efficient management of children, tests must focus on the important questions. When referring for an assessment, the audiologist needs to know if the purpose of the evaluation is to monitor ventilation tubes, for example, or to rule out a central auditory processing disorder. The audiologist, in turn, has an obligation to rule out any significant loss of hearing in children, who cannot communicate the nature of their hearing status. In this author's mind, the pediatric otolaryngologist has an obligation to determine and manage the physiologic status of the ear and the audiologist to determine and manage the functional status of the auditory system (hearing status). These two things are very closely entwined. As such, the two professions must work together as a team.

Audiologists who work with infants and toddlers need specific training and experience with the test procedures and with young children. The American Board of Audiology has recently instituted Pediatric Specialty Certification which will provide audiologists with a mechanism for establishing credentials and expertise in the area. The need for specialized training for pediatric audiologists has been heightened by the development of newborn hearing screening programs in every state. Every program relies on accurate assessment of newborns who fail the screening tests. Full audiologic assessments of two-week-old infants are now commonly needed and, thanks to objective test procedures, accurate hearing measures can be obtained even on the youngest patients. The assessment procedures used are determined, in part, by the capacity of the patient to participate and provide information. Some objective measures, for example tympanometry or otoacoustic emissions, are applied regardless of age. In general, a child must be approximately six months of age and have head and trunk control, before a reliable head-turn response can be used for determination of hearing thresholds. Before that age, electrophysiological measures, such as the auditory brainstem response (ABR) or auditory steady state response (ASSR) can usually be used to accurately predict hearing thresholds and to estimate an audiogram. The broad skill set required for assessment of infants and toddlers may not be found in all audiologists who do not have specific training and experience. In the future, specialty certification should indicate which professionals have the skills for pediatric audiologic assessment but, for the present, care must be used in referring to those professionals who have the training and experience.

## NEWBORN HEARING SCREENING

Throughout the US and in many of the developed countries of world, it is accepted practice to screen all infants during the newborn period for hearing loss. In the past, infants who were "at risk" for hearing loss were screened in some hospitals but current standards call for all infants to be screened in "universal" hearing screening programs. All 50 of the states have established programs that screen the vast majority of infants, either by law or just by convention. In the US, infants are screened before discharge from the birthing hospital using either an automated screening auditory brainstem response (ABR) or an otoacoustic emission (OAE) procedure. The screenings are designed to identify bilateral or unilateral hearing loss that is mild (about 35–40 dB) or greater and the tests have been found to have high sensitivity and specificity for detecting hearing loss.[1]

While the goal of newborn hearing screening (NHS) is to identify sensorineural or permanent conductive hearing loss, children with transient conductive losses of sufficient degree will also fail NHS. While this is unavoidable, proper audiologic follow up can determine which infants fall into this category. According to the Joint Committee on Infant Hearing (JCIH)[2] the primary goals of NHS systems are: (1) to screen all babies using a physiologic measure by one month of age, (2) to provide comprehensive medical and audiological evaluations of all infants who fail the initial screening by three months of age, and (3) to begin intervention for all children with permanent hearing loss by six months of age. The need and urgency for early detection and intervention are based on research that clearly demonstrates the significant advantages in communication ability for infants with hearing loss who meet these timelines.[3–6]

The otolaryngologist plays a crucial role in the NHS process and should be a strong advocate for early intervention for infants with hearing loss including fitting of amplification as soon as possible and early enrollment in intervention programs. By law, any child determined to have hearing loss of any degree must be referred for appropriate early intervention within 48 hours of such determination. During the time when educational intervention is in process, the otolaryngologist should conduct a thorough examination children with hearing loss identified through NHS programs. The JCIH suggests the otolaryngologist provide a full head & neck evaluation of children referred from NHS that documents any defects of the auricle or ear canal or any signs of hearing related syndromes. A family history can help to reveal other possible genetically based hearing loss which is thought to be a factor in up to 50% of congenital hearing loss.[7] As recommended by JCIH 2007, if etiology remains undetermined, further testing including electrocardiogram, urinalysis, CMV testing or radiologic studies may be prudent.[2] During this process, the otolaryngologist will issue medical clearance for the fitting of hearing aids, which should proceed with all haste. With rare exception, binaural hearing aids should be fit to children with all degrees of hearing loss, even mild loss. Finally, physicians play a critical role in reassuring families and encouraging active and early management of hearing loss.

## AUDIOLOGIC TEST PROCEDURES

### Pure Tone Audiometry

The basic audiologic measure is the audiogram which is a graphic representation of hearing thresholds for pure-tones obtained individually in each ear with presentations of air conducted and bone conducted stimuli. The X axis of the audiogram is frequency in Hz and is generally a logarithmic scale with 1000 Hz in the center and a range from about 125 to 8000 (occasionally up to 12,000) Hz. The Y axis is in decibels (dB) in Hearing Level (HL). The Y axis ranges from approximately –20 to 120 dBHL with the lowest levels at the top of the graph. To maintain a standard aspect ratio, audiograms should have a frequency scale with 1000 Hz in the center and each octave on the X axis should be the same size as 20 dB on the Y axis. Hearing Level is defined as average normal threshold and these values (in dB Sound Pressure Level or SPL) are determined for each frequency and published at regular intervals by the American National Standards Institute (ANSI) Standard 3.6–89. Hearing Level therefore refers to the level relative to normal hearing. Audiometers, used to present stimuli to measure audiograms, are calibrated to ANSI or ISO (International Standards Organization) standards.

Hearing thresholds are measured by air conduction when using stimuli that are presented through earphones, either headphones or inserts (small transducers connected to the ear by tubing and foam earplugs). This simulates the natural hearing condition and air conduction thresholds give an estimate of the degree of hearing loss experienced by the listener. Hearing thresholds are also measured using a vibrator that is coupled to the mastoid with a headband. The bone conduction vibrator can stimulate the cochlea directly and bypass the tympanic membrane and middle ear. Bone conduction thresholds are useful because they can essentially determine cochlear sensitivity directly and by comparison with air conduction thresholds, determine the ability of the TM and ossicular mechanism to conduct sound pressure through the middle ear.

An example of an audiogram is shown in Fig. 1. In some instances it is necessary to use a noise masker in one ear to isolate the responses of the other if hearing loss exists. If the air conduction thresholds differ by more than about 60 dB (using insert earphones) the better, non-test ear must be masked to insure that the presentation is heard in the test ear alone without "crossing over" to the better ear. When testing by bone conduction the stimulus cross over is close to zero dB so any difference in bone conduction threshold with air or bone conduction in the better ear requires masking. In the example audiogram the right ear has a 20–40 dB (mild) hearing loss by air and bone conduction but only the bone conduction required masking. Symbols will change with masking condition and should be noted on a legend. When color is used, all left ear symbols are in blue and right ear in red.

When air conduction and bone conduction thresholds are similarly elevated, a sensorineural loss is identified and when bone

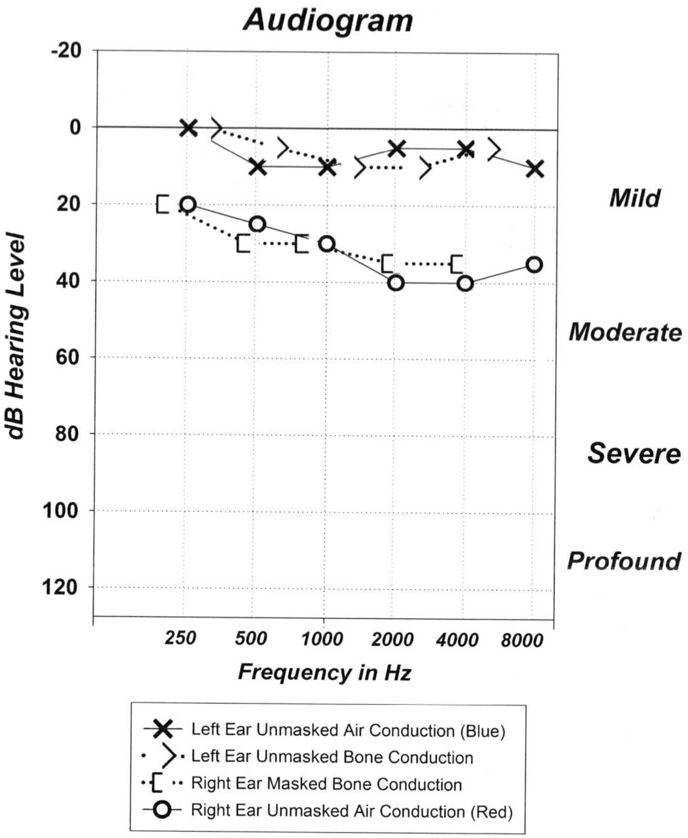


**Fig. 1.** Audiogram depicting pure tone thresholds for the right ear (open circles) and left ear (x) showing a mild to moderate, hearing loss in the right ear. Masked bone conduction thresholds ([) are equal to air conduction in the right ear indicating a sensorineural hearing loss.

conduction thresholds are significantly better than air, a conductive component is contributing to the loss. It is possible to have both elevated bone thresholds and an air-bone gap producing a mixed hearing loss. There are general categories for the degree of hearing loss and these are shown on the figure at the right of the audiogram. The right ear would be considered to have a mild sensorineural hearing loss and the left is within normal limits, which in children should be about 15 dB or better.

## Speech Audiometry

Speech stimuli are also used in the routine audiometric assessment and results of speech tests are often reported on the audiogram along with pure tone thresholds. A threshold in dB can be established for speech revealing the speech reception threshold (SRT). The SRT is important as a second measure to support pure tone audiometry in the determination of the degree of loss. SRT measures involve presentation of two syllable words called spondees to which the patient replies usually by repeating the word verbally. The second standard measure using speech stimuli is known as speech intelligibility, often referred to as speech discrimination. For this test, the speech, generally monosyllabic words, is presented at a level that should be audible (suprathreshold) and the percentage of words that can be correctly repeated is reported. This measure helps to determine the degree of handicap for processing and understanding conversational speech. The lists used for speech intelligibility are made of words that represent the natural occurrence of speech sounds in the lexicon. The word lists are consequently referred to as phonetically balanced or PB.

Obvious limitations exist in the use of speech audiometry with children. Words cannot legitimately be used as a measure of hearing unless the words are within the vocabulary of the patient. The use of speech audiometry depends on the individual linguistic sophistication of the child. The child's ability to understand a word also will precede their ability to produce the word intelligibly.

Spondee lists used for children are often made up of selected words that may be understood by children such as "hotdog," "airplane" or "toothbrush." If the child understands but does not naturally produce these words, a picture selection task in employed. The child is shown a board with four to six pictures and told "Show me popcorn." Generally the child is familiarized with the names of the objects before testing. A threshold for speech is obtained by determining the lowest level of presentation that will reveal an accurate response 50% of the time.

A similar procedure is used for speech intelligibility. The monosyllable word lists are chosen based on average vocabulary and minimum ages are set for use of the tests. One popular test is the Word Intelligibility by Picture Identification (WIPI) test.[8] This test provides sets of six color pictures in a closed set task in which the child has to point to the item that is heard. This test is appropriate for children as young as four years old. Another, the Phonetically Balanced Test of Speech Discrimination for Children (PBK-50) does not employ a picture pointing response but the vocabulary and the task are appropriate for children as young as six years of age.[9]

For children with hearing loss who may have significant compromises in language and speech development, a variety of specialized assessments are available to determine how well the child can hear and understand speech. The scope of this chapter does not allow for a full description of these tests.

## Audiometry Across Age Groups

Cooperative children with a developmental age of five to six months and older can participate to provide accurate threshold measurements for a pure tone audiogram. The audiologist presents the discrete pure tones for about one second each and varies the level, looking for a prescribed response after each presentation. By bracketing the stimulus level a threshold is determined as the lowest level, in 5 dB increments, to which the child can consistently respond at least 50% of the time. For children between two and five years of age, audiometric testing will often enlist a game, and the procedure is termed conditioned play audiometry or CPA. The child is taught to respond to sounds with a play response such as dropping a block in a bucket or putting a peg into a slot on a board. Older children and adults will generally push a button or raise their hand when they hear a sound.

Infants of about five to six months of age, who can sit unattended and have good head control, are tested using a procedure known as visual reinforcement audiometry (VRA). This procedure adapts the audiometric procedure for use with children up to about 24 months of developmental age. In VRA the child is trained to expect an attractive visual stimulus (lighted animated toy, cartoon video clip) when a sound is heard. The visual reinforcer is placed to the side of the child so that when the child seeks the reinforcement, a clear head turn is required. The head turn is judged as the response to the sound presentation. The child is seated in the test booth and a test assistant is used to keep the child's attention on some activity other than the reinforcer between trials. The test assistant often is the person making judgments regarding the presence of a valid head turn response.

This procedure is often conducted in a "sound field" situation in which the stimuli are presented through wall-mounted speakers, generally near the reinforcement presentation. However, the sound field test has a *significant* limitation in that it does not isolate the ears for testing. Results of sound field testing can only indicate the hearing in the better hearing ear but it will not be clear which ear is responding. In the past, young children rejected headphones strenuously. However, the small insert earphones presently used can be attached to the child's back and, at least for children who are not old enough to pull them out, can provide a way to present stimuli to the ears individually without significant discomfort to the child. Using insert earphones allows each ear to be assessed individually.

For children below the developmental age of six months, behavioral observation is often employed. Very young infants may not be able to demonstrate a reliable head turn but will often show consistent response such as a startle or eye widening in response to sound. This information provides useful qualitative information. Behavioral observation has the limitation that responses will be seen only for supra-threshold level stimuli. Therefore, behavioral observation cannot be used to determine the degree of hearing loss or to rule out a mild-moderate hearing loss. For these infants, threshold determination requires an objective electrophysiologic response such as the ABR (see section below).

## TYMPANOMETRY AND MIDDLE EAR MUSCLE REFLEX

Tympanometry is an objective and fast measure of tympanic membrane and middle ear compliance that can provide important information regarding the middle ear status of children. The tympanometer is a device that includes an air pressure pump, a sound source and a microphone all of which are connected by plastic tubing to an ear probe. The probe is fitted to the ear with a compliant ear tip that must form a pressure seal in the ear canal. A variety of ear tips are available that can fit all sizes of ear canal.

The physical and acoustic principles of tympanometry are related to the measurement of energy flow through a mechano-acoustic system. Basically, the ear drum and middle ear system have known mechano-acoustic properties, and various pathologies cause deviations from those properties, that can be quantified. Most clinical systems measure acoustic admittance ($Y_a$) (the inverse of acoustic impedance), at one probe-tone frequency, generally 220 or 226 Hz. The low probe tone frequencies are not optimal for all types of measures of middle ear function, but 220–226 Hz will be highly influenced by the stiffness of the tympanic membrane (TM) and middle ear and therefore can be useful for assessing the possibility of otitis media and/or middle ear effusions. Single frequency acoustic admittance tympanometry produces results that are informative but this technique has limited capacity to differentiate specific tympanic membrane and middle ear pathologies, particularly for infants under the age of four months. In the near future, audiologists may be using a more sophisticated technique known as wide-band reflectance which utilizes a full range of audiometric frequencies in a non-pressurized measurement and can potentially provide more specific information regarding middle ear function and dysfunction.[10]

To measure the tympanogram, an ear probe is securely fit into the ear canal and a probe tone is introduced. The ear canal is a mostly a hard-walled cavity but the TM at the end of the cavity will vibrate and, in the normally functioning ear, the majority of the applied sound energy will pass via the TM into the middle ear and very little will be reflected. In this instance the microphone in the ear probe will record very little reflected sound.

For tympanometry, pressure is introduced into the sealed ear canal. The pressure pump can apply a continuum of positive and negative pressure, which is generally varied between +200 and −400 mm $H_2O$, also referred to as dekaPascals (daPa). With 200 daPa-applied pressure, the eardrum is essentially stiff and the enclosed ear canal and TM now resembles a hard-walled cavity. In this instance, most of the applied sound will be reflected and the microphone will record a relatively high sound level. With the TM essentially stiff, because the applied sound level is known, the measured sound level can be used to give an estimate of the ear canal volume. This is one of the important measures provided by the system. Very high values of "equivalent volume" generally indicate a TM membrane perforation or patent ventilation tube.

It must be noted that the probe tone frequency that is best used in immittance measures changes with age. This is because of the rapidly changing acoustic transmission properties of the neonatal ear. In general, infants up to six months of age should be evaluated with a 1000 Hz probe tone but after six months of age, a lower frequency, 226 Hz is appropriate.[11–13]

As the applied pressure is changed, either positive to negative or vice versa, the amount of reflected sound is measured and is converted into units of ear drum compliance (or admittance) in millimhos (mmhos). The admittance in mmhos of a column of air is equivalent to the volume of air in cc's. Depending on the machine used, the compliance in cc's or admittance in mmhos will be provided but, with a 226 Hz probe tone, these are equivalent.

In an ear with normal Eustachian tube function, the TM will be most compliant (and the least sound reflected) when the pressure applied by the tympanometer is near atmospheric pressure (equal to the middle ear pressure). Equalizing the pressure on each side of the TM allows it to vibrate in the normal position. In this instance the TM is neither retracted nor inflated and its mobility or compliance is maximized. The tympanogram is a plot with the applied pressure on the X-axis and the TM compliance on the Y (see Fig. 2). The point of maximum compliance or admittance is the assumed middle ear pressure. This value allows the clinician to monitor Eustachian tube (ET) function. Persistent negative middle ear pressure is indicative of ET dysfunction. Tympanograms performed

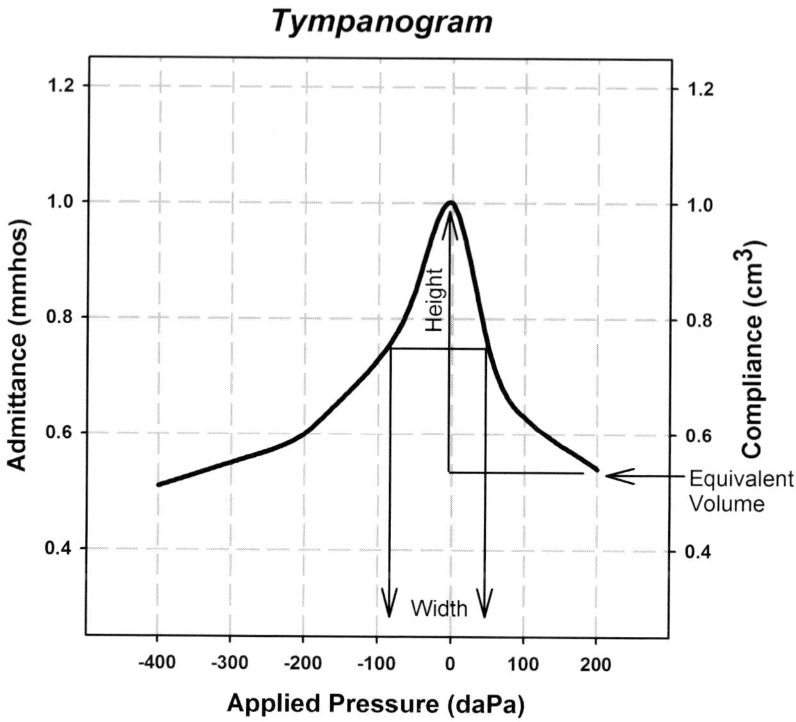


**Fig. 2.** Normal tympanogram is depicted. Equivalent ear canal volume in cc's is assumed as the reading at +200 daPa. Measurements for tympanometric height (static compliance or admittance) and width are shown.

before and after a Valsalva maneuver or swallowing can also be used to evaluate ET function.

The figure shows a normal tympanogram. Several important measurements are taken. The first is the Peak Pressure in daPa. The peak is found where the compliance reaches maximum and then reverses at a particular applied pressure. In this example the peak pressure is 0 daPa. The height of the tympanogram on the Y-axis (also called Static Compliance or Static Admittance) is measured in cc's (compliance) or millimhos (mmhos for admittance) and indicates the overall mobility of the TM (and ossicular chain). The admittance at the applied pressure of 200 daPa allows the system to measure the Equivalent Volume of the ear canal cavity. This is possible because, at this pressure the TM is distended and essentially immobile and therefore not contributing to the overall admittance. In most clinical systems, the admittance of the ear canal is disregarded in the reporting of the static admittance. That is, the contribution to the peak admittance from the ear canal is subtracted to provide the admittance of the middle ear (Ya) often referred to as "compensated." In Fig. 2 the equivalent volume is approximately 0.55 cc. The "height" of the tympanogram is measured from the point of compliance at +200 daPa and therefore represents the "compensated" admittance or compliance. The admittance of the tympanogram in Fig. 2 is 0.45 mmhos.

The shape of the tympanogram, or "steepness" of the peak, can be indicated by the Tympanic Width. This is the width of the tympanogram in daPa at the point of half of the height of the tympanogram. This measure is also highly correlated with the admittance or height of the tympanogram. As illustrated in Fig. 3, as the height of the tympanogram degreases, the width at half-height increases. Another measure that is often reported but used less often clinically is the tympanic gradient. This measure relates to the steepness of the peak.

A normal tympanogram will have an admittance peak and that peak will be found at or near 0 daPa. When the peak occurs at a significant negative pressure (<–150 daPa), Eustachian tube dysfunction, and sometimes middle ear effusions are indicated. Figure 3 illustrates a typical progression of tympanograms from normal function (#1) through successively negative pressure and reduced compliance (#2 and #3) to the "flat" tympanogram (#4). While this is stylized data, such a progression in tympanometric results over time would not be unusual in a patient with persistent ET dysfunction.

Few studies actually validate the relationship between tympanometry, middle ear pressure and effusions with myringotomy and tympanocentesis and therefore it is not possible to know exactly how much negative middle ear pressure is associated with fluid. Effusions are best predicted by a flat tympanogram, for example tympanogram #4 in Fig. 3. Smith *et al.*,[14] found that 80% of subjects with a "flat" tympanogram, one with no obvious peak and poor compliance, were

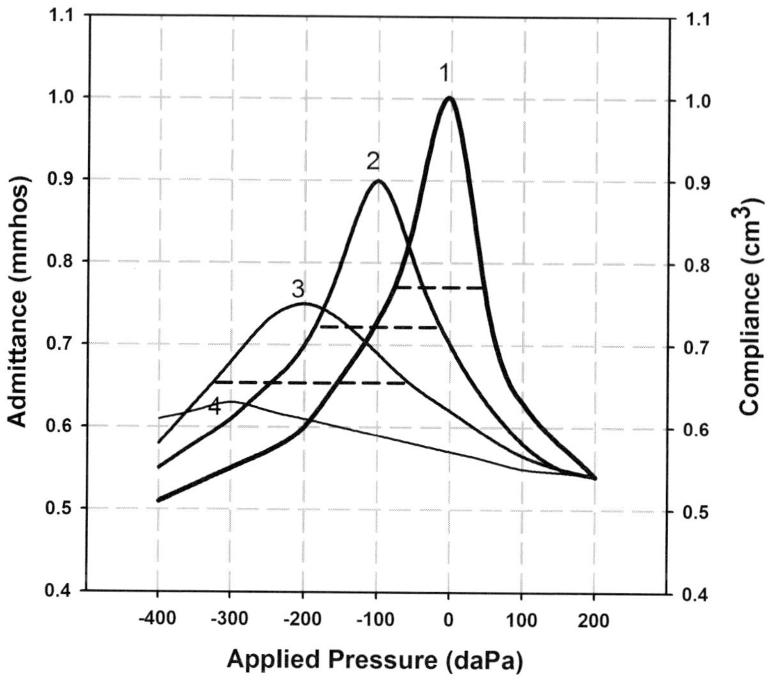


**Fig. 3.** Progression of abnormality in tympanograms as might be seen in a patient with Eustachian tube dysfunction.

found to have middle ear effusions (MEE). They conclude, "For tympanograms generally, the lower the height and the greater the width, the greater was the probability of associated middle-ear effusions (page 1)." Clearly effusions cannot be ruled out in children with negative pressure, peaked tympanograms but when a pressure peak is seen, the TM must still have regions of partial mobility.

Published normative data for ranges of equivalent volume, middle ear pressure, tympanometric height in mmhos and width in daPa are summarized in Table 1.

## OTOACOUSTIC EMISSIONS

Otoacoustic emissions or OAEs are acoustic signals that are generated by outer hair cells in the cochlea as part of the normal

**Table 1. Tympanometric normative data (fifth to 95th percentiles) by age and probe frequency.**

| Study | Age | Probe (Hz) | Equivalent volume I (cc's) | ME pressure (daPa) | $Y_a$ (mmhos) compensated at pressure (daPa) | Width (daPa) |
|---|---|---|---|---|---|---|
| Kei *et al.* (2003)[15] | 1 to 6 days | 1000 | N/A | −58 to +86 | 0.39 to 2.28 (+200) | 46.1 to 154 |
| Margolis *et al.* (2003)[16] | Birth to 4 wks | 1000 | N/A | −133 to +113 | 0.6 to 4.3 (−400) | |
| Alaerts *et al.* (2007)[11] | 3 to 9 mo | 226 | 0.35 to 0.74 | −91 to +49 | 0.22 to 0.49 (+200) | 94 to 192 |
| Alaerts *et al.* (2007)[11] | 9 to 32 mo | 226 | 0.38 to 0.74 | −237 to +50 | 0.22 to 0.82 (+200) | 68 to 173 |
| Roush *et al.* (1995)[17] | 6 to 30 mo | 226 | | −174 to +18 | 0.20 to 0.70 | 102 to 204 |

processing of sound during audition, first described by Kemp.[18] OAEs are elicited by soft to moderate sounds presented to the ear through an ear canal probe and measured with a small microphone in the same probe. OAEs are particularly important for use in the pediatric patient population because the measure is fast, requires minimal cooperation and provides an objective measure of auditory function (including an indirect measure of middle ear function) with no overt response needed from the patient. OAEs are often used in an automated screening mode in screening neonates for hearing loss.

OAEs are an outward reflection of the unique motile properties of outer hair cells. As the basilar membrane is deflected in response to incoming sound energy, the stereocillia of hair cells that are seated on the membrane are deflected which, in turn, opens transduction channels in the cells allowing an influx of potassium and calcium which depolarizes the cells. Outer hair cells respond to the depolarization by physically expanding and contracting due to prestin motor-like molecules incorporated in the cell wall. This energy is imparted to basilar membrane and amplifies the original motion. Inner hair cells are also depolarized by deflection of their stereocillia leading to the release of neurotransmitter activating the auditory nerve. The motile properties of the adjacent outer hair cells provides the additional energy needed for the inner hair cell to be activated by very soft sounds. The active amplification properties of the outer hair cell are responsible for the sensitivity of the inner hair cells to the softest sounds (below about 50 dB).

The active energy produced by the motility of the outer hair cells is dissipated through the fluids in the cochlea and will drive the auditory system in reverse, sending energy into the middle ear via the ossicular chain and eventually the tympanic membrane producing a energy wave front (sound) in the ear canal. The energy has much the same properties of the acoustic signal that was used to activate the ear but also reflects the processing, such as traveling wave delay, in the cochlea itself.

OAEs are routinely measured in one of two ways. A transient emission (TEOAE) is elicited with a short duration signal, usually a click or a tone burst. The click has a wide range of frequencies and will activate the majority of the basilar membrane, starting with high frequencies and progressing to lower frequencies. The OAE that results reflects this basilar membrane motion pattern and delay time. The response is broad band but the OAE acoustic waveform can be tested for reliability (reproducibility) and a spectral analysis can be performed to determine which frequency regions are responding reliably.

The other common method of measuring emissions is known as Distortion Product (DP) OAE. Because of naturally occurring distortions in the amplification process, when two primary pure tones with properly spaced frequencies of $F_1$ and $F_2$ are presented to the ear, a third tone (distortion) will be produced in the cochlea at a predictable frequency. The most prominent distortion in the human ear is one produced at the frequency computed as $2F_1 - F_2$. For example, primaries of 2000 and 2400 Hz will produce distortion at 1600 Hz. In this case, the auditory system is being tested in the region near $F_2$ (2400 Hz). The ear can be tested at multiple audiometric frequency regions by changing the tone pairs and the results are often termed a DP-gram. Detection of the response is based on the response energy at the distortion frequency being significantly larger than any background noise (surrounding frequencies). Also, while TEOAEs and DPOAEs may have different modes of transmission through the inner ear,[19] they are both used commonly and essentially interchangeably for clinical use at the current time. For both measures, many stimuli are presented and averaging is used to reduce noise in the response. Because the level of the acoustic emission is often quite low (less than 20 dB SPL) these measurements must be performed in a quiet environment and usually in a sound treated room.

### Interpretation of OAEs

Any difficulty with transmission through the middle ear, Eustachian tube dysfunction or middle ear effusions, can impede the transmission of the eliciting sound or the transmission of the emission, which must travel through the middle ear. Therefore, regardless of the condition of the cochlea or the cochlear amplifier, OAEs can be absent if the middle ear is not functioning normally. Conversely, when an OAE is present, one can assume that middle ear function is close to normal. In any regard, a tympanogram should always be performed along with OAEs to aid in interpretation.

Current clinical application of OAEs does not involve a threshold search of any sort. Rather the stimulus level is fixed at 80–85 dB SPL for transients and generally around 50–60 dB SPL for distortion product tones. The response is determined as the amplitude of the response relative to a measure of the background noise also known as the signal to noise ratio (SNR). No fixed normative value exists for response determination but generally, when the SNR is minimally between 3 and 6 dB, an OAE is judged to be present. When a response is present, the exact threshold of hearing cannot be predicted. Rather, when a clear OAE is present, hearing thresholds are assumed to be better than about 40 dB HL. However, a major precaution exists when any retrocochlear lesions may exist, for example auditory neuropathy (see discussion later). Because the OAE is a preneural response (it can exist even when innervation of the cochlea is interrupted[20]) only the cochlear amplifier function of the outer hair cell is assessed by this test.

## ELECTROPHYSIOLOGIC MEASURES OF HEARING: ABR AND ASSR

Along with universal newborn hearing screening has come an urgency to be able to accurately predict hearing thresholds in very young infants. As previously mentioned, standard behavioral measures of hearing will not produce accurate thresholds until an infant has the developmental age of five to six months. Infants are failing hearing screenings at birth and it is critically important to determine hearing levels and begin rehabilitation as soon as possible. In addition, procedures must be in place to identify hearing loss in children with developmental delays that may preclude them from being able to give reliable responses for significant periods of time.

The goal of hearing testing in infants who fail NBHS is to first determine if hearing loss truly exists. If thresholds are elevated, a determination must be made if the loss is due to conductive factors or is sensorineural in nature. If the loss is not amenable to treatment, the next step in rehabilitation is to fit the infant with appropriate hearing aids. To do so requires frequency and ear specific thresholds. The JCIH 2007[2] statement states specifically "The initial audiologic test battery to confirm a hearing loss in infants must include physiologic measures and, when developmentally appropriate, behavioral methods (page 13)." They go on to state that the audiologic test battery for infants who fail NHS must include frequency specific ABR using air and bone conducted stimuli, otoacoustic emissions, tympanometry using a 1000 Hz probe tone and age-appropriate behavioral observation of auditory behaviors.

## ABR

The ABR is an evoked auditory potential that is generated in the auditory nerve and brainstem pathway. ABR measures neural activity that is time-locked to the auditory stimulus but the response from the brainstem is small when recorded from the scalp and requires response averaging and tightly synchronized neural response to be recorded. The auditory nerve is activated by the inner hair cells and is the basis of the first of the three to five waves or peaks. The ABR is most robust when a broad band short duration stimulus is used, activating many of the cochlear nerve fibers. Generally this is done with a click. However, to predict the audiogram, the response can be generated with tonal stimuli that activate frequency specific regions of the cochlea.

The ABR of infants under about two years of age has a slightly different morphology and longer peak latencies than those of adults but the response is present in full term newborns. ABRs can be used with tonal stimuli to accurately predict audiometric thresholds in infants and toddlers.[21,22] One significant caution regarding the use of ABR for hearing threshold prediction comes when any compromise is suspected to the activation or neural conduction in the auditory nerve such as in the condition known as "Auditory Neuropathy.[23] This will be discussed in a later section.

The ABR is represented by a series of voltage fluctuations, occurring in the first 10–20 ms following stimulation. The response is time-locked to short duration stimuli and is recorded from pairs of electrodes on the scalp. Because these potentials are very small, responses are elicited to thousands of stimuli and averaged. The time-locked nature of the response allows the averaging to enhance the evoked potential relative to random background noise (muscle activity and non-synchronous EEG). The response is present in sleeping subjects and is highly reliable.

ABR testing is used for neurological diagnosis and for infant hearing screening. These procedures are performed using click stimuli. The click is short duration (100 ms) and contains a broad range of frequencies. Therefore the click synchronously initiates activity in a wide range of cochlear neurons from the base to the apex. While the click is excellent for some purposes, it cannot be used to isolate specific frequency regions as needed to predict an audiogram. Therefore, for audiometric use with children, the test must be performed using short duration tones known as tone bursts or tone pips. Tone bursts contain a few cycles of the nominal frequency tapered at the ends and are a few milliseconds in duration.

Examples of averaged ABRs are shown in Fig. 4. These are responses from a normally hearing infant. The top set are recorded using 500 Hz tone bursts and the major response peak, known as Wave V is indicated by the arrow. The level of stimulus used is shown at the right. The stimuli are calibrated in "normalized" hearing level, meaning that they are relative to the level needed to find a psychophysical threshold with the same stimulus. In this example a response to the 500 Hz stimulus is seen at 20 dB but not at 10 dB and therefore the threshold for this patient would generally be interpolated as 15 dB. This considered to be within normal limits.

The response to 4000 Hz stimuli is shown below. Note that the Wave V peak is earlier than for 500 Hz. This is because 4000 Hz

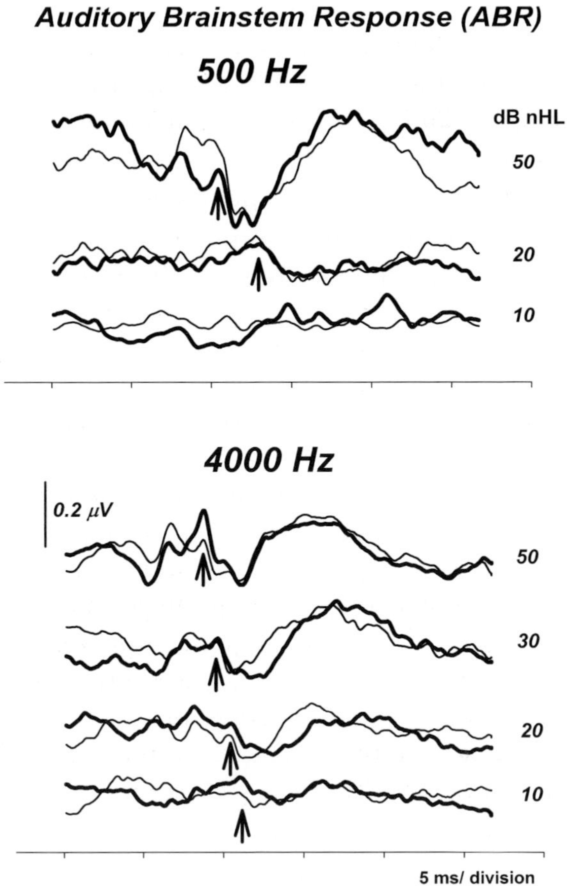


**Fig. 4.** ABRs recorded from two electrode channels are overlaid. These responses are from a normally hearing infant. Stimuli for top panel are 500 Hz tone bursts and for bottom are 4000 Hz tone bursts with stimulus level in dB nHL indicated on the right.

stimulates the basal region of the cochlea, which is activated first by the cochlear traveling wave. The 500 Hz region is activated a few milliseconds later and this difference is reflected in the response latencies. A clear response is seen at 10 dB for the 4000 Hz ABR. Also note that the latency of the response increases as the stimulus level decreases. This is expected and can be helpful in identifying the response threshold.

A typical ABR assessment will use stimuli ranging from 500 to 4000 Hz in octave steps. It is not always possible or necessary to test all frequencies in both ears for a variety of reasons. First, it is important for the infant/child to be sleeping during the testing to reduce interference from movement. For infants under six months of age, natural sleep is preferred but older infants often need to be sedated for testing. In any regard, the amount of time available for testing is quite limited and the audiologist must be innovative with the use of test time.

Unless air conducted thresholds are normal, bone conducted stimuli are also used to determine threshold for at least one frequency. This will aid in determining the type of hearing loss.

All assumptions regarding the threshold of the ABR being predictive of hearing as well as assumptions regarding the presence of an OAE being indicative of normal hearing are challenged when evidence of auditory nerve dysfunction is suspected. The disorder that has been termed "auditory neuropathy."[23] This condition is felt to exist when cochlear function is reasonably normal and the peripheral auditory nerve is either not adequately activated when neural conduction is disrupted. Infants and toddlers with this disorder may have a history of hyperbillirubinemia, or low birthweight or may have a genetic disorder. The classic audiologic findings in these cases include: (1) an abnormal or absent ABR to high level click stimuli, (2) evidence of hair cell functionality in the form of a normal OAE or a prominent cochlear microphonic potential in the ABR recording, (3) any degree of hearing loss (normal to profound), and (4) reduced speech perception ability.

An example of an ABR from a child with suspected auditory neuropathy is shown in Fig. 5. Two averages are overlaid, each performed with a click stimulus but one using a positive polarity pulse and the other negative. The cochlear microphonic from the hair cells will change polarity with the stimulus and the result is the mirror image section of the recording during the first 7 ms. The neural response including Wave V which would not change phase with the stimulus, is absent in this recording. This child also shows a moderate flat hearing loss on pure tone testing and a normal

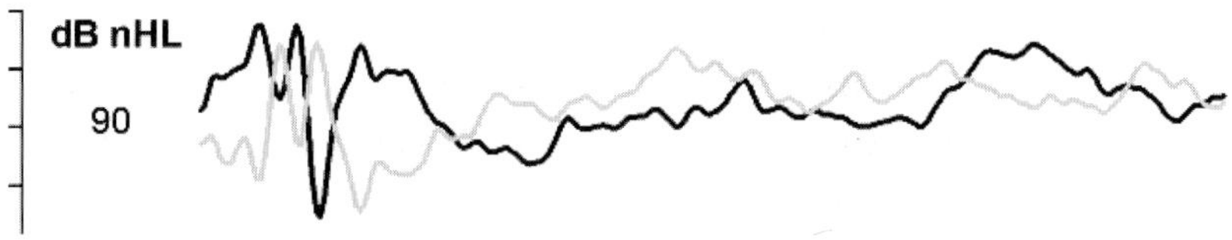


**Fig. 5.** ABR elicited with 90 dB nHL click stimuli; positive polarity and negative polarity click responses overlaid. The amplitude scale at left is 100 nV/division. The recording duration is 25 ms. The mirror-image section of the recording during the first 7 ms is considered cochlear microphonic.

otoacoustic emission. The child's history includes fetal distress, multiple transfusions and ten days in the neonatal intensive care unit. Care must be taken to determine when auditory neuropathy may be present because in these cases, both the ABR and the OAE would be inaccurate in predicting hearing results.

## ASSR

The auditory steady state response (ASSR) is also an electrophysiologic measure that can be used to predict hearing thresholds in infants and toddlers. The stimulus for the ASSR involves a steady state tone or noise that is amplitude modulated. The amplitude modulation slowly ramps the amplitude of the tone up and down with a sinusoidal envelope. The best frequency range for amplitude modulation envelope when testing infants and toddlers is 80–100 Hz. Pure tones in the range of 250–8000 Hz can be used as the carrier frequencies, thereby providing an estimation of the pure tone audiogram. Detection of an ASSR for the carrier tone or audiometric frequency is based upon detection of neural energy (in the EEG) at the modulation rate. In other words, the cochlea responds at the carrier frequency, the auditory nerve and brainstem respond at the modulation frequency. If there is no response at the level of the cochlea, then there will be no evidence of the neural response at the modulation frequency. Detection of the ASSR is "objective," that is, based upon a computerized detection algorithm. Specifically, the EEG is subjected to an online frequency (spectral) analysis. If there is energy at the modulation rate (e.g. 80 Hz) that is significantly larger than background EEG noise, then a neural response to the carrier tone (presented at that modulation rate) is apparent. A frequency or spectral analysis is performed and a spike in the spectrum at the modulation frequency that is sufficiently larger than the background, is indication that modulated activity is detected in the neurons conducting the carrier frequency.

The potential advantage of the use of the ASSR technique is that multiple carrier tones can be presented simultaneously to assess hearing by using unique modulation frequencies applied to each tone. The detection software can search for multiple peaks in the EEG frequency spectrum corresponding to multiple modulation frequencies. Some applications have shown that testing of four frequencies in each ear simultaneously is possible. Because test time is a major limitation in assessment of audiometric thresholds in infants, the ASSR may offer a significant time advantage. Currently, only the ABR is recommended for audiometric predictions by the JCIH 2007 because the ASSR thresholds have not been shown to be as accurate as ABR in hearing level prediction when thresholds are in the normal to moderate range of hearing loss. Also, the published data on ASSR has been sparse until recently. Differences in threshold may be related to technical aspects of the response detection and newer systems may well improve on the ability of the ASSR to assess normal or mild-to-moderately elevated thresholds. This technique shows tremendous promise and should soon be used in many clinical settings for hearing threshold predictions in children.

## SUMMARY AND CONCLUSIONS

The tests described here constitute a basic audiologic assessment. Not all audiologic test categories are described. Other tests are used to assess performance with hearing devices such as hearing aids, FM systems or cochlear implants. In addition, audiologists will use other assessment tools to evaluate "central auditory processing" abilities in children who may have normal sensitivity but difficulty with listening, auditory memory, hearing in noise and other "high-level" auditory functions that may be crucial for normal classroom performance. Cortical auditory evoked potentials (AEPs) are also not described here because they are not commonly used to assess infants and toddlers or even school aged children. However, cortical AEPs provide valuable information and may soon be seen in a standard pediatric audiologic test battery.

The assessments discussed in this chapter are rarely used alone, rather are combined in test batteries to provide a more complete picture of the child's auditory function. A tympanogram, for example, may look exactly the same in a child with mild conductive loss and one with profound deafness. Clearly neither OAE nor ABR results should be interpreted alone, without the risk of serious misinterpretation, such as might be found in auditory neuropathy. Finally, new assessment tools are constantly emerging and the "typical" audiologic test battery for children will look very different in ten years than it does today.

## REFERENCES

1. Norton SJ, Gorga MP, Widen JE, *et al.* Identification of neonatal hearing impairment: summary and recommendations. *Ear Hear* 2000;21: 529–535.
2. Joint Committee on Infant Hearing. Year 2007 Position Statement: principles and guidelines for early hearing detection and intervention programs. *Pediatrics* 2007;120:898–921.
3. Yoshinaga-Itano C, Sedey AL, Coutler DK, Mehl AL. Language of early-and later-identified children with hearing loss. *Pediatrics* 1998;5: 1161–1171.
4. Moeller MP. Early intervention and language development in children who are deaf and hard of hearing. *Pediatrics* 2000;106:1–9.
5. Kennedy CR, McCann DC, Campbell MJ, *et al.* Language ability after early detection of permanent childhood hearing impairment. *N Engl J Med* 2006;354:2131–2141.
6. Sininger YS, Grimes A, Christensen E. Auditory development in early amplified children: factors influencing auditory-based communication outcomes in children with hearing loss. *Ear Hear* 2010;31:166–185.

7. Nance WE. The genetics of deafness. *Ment Retard Dev Disabil Res Rev* 2003;9:109–119.
8. Ross M, Lerman J. A picture identification test for hearing-impaired children. *JSHR* 1970;13:44–53.
9. Sanderson-Leepa ME, Rintelmann WF. Articulation functions and test-retest performance of normal-hearing children on three speech discrimination tests: WIPI, PBK-50, and NU auditory test no. 6. *J Speech Hear Disord* 1976;41:503–519.
10. Feeney MP, Grant IL, Mills DM. Wideband energy reflectance measurements of ossicular chain discontinuity and repair in human temporal bone. *Ear Hear* 2009;30:391–400.
11. Alaerts J, Luts H, Wouters J. Evaluation of middle ear function in young children: clinical guidelines for the use of 226- and 1,000-Hz tympanometry. *Otol Neurotol* 2007;28:727–732.
12. Baldwin M. Choice of probe tone and classification of trace patterns in tympanometry undertaken in early infancy. *Int J Audiol* 2006;45: 417–427.
13. Kei J, Levick JA, Dockray J, *et al.* High frequency (1000 Hz) tympanometry in normal neonates. *J Am Acad Audiol* 2003;14:20–28.
14. Smith CG, Paradise JL, Sabo DL, *et al.* Tympanometric findings and the probability of middle-ear effusion in 3686 infants and young children. *Pediatrics* 2006;118:1–13.
15. Kei J, Allison-Levick J, Dockray J, *et al.* High-frequency (1000 Hz) tympanometry in normal neonates. *J Am Acad Audiol* 2003;14:20–28.
16. Margolis RH, Bass-Ringdahl S, Hanks WD, Holte L, Zapala DA. Tympanometry in newborn infants — 1 kHz norms. *J Am Acad Audiol* 2003;14:383–392.
17. Roush J, Bryant K, Mundy M, Zeisel S, Roberts J. Developmental changes in static admittance and tympanometric width in infants and toddlers. *J Am Acad Audiol* 1995;6:334–338.
18. Kemp DT. Stimulated acoustic emissions from within the human auditory system. *J Acoust Soc Am* 1978;64:1386–1391.
19. Shera CA, Guinan JJ. Evoked otoacoustic emissions arise by two fundamentally different mechanisms: a taxonomy for mammalian OAEs. *J Acoust Soc Am* 1999;105:782–798.

20. Siegel JH, Kim DO. Vulnerability to acoustic trauma and other alterations as seen in neural responses and ear-canal sound pressure. In: Hamernik D, Henderson D, Salvi R, eds. *New Perspectives on Noise-Induced Hearing Loss.* New York: Raven Press, 1982, pp. 137–151.
21. Stapells DR, Gravel JS, Martin BA. Thresholds for auditory brainstem responses to tones in notched noise from infants and young children with normal hearing or sensorineural hearing loss. *Ear Hear* 1995;16:361–371.
22. Sininger YS, Abdala C, Cone-Wesson B. Auditory threshold sensitivity of the human neonate as measured by the auditory brainstem response. *Hear Res* 1997;104:27–38.
23. Starr A, Picton TW, Sininger Y, Hood LJ, Berlin CI. Auditory neuropathy. *Brain* 1996;119:741–753.

# RHINOLOGY

5

# Acute and Chronic Rhinosinusitis

*Scott C. Manning*

## INTRODUCTION

The mucosal linings of nose and sinus cavities are contiguous and imaging studies demonstrate that even acute viral upper respiratory infections are characterized by inflammation of the entire system. Thus, the term rhinosinusitis is probably more descriptive than the term sinusitis for most conditions involving sinus inflammation. Viral illness is the most common predisposing factor and young children can average six to eight viral upper respiratory infections per year. Other potential predisposing factors include allergic rhinitis, adenoidal hypertrophy (inflammation), immunodeficiency, ciliary dyskinesia, aspirin exacerbated respiratory disease, cystic fibrosis and environmental pollution. Thus, acute and chronic rhinosinusitis accounts for a large percentage of pediatric primary care visits. And from a clinical standpoint, pediatric rhinosinusits represents more of an endpoint of different interacting conditions rather than one specific disease.

## INFLAMMATION

By some estimates, up to 5% of viral upper respiratory infections become secondarily infected with bacteria resulting in a more protracted and symptomatic clinical course. The pendulum is shifting away from a primary focus on the bacteria towards the view that most patients with chronic or refractory disease have an underlying hyperinflammatory state which is not always allergy.[1]

Studies of baseline incidence of asthma and allergic rhinitis in developed countries indicate an increasing incidence possibly related to the "hygiene hypothesis." Specifically, small families, vaccination, clean water and sanitation, early introduction of food antigens and possibly even high fat diet all may contribute to an overall Th1 to Th2 shift. Older studies that failed to demonstrate a strong association between refractory pediatric rhinosinusitis and allergy were no doubt hampered by the insensitivity of skin testing in young children and the non-specific symptoms with overlap with other predisposing conditions. Some newer studies have shown a stronger association between chronic rhinosinusitis and allergy in children than in adults. Unanswered questions include how prevalent is true allergy in young children, how much IgE, mast cell and eosinophil response is due to non-atopic antigens (bacteria, fungi) in the setting of prior breakdown of epithelial defense (viruses or eosinophilic degranulation) and how much mast cell and eosinophil response is not related to IgE?[2]

The "superantigen theory" holds that bacterial or fungal antigens could act as superantigens in patients with underlying hyperinflammatory states and bypass normal antigen processing with rapid recruitment of eosinophils and rapid onset of symptoms.[3] This theory may explain the clinical picture, especially in asthmatic children, of onset of severe congestion, culture-positive green rhinorrhea and cough within less than one day of onset of other viral symptoms. Staphylococcal organisms that may be normal flora could potentially act as superantigens in a susceptible patient with acute viral illness as the trigger. And because streptococcus pneumonia is a strong competitive inhibitor of staphylococcal colonization, the newer polyvalent pneumococcal vaccines may have added to the problem of increased staphylococcal colonization. And finally, methicillin resistant *Staphylococcus aureus* may be a more virulent superantigen source than non-resistent *Staphylococcus aureus.*

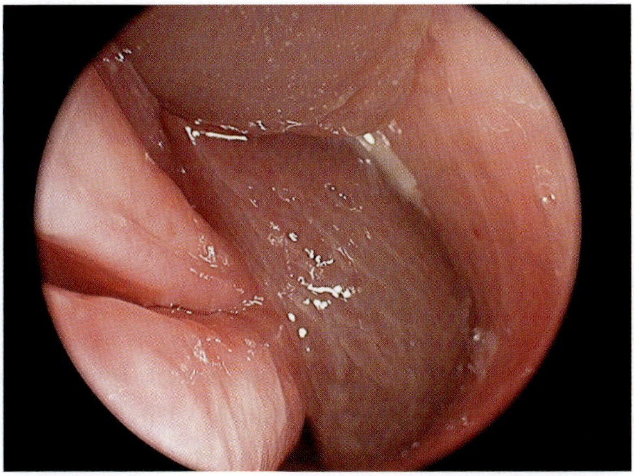

**Fig. 1.** Spheno-ethmoid polyps extending to the right nasal floor in a 12-year-old boy with aspiring exacerbated respiratory disease.

Aspirin exacerbated respiratory disease (AERD) is an updated term for the aspirin triad of aspirin sensitivity, asthma, and nasal polyposis (Fig. 1). This condition represents an abnormal regulation of arachadonic acid metabolism with elevated cysteinyl leukotrienes and it is not always associated with allergic rhinitis. By some estimates up to 20% of steroid dependent asthmatic patients without overt nasal polyps may have some degree of AERD and children usually have never been exposed to aspirin because of the concern for developing Reye's Syndrome. Once cystic fibrosis has been ruled out, any patient with refractory nasal polyps should be tested for aspirin sensitivity in a controlled setting (with available treatment for potential anaphylaxis). Aspirin desensitization therapy has been beneficial in uncontrolled studies of adult chronic rhinosinusitis patients with AERD.[4]

Some authors have postulated a relationship between gastroesophageal reflux or even eosinophilic gastritis and pediatric chronic rhinosinusitis but studies to date have failed to show any causality. It is likely however that those two entities are co-associated with chronic rhinosinusitis as part of the overall picture of hyperinflammatory state. Other potential hyperinflammatory co-morbid associations with chronic rhinosinusitis may include eczema, asthma, adenoidal hypertrophy, recurrent croup and migraine headache. A detailed history of any patient with refractory or recurrent rhinosinusits will usually turn up a surprisingly large percentage of these associated problems.

## BIOFILMS

The ability of bacteria to form organized structures on surfaces including mucous membranes with increased resistance to local and systemic immune defenses probably explains at least some of the relative lack of culture results and antibiotic efficacy in many patients with chronic rhinosinusitis. In humans, respiratory biofilms have been most extensively demonstrated in lung mucosa of cystic fibrosis patients with gram negative infection. Sinus and middle ear biofilms have also been demonstrated in humans and in laboratory animal models but their significance in chronic rhinosinusitis has yet to be determined.[5]

## CYSTIC FIBROSIS

Any child with nasal polyposis of otherwise unknown etiology should undergo evaluation to rule out cystic fibrosis starting with a sweat chloride evaluation. Chronic rhinosinusitis in patients with CF is heterogeneous with perhaps 90% of CF patients showing sinus mucosal inflammation radiographically, 70% flareups of symptomatic sinusitis and only 20% with overt nasal polyposis. Also, CF patients may present later in life, even in adulthood, with chronic rhinosinusitis with or without polyposis as their only complaint. This is especially true for some heterozygotic genetic patterns. Some authors also feel that CT carrier state (one gene) can itself be a risk factor for chronic rhinosinusitis. Clinicians should have a low threshold for evaluating for CF even in older patients if the degree of inflammation, recurrence or polyposis is unusual. There is no distinct histologic criteria for diagnosis of sinus CF but a finding of dilated mucosal glands in a patient with unusually severe disease should be another trigger for evaluation with sweat chloride testing.

Treatment decisions for CF patients with CRS are fundamentally no different than for other patients. Studies usually show no significant improvement of lung function with sinus surgery so the primary goal is improved quality of life. As with non-CF patients, surgery for extensive polyposis with significant nasal airway obstruction will predictable result in the greatest improvement in quality of life. Chronic rhinosinusitis without overt polyposis and nasal obstruction can be expected to show lesser but still significant quality of life improvement after surgery.[6] Patients with extensive polyposis and CF have high rates of polyp recurrence after surgery and should be maintained on topical nasal therapy with saline and topical steroids in order to reduce recurrence rates.

## PRIMARY CILIARY DYSKINESIA

Primary ciliary dyskinesia is a rare cause of failure of epithelial immune defense estimate at approximately one in 30,000 live births. Inheritance is autosomal recessive and at least eight associated genes have been identified. Most affected patients have a history of neonatal respiratory distress and almost all young pediatric patients have persistent middle ear effusions. Only 50% of patients demonstrate situs inversus (Kartagener's Syndrome). Chronic rhinosinusitis and chronic cough are near universal symptoms and families will often describe the presence of unusually thick and stringy nasal mucous. Most patients will eventually progress to some degree of bronchiectasis.[7]

Usually the first step in evaluation of a pediatric patient with suspected primary ciliary dyskinesia (without situs inverse) is to rule out cystic fibrosis. The next step for moderate levels of clinical suspicion, if available, can be to measure nasal nitric oxide with a nasal probe. Levels under 100 parts per billion are considered diagnostic. For patients with a high index of suspicion, a nasal brush biopsy for electron microscopic histopathologic examination is the first step. This procedure can generally be performed in the outpatient clinic. Positive biopsies are usually defined as at least 80% ciliary dysmorphology of outer or inner dynein arms, central apparatus defects or combinations thereof. Treatment of chronic rhinosinusitis in patients with primary ciliary dyskinesia consists mainly of prophylactic antibiotics, potentially in the form of topical nasal sprays. Sinus surgery may help patients with refractory disease but some degree of rhinorrhea usually persists.

## ANATOMY AND IMAGING

A common story from parents of children with chronic rhinosinusits is that they have been told that the fundamental problem is that the sinuses are "too small." In fact, there is no correlation between sinus size or almost any other normal anatomic variation and sinusitis.[8] Nasal polyposis (inflammation not anatomy) does correlate with more disease burden by quality of life studies in adults. The relatively common (up to 10%) finding of a small or "hypoplastic" maxillary sinus almost never causes pain or other direct symptom but may sometimes be associated with a greater likelihood of night time cough (Fig. 2). Radiologists sometimes invoke consternation among parents and primary care referring physicians by noting

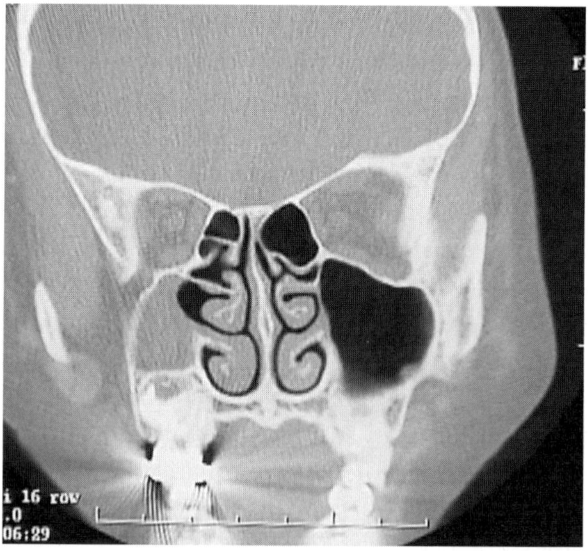


**Fig. 2.** A hypoplastic right maxillary sinus in a patient with migraine headache. No sinus treatment was undertaken.

"absence of frontal sinuses" but this is a normal finding in young children and in fact, about 8% of people never fully develop frontal sinuses (more common in cystic fibrosis patients). Acute and chronic rhinosinusitis in children is a consequence of problems with mucosal defense (viral illness in conjunction with underlying inflammatory state) rather than anatomic abnormalities.

Computed tomography for rhinosinusitis has no doubt contributed greatly to the exponential increase in imaging studies seen in the Unitied States over the last several years. New technologies allowing office based CT imaging as potential profit sources has probably added to the incidence of sinus imaging. It is important to keep in mind that young children have six to eight viral upper respiratory infections per year and that these infections can result in sinus mucosal inflammation that persists radiographically for up to eight weeks. It is no surprise therefore that analysis of head CTs in children under age eight in winter and spring presenting for other reasons without sinus symptoms show up to 70% with sinus mucosal inflammation.[9] Also, mucosal inflammation by CT correlates poorly if at all with symptoms of rhinosinusitis in general. Symptoms of facial pain and headache in particular fail to correlate with CT findings (in fact headache as the primary symptom probably correlates with an increased likelihood of complete lack of mucosal inflammation on CT). Air-fluid levels, and significant opacification of frontal and sphenoid sinuses (as opposed to peripheral mucosal inflammation of ethmoid and maxillary only) may correlate better with symptom scores in older patients. Adenoidal hypertrophy, inferior turbinate hypertrophy (allergic rhinitis) and severe septal deviation (unusual in children) can obviously correlate with nasal obstruction as a primary symptom (Fig. 3). The latter findings are often not remarked upon by radiologists examining images with "sinusitis" as the primary diagnosis. It is important therefore for the clinician to review the images themselves rather than to rely solely on the written report.

As with any diagnostic test, imaging should be considered when it is likely to result in a change in therapy. The strongest indications for CT imaging for sinus disease are unusual nasal polyposis (rule

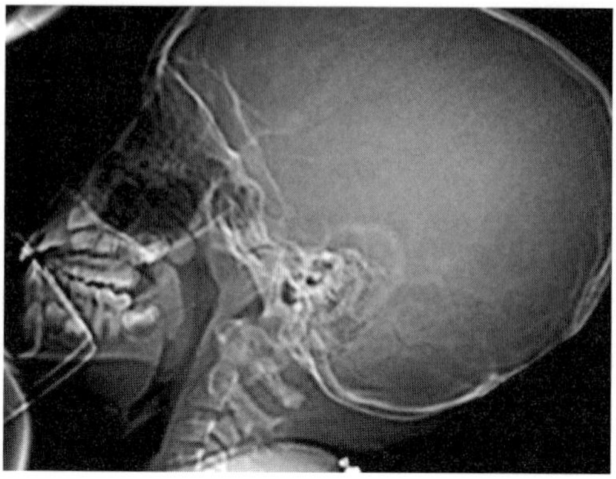

**Fig. 3.** A computed tomography sinus scout view demonstrating large inferior turbinates projecting into the nasopharynx and moderate adenoidal hypertrophy in a patient with a principal complaint of nasal congestion. The sinuses were normal.

out tumor) and concern for complication such as periorbital cellulitis or intracranial abscess. Imaging can also be useful in order to rule out sinus disease in patients with principal complaints of headache or nasal obstruction. Plain films can be advantageous for that purpose with no need for sedation in young children, less cost and less radiation. The relative insensitivity of plain films versus CT in patients with minimal mucosal inflammation may be an advantage in terms of better specificity (not being positive for clinical irrelevant "disease") as an initial screen.

In adult studies with validated quality of life measures, CT findings correlate poorly with symptom scores.[10] Therefore, with the exception of tumors or suppurative complications, CT findings alone do not define a need for surgery, especially in children. CT imaging provides necessary landmarks for safe sinus surgery but the decision for surgery is generally based upon lack of response to medical therapy in patients with imaging proven sinus disease.

## ACUTE RHINOSINUSITIS

Up to 2%–5% of viral upper respiratory infections in childhood may progress to acute bacterial rhinosinusitis (ABRS). Historically, the most common bacterial pathogens were the same as with acute otitis media specifically *Streptococcus pneumoniae*, *Moraxella catarrhalis* and non-typeable *Hemophilus influenzae*.

With the advent of newer polyvalent vaccines for *Streptococcus pneumoniae*, non-typeable *Hemophilus influenzae* has become the most commonly encountered organism in both acute and chronic pediatric rhinosinusitis. Also, *Staphyloccus aureus* and in particular, methicillin resistant *Staphylococcus aureus* (MRSA), appear to be increasing in incidence for both acute and chronic rhinosinusitis perhaps due to loss of competitive inhibition from *Streptococcus* species.[11] In terms of empiric antibiotic decision making, an increasing percentage of *streptococcus pneumoniae* isolates show intermediate penicillin resistance and an increasing percentage of *Hemophilus* isolates are beta-lactamase positive.

Symptoms of ABRS overlap with those of viral illness and allergy and it is not surprising that studies using vague symptom criteria alone to define disease often show no difference in outcomes between antibiotics and placebo. A Cochrane review of studies with radiologic confirmation of ABRS concludes that antibiotics can accelerate the time to symptom resolution although no differences among antibiotics were evident.[12] However, in an age of increasing MRSA, it is prudent to perform nasal culture whenever feasible. A culture swab of purulent nasal secretions using an otoscope for visualization can be instrumental in making the correct antibiotic choice. When MRSA is ruled out or not suspected, the most commonly recommended current empiric antibiotic choices for children with ABRS are amoxicillin-clavulanate or cefuroxine.

## CHRONIC RHINOSINUSITIS

The most common problem presenting to otolaryngologists is that of rhinosinusitis symptoms which respond, at least in part, to medical therapy but then recur. Common symptoms reported by parents and pediatric patients include night time cough, purulent rhinorrhea, fatigue, asthma exacerbation, and congestion. Headache or localized pain as the dominant persisting symptom often correlates with lack of sinusitis on imaging and warrants a neurology referral for migraine or pre-migraine especially if family history is positive for migraine. Persisting congestion as the dominant symptom is more often associated with adenoid or inferior turbinate hypertrophy — themselves often associated with allergic rhinitis. It is important to match the predominate symptom to the right diagnosis and treatment plan in order to achieve family satisfaction. "Sinusitis" can mean many different things to families and referring physicians but operating on clear sinuses for the primary symptom of headache is unlikely to result in a successful outcome.

Interestingly, culture studies of adults with chronic rhinosinusitis (CRS) often show little difference between cases and controls with a predominance of staphylococcal species, some streptococcus pneumonia and sometimes gram-negative bacteria in patients who have received extensive course of antibiotics. However, patients with CRS will usually show more evidence of inflammation in terms of polymorphonuclear leukocytes, eosinophils and cytokines versus controls. This fact supports the notion that CRS patients tend to be intrinsically hyper-inflammatory though not necessarily positive for inhalant allergies.

Meta-analyses of placebo-controlled studies of CRS have failed to demonstrate efficacy for standard antibiotic therapies. A fundamental problem with CRS studies lies in the ambiguities of defining the "disease" (probably more of a common endpoint of many different pathways) and, in fact, the United States Food and Drug Administration only recently (2006) attempted to define CRS for the purpose of comparative drug trials.

## MEDICAL TREATMENT OF CHRONIC RHINOSINUSITIS — DEMONSTRATED EFFICACY IN CLINICAL TRIALS

### Topical Glucocorticoids

Placebo controlled studies of topical glucocorticoids have shown consistent benefit for acute and chronic rhinosinusitis symptoms and for rhinosinusitis with polyps[13] Steroids can potentially block inflammatory pathways in both allergic and non-allergic patients the their efficacy underscores the concept of hyper-inflammatory state in most patients with chronic or recurrent disease. Topical glucocorticoids are often used in conjunction with other therapies such as antibiotics and topical saline.

**Nasal Saline Lavage**

Meta-analyses of trials involving saline spray or lavage have consistently shown benefit. Saline is usually used in conjunction with other therapies.[14] The treatment benefit of saline must be kept in mind when interpreting comparative studies using saline as a "control."

**Long-Term Macrolide Therapy**

Long-term macrolide therapy has been demonstrated to have an anti-inflammatory effect independent of any antimicrobial effect. Macrolide therapy can reduce cytokine production, neutrophil inflammation and production of biofilms according to recent studies. It is becoming standard therapy for some cystic fibrosis populations and for adults who have failed standard antibiotic therapy.[15]

**Oral Glucocorticoids**

Systemic steroids have shown a strong treatment effect in comparative studies of adults with CRS and polyposis and a lesser effect for CRS without polyps. In children, systemic glucocorticoids are usually given for brief periods at the onset of therapy to reduce nasal congestion while topical glucocorticoids start to take effect. They are also commonly utilized in the perioperative period for patients with polyposis.

**Allergy Immunotherapy**

While allergic rhinitis does not seem to be more common in adults with CRS versus controls, several studies have found an increased prevalence of allergy in pediatric CRS patients. Comparative trials are lacking but retrospective studies support the concept that immunotherapy can reduce the incidence of rhinosinusitis in selective children. From a practical standpoint, immunotherapy in children is usually considered in older patients with demonstrated atopy often with asthma who have failed other forms of medical therapy.

### Aspirin Desensitization, Antivirals, Antihistamines

Aspirin desensitization has proven beneficial for aspirin exacerbated respiratory disease patients with polyposis in non-comparative trials. Antivirals such as dipyridamole can shorten the course of common upper respiratory infections but their side effects can be significant. Antihistamines are obviously effective for histamine symptoms of allergic rhinitis but they do not affect the time course of CRS.

### Leukotriene Modifiers

Leukotriene receptor antagonists have shown benefit for adult patients with polyposis in a few open studies. Leukotriene modifiers in conjunction with antihistamines can be equivalent to nasal steroids for symptoms of allergic rhinitis.

### Topical Antibiotics

Topical antibiotics potentially provide a mechanism to deliver high dose therapy while minimizing side effects and pressure for development of resistance. Mupirocin was developed in the 1980s as a water soluble topical treatment for nasal carriers of *Staphylococcus aureus* and it is commonly used now for treatment of nasal MRSA. Studies have shown that it is effective in treating staphylococcus carrier state at least for the short term of a few months.[16] Some clinicians use it empirically for CRS as a 0.4% solution in saline hoping to eliminate *Staphylococcus aureus* as a superantigen in a predisposed patient. At least one placebo controlled trial of topical tobramycin versus saline failed to show any significant difference in outcomes.

### Intravenous Antibiotics

Retrospective reviews have demonstrated short-term clinical response but high relapse rates and high complication rates. Intravenous antibiotics are probably best utilized for treatment of suppurative complications or resistant organisms.

### Intravenous Immunoglobulin (IVIG)

Intravenous immunoglobulin has shown benefit in non-comparative retrospective reviews of patients with primary immunodeficiency and CRS.

## MEDICAL TREATMENT OF CHRONIC RHINOSINUSITIS — NO DEMONSTRATED EFFICACY OR INSUFFICIENT EVIDENCE

### Gastroesophageal Reflux

Proton pump inhibitor therapy has not shown benefit for CRS in studies to date. Gastroesophageal reflux may be a non-causal co-morbid state in cases of association with CRS.

### Topical or Systemic Antimycotics

Much excitement has been generated over the hypothesis that a large percentage of CRS in immunocompetent patients was possible due to hypersensitivity to inhaled fungal antigen. Trials to date have shown no benefit for topical or systemic antifungals over topical saline as placebo.[17]

## SURGICAL THERAPY FOR NASAL CONGESTION

Many pediatric patients presenting with a diagnosis of "sinusitis" have chronic nasal congestion refractory to medical therapy as their principal complaint. Nasal endoscopy possibly supplemented with imaging often demonstrates adenoid hypertrophy and/or significant inferior turbinate hypertrophy. This subset of patients and families probably experiences the greatest overall symptom improvement with intervention within the overall spectrum of rhinosinus symptomatology (Fig. 4). Adenoidectomy can not only relieve nasal obstruction but can also reduce the incidence of other rhinosinusitis symptoms presumably by eliminating an important target for inflammation in general. Conservative inferior turbinate reduction by radiofrequency ablation, microdebrider excision or other techniques not only relieves obstruction but also acts as an adjunct to medical therapy by allowing better application of topical therapy such as saline. The clinician must keep in mind that patients with allergic rhinitis may have significant adenoidal hypertrophy even into young adulthood and are more likely to experience significant regrowth after adenoidectomy. Conservative nasal septoplasty is indicated for

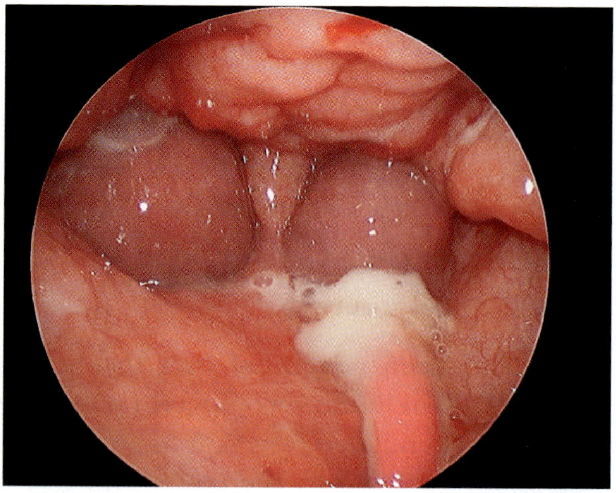

**Fig. 4.** A mirror nasopharyngoscopy view of large inferior turbinates projecting through the choanal openings and purulent nasal secretions.

older patients with severe obstruction due to septal deviation but it is not likely to reduce the incidence of rhinosinusitis.

## SURGICAL THERAPY FOR RHINOSINUSITIS

### Adenoidectomy

As mentioned previously, pediatric rhinosinusitis is a result of problems with mucosal defense, not anatomy. Direct sinus surgery changes anatomy and therefore is not the logical starting place in therapeutic decision making. Adenoidectomy is the logical first step in young children with image proven rhinosinusitis refractory to medical therapy and studies consistently demonstrate efficacy although large comparative trials are lacking. Adenoidectomy probably benefits more by reducing the target for allergic, bacterial and viral inflammation than by making more "room" in the nasopharynx in cases of CRS.

### Ethmoidectomy and Maxillary Antrostomy

Interestingly, though classically viewed as beneficial by improving ventilation, ethmoidectomy may actually help by decreasing the target for inflammation by reducing the overall mucosal surface area in the process of coalescing the honeycomb of ethmoid cells into one main space (Fig. 5). Most pediatric rhinosinusitis improves with time presumable due to maturation of systemic immunity. Patients who have first failed medical therapy then adenoidectomy and who have image documented significant sinusitis on imaging with an important impact on quality of life or health (asthma exacerabation) are candidates for ethmoidectomy/antrostomy. This appears to be a very small percentage of pediatric patients overall presenting with CRS. As with adult patients, uncontrolled studies show significant improvement in quality of life with both adenoidectomy and endoscopic ethmoidectomy with nasal antral windows. Randomized studies comparing medical therapy to surgery in children with CRS

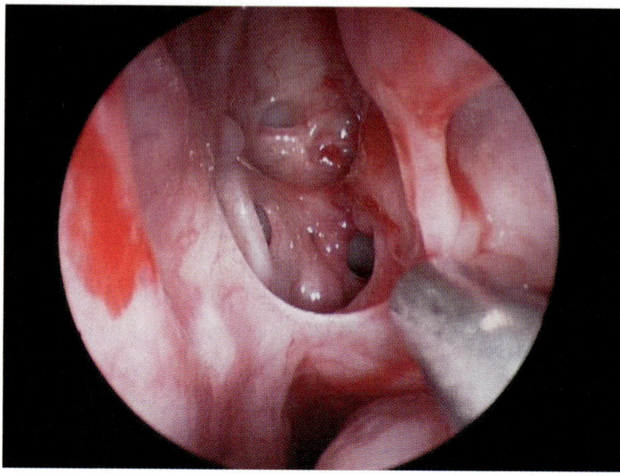

**Fig. 5.** A right endoscopic view of a healed ethmoid cavity after ethmoidectomy demonstrating the concept of reducing the amount of mucosal inflammatory target surface area.

are lacking but adult comparative trials not surprisingly show more quality of life improvement in the domain of congestion in surgical patients with polyposis.

The incidence of pediatric sinus surgery appears to be diminishing as the initial exuberance of the late 1980s and early 1990s is tempered with experience. Surgeons should be especially circumspect in decision making for patients under age seven and sinus surgery could potentially impact facial growth and because those patients are potentially still improving with maturation of immunity. Patients and families considered for endoscopic sinus surgery should be counseled that the realistic expectation is to reduce the frequency and severity of symptom recurrence. It is not a cure for allergy or viral illness and long term results are improved by continued use of appropriate topical nasal medical therapy.

## Suppurative Complications — Periorbital Cellulitis

Periorbital cellulitis is the most common significant suppurative complication of pediatric rhinosinusitis. Preseptal cellulitis is much less common than before the introduction of the Hemophilus influenza B vaccine in 1991 and these patients are generally easily managed with systemic antibiotics. Postseptal cellulitis is defined by signs of chemosis and proptosis and the most common imaging finding is a medial subperiosteal abscess or phlegmon. Children under age seven have a more favorable prognosis in terms of responding to intravenous antibiotics and are more likely to culture a single organism such as non-typeable *Hemophilus influenzae*. Patients older than age 15 are more likely to have polymicrobial synergistic infection with progression on systemic antibiotic therapy leading to a need to surgical drainage. Relative indications for surgery include progression of disease on antibiotics in general, decreasing visual acuity, large abscess, and immunodeficiency. The "correct" surgical approach is defined by surgeon experience but there is an overall trend away from external ethmoidectomy towards endoscopic ethmoidectomy with opening of the adjacent lamina papyracea.

**Suppurative Complications — Epidural Abscess**

Young teenage males with small developing frontal sinuses constitute the greatest risk group for intracranial complications of sinusitis. Allergic rhinitis, severe viral upper respiratory illness and sudden pressure changes from diving or flying are often in the historical background. The initial symptoms may be difficult to detect such as subtle changes in affect, gait and behavior and a high index of suspicion for imaging decisions is appropriate for the high risk demographic patients. Magnetic resonance imaging with contrast is more sensitive than computed tomography for demonstrating small epidural or subdural abscesses. These patients are managed in conjunction with the neurosurgery service and once again the "correct" approach is defined by institutional culture and experience. In general, as sinus surgeons have become more comfortable with endoscopic drainage of frontal sinuses, these cases are managed more frequently with frontal burr hole and endoscopic sinus drainage versus frontal sinus cranialization or obliteration (Fig. 6).

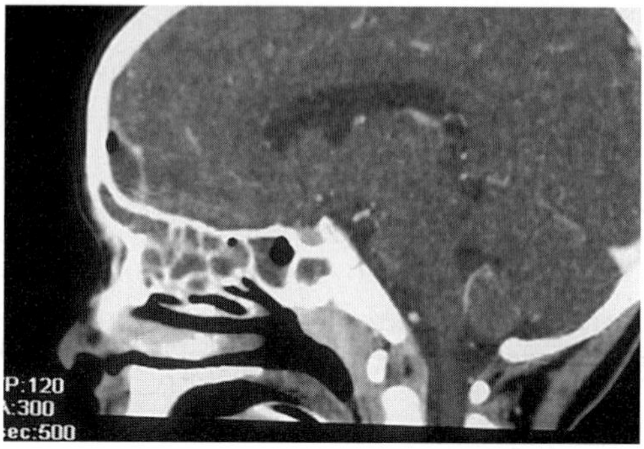


**Fig. 6.** A sagital computed tomography showing an epidural abscess and sinusitis in a teenage boy. The patient was successfully treated with a burr hole by neurosurgery service and endoscopic ethmoidectomy and frontal sinusotomies by otolaryngology service.

## Decision Making for Endoscopic Sinus Surgery

The strongest indications for surgery are the least frequently encountered problems namely suppurative complication refractory to intravenous antibiotics and sinus tumor or rule out tumor. The next strongest indication is arguably refractory nasal polyposis, often cystic fibrosis, and this is probably the population experiencing the strongest immediate improvement in quality of life. Rule out tumor such as unilateral polyposis with negative sweat chloride (rhabdomyosarcoma) and refractory frontal or sphenoid sinusitis (especially in a young teenage male) constitute infrequent but strong indications for immediate surgery.

The most common clinical problem, CRS in otherwise healthy patients, is probably the weakest indication for surgery as most of these patients can be managed with medical therapy. Most young children will experience an overall decreasing incidence of upper respiratory infection as they age and their immune system matures. Age seven is a good clinical benchmark for an expected normal reduction in upper respiratory viral infection and patients under this age may be at risk for effects on facial growth and development with aggressive surgery (Fig. 7).

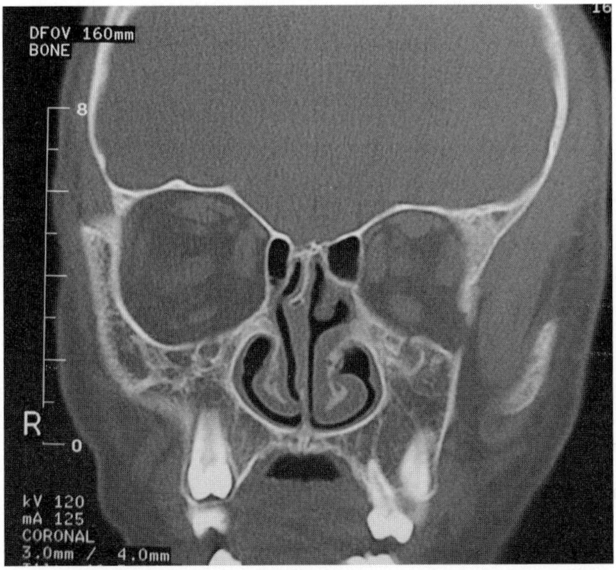


**Fig. 7.** Extremely underdeveloped sinuses in a 16-year-old imaged because of headaches (now resolved). The parents recalled a history of endoscopic ethmoidectomy and nasal antral windows at age 12 months for chronic rhinorrhea.

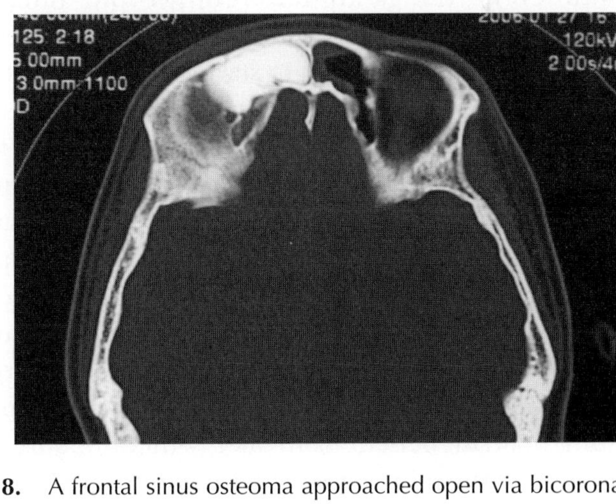


**Fig. 8.** A frontal sinus osteoma approached open via bicoronal flap.

A recent review of our 300-bed regional pediatric hospital experience showed an average of 70 endoscopic sinus cases per year with about 40% for the indication of CRS in a "hyper-inflammatory" patient usually with asthma, refractory to medical therapy. The next most common indication was cystic fibrosis with polyposis (regional CF center) followed by rule out invasive fungal sinusitis in immunodeficient patients (regional bone marrow transplant center). Endoscopic drainage of medial subperiosteal abscess (seven cases), tumor excision (seven cases: pituitary adenoma, osteoma, aneurismal bone cyst, olfactory neuroblastoma), and frontal sinusotomy for epidural or subdural abscess (five cases) finished out the list (Fig. 8).

## CONCLUSION

Rhinosinusitis is not a single diagnosis but rather the endpoint of many potential pathways including allergic rhinitis, adenoidal hypertrophy, recurrent viral illness and non-atopic inflammatory diathesis. Rhinosinusitis is not even a "common" endpoint as the term "sinusitis" means different things to different people ranging from synonymous with headache to chronic congestion. In order to make an effective treatment plan, it is vital to start with an understanding of what symptoms are most important to resolve for patients and parents. For image proven chronic rhinosinusitis, the logic of treatment is to start with the least expensive and invasive therapies usually combining an anti-inflammatory medication such as topical nasal steroids with an antibacterial medication such as topical 0.4% mupirocin in saline solution for a time period sufficient to break the cycle of recurrence, such as three weeks minimum. Allergy evaluation and appropriate treatment is critical keeping in mind that allergy testing is insensitive in young children but those with clinical symptoms and negative testing may still benefit from allergy therapy. Surgery is considered generally for the minority of older patients with image proven refractory disease with the realistic expectation of improvement rather than cure.

## REFERENCES


1. Weldin DR. What drives the inflammatory response in rhinosinusitis? *Allergy Asthma Proc* 2006;27:441–446.
2. Pant H, Ferguson BJ, Macardle PJ. The role of allergy in rhinosinusitis. *Curr Opin Otolaryngol Head Neck Surg* 2009;17:232–238.
3. Ferguson BJ, Seethala R, Wood WA. Eosinophilic bacterial chronic rhinosinusitis. *Laryngoscope* 2007;117:2036–2040.
4. Culp JA, Borish L, Mozena JD. Aspirin-exacerbated respiratory disease: an easy-to-overlook diagnosis. *J Respir Dis* 2006;27:282–290.
5. Singhal D, Psaltis AJ, Foreman A, Wormald P-J. The impact of biofilms on outcomes after endoscopic sinus surgery. *Am J Rhinol Allergy* 2010;24:169–174.
6. Khalid AN, Mace J, Smith TL. Outcomes of sinus surgery in adults with cystic fibrosis. *Otolaryngol Head Neck Surg* 2009;141:358–363.
7. Leigh MW, Pittman JE, Carson JL, Ferkol TW, Dell SD, Davis SD, Knowles MR, Zariwala MA. Clinical and genetic aspects of primary ciliary cyskinesia/Kartagener syndrome. *Genet Med* 2009;11:473–487.
8. Kim HJ, Jung Cho M, Lee JW, Tae Kim Y, Kahng H, Sung Kim H, Hahm KH. The relationship between anatomic variations of paranasal sinuses and chronic sinusitis in children. *Acta Otolaryngol* 2006;126: 1067–1072.
9. Manning SC, Biavati MJ, Phillips DL. Correlation of sinusitis signs and symptoms to imaging findings in pediatric patients. *Int J Pediatr Otorhinolaryngol* 1996;35:97–105.
10. Holbrook EH, Brown CL, Lyden ER, Leopold DA. Lack of significant correlation between rhinosinusitis symptoms and specific regions of sinus computer tomography scans. *Am J Rhinol* 2005;19:382–387.
11. Brook I, Foote PA, Hausfeld JN. Increase in the frequency of recovery of methicillin-resistant *Staphylococcus aureus* in acute and chronic maxillary sinusitis. *J Med Microbiol* 2008;57:1015-1017.
12. Fokkens WJ, Lund VJ, Mullol J, *et al.* European position paper on nasal polyps 2007. *Rhinology* 2007;45(suppl 20):1–139.
13. Joe SA, Thambi R, Huang J. A systematic review of the use of intranasal steroids in the treatment of chronic rhinosinusitis. *Otolaryngol Head Neck Surg* 2008;139:340–347.

14. Harvey R, Hannan SA, Badia L, Scadding G. Nasal saline irrigations for the symptoms of chronic rhinosinusitis. *Cochrane Database Syst Rev* 2007;(3):CD006394.
15. Wallwork B, Coman W, MacKay-Sim A, Greiff L, Cervin A. A double-blind, randomized, placebo-controlled trial of macrolide in the treatment of chronic rhinosinusitis. *Laryngoscope* 2006;116:189–193.
16. Casewell MW, Hill RL. Elimination of nasal carriage of *Staphylococcus aureus* with mupirocin ('psedomonic acid'): a controlled trial. *J Antimicrob Chemother* 1986;17:365–372.
17. Kennedy DW, Kuhn FA, Hamilos DL, Zinreich SJ, Butler D, Warsi G, Pfister PJ, Tavakkol A. Treatment of chronic rhinosinusitis with high-dose oral terbinafine: a double-blind, placebo-controlled study. *Laryngoscope* 2005;115:1793–1799.

6

# Pediatric Epistaxis

*Brian F. McGettigan and Udayan K. Shah*

## INTRODUCTION

Epistaxis is hemorrhage from any segment of the nasal airway, from the anterior nares to the nasopharynx. Epistaxis is commonly experienced by persons of all ages and, for children, is problematic because it may limit physical activity, school, and social participation, and at worst may lead to hemodynamic compromise. This chapter will address the etiology, evaluation, and management of this condition.

## EPIDEMIOLOGY

While the population prevalence of epistaxis is unknown because most cases are self-limited and are cared for by parents or caretakers, Emergency Department (ED) statistics from 1992 to 2001 showed that epistaxis accounted for approximately one visit out of 200 for the general population. Epistaxis accounted for 0.40% of visits in children age ten or younger and 0.36% of visits in children/adolescents age ten to 19.[1] The incidence of epistaxis is increased during cold weather and low humidity and in areas with increased concentrations of atmospheric pollutants such as London, England.[2,3]

Epistaxis has a bimodal incidence, with the majority of cases occurring in children younger than ten years and in adults age 65 years and older. Epistaxis occurs at least once in 30% of children age five years or younger and 56% of children age six to ten.[4] Epistaxis is rare (1/10,000) in children younger than two years.[1]

## ANATOMY/PHYSIOLOGY

The nose has a rich vascular supply from both the internal and external carotid artery systems. Branches from the external carotid include the internal maxillary artery and the facial artery. The facial artery courses up from the neck over the body of the mandible, past the oral commisure, to the side of the nose. It gives off the superior labial artery which provides septal and alar branches that supply the anterior nasal floor and anterior septum (Figs. 1a and 1b). The internal maxillary artery passes from the external carotid artery into the pterygomaxillary fossa and divides into six main branches. Two of these branches, the descending palantine and the sphenopalantine arteries, provide blood supply to the nose.

The descending palatine artery divides into the greater and lesser palantine arteries and follows through the greater palantine canal to supply the lateral nasal wall and palate. A smaller branch from this artery ascends through the incisive foramen to supply the anterior septum. The sphenopalantine artery is the terminal branch of the internal maxillary artery and enters the nose through the sphenopalantine foramen posterior to the attachment of the middle turbinate. It has posterior septal and lateral nasal branches that supply the lateral nasal wall and the septum, especially the posterior aspect.[5]

The ophthalmic artery is the primary blood supply to the nose from the internal carotid artery. It passes from the intracranial space to the orbit via the superior orbital fissure and divides into several branches, including anterior and posterior ethmoid arteries. Both arteries pass into the nasal cavity through bony foramina along the frontoethmoid suture line to supply the superior lateral and medial nasal walls. They re-enter the cranial cavity via the cribiform plate.[5]

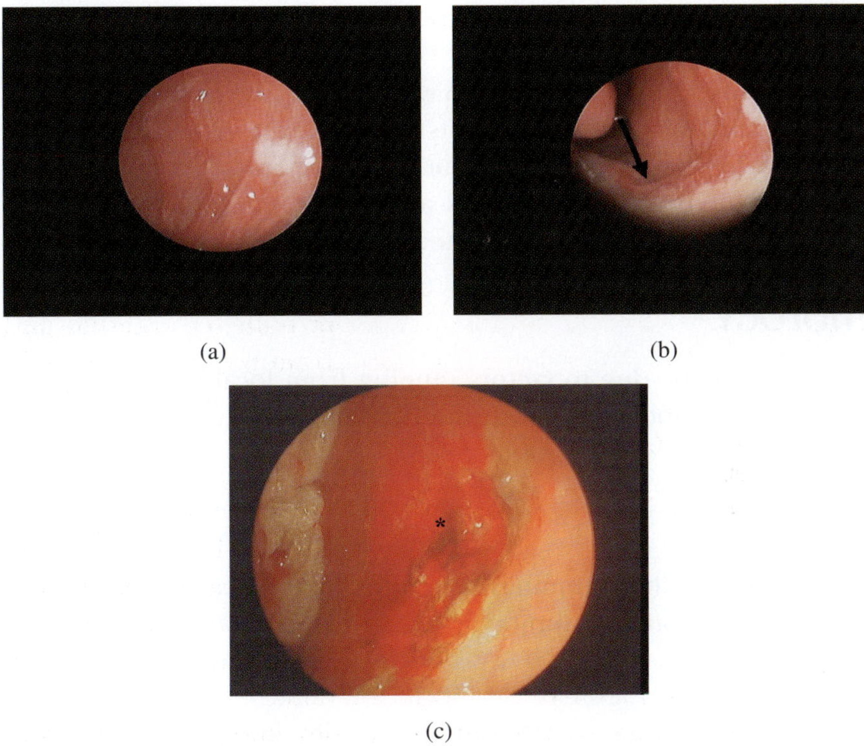


**Fig. 1.** Vessels.

**(a)** Kiesselbach's plexus over Little's area.

**(b)** Vessel (arrow) from lateral nasal floor along sill.

**(c)** Anterior epistaxis (asterisk).

Venous drainage parallels the arterial supply, with blood passing to both internal and external jugular venous systems.[5]

Two anatomic areas of the nose contribute to most episodes of epistaxis. Most epistaxis is anterior, due to Kiesselbach's plexus (Fig. 1c). This arterial confluence of the superior labial, greater palantine, anterior ethmoidal and sphenopalantine arteries is located on the anterior septum over an area called Little's area.[5,6] More posteriorly is Woodruff's plexus, located posterior to the attachments of the inferior and middle turbinates in the region of the sphenopalatine foramen. While historically, Woodruff's area has been considered to be arterial, recent cadaveric studies suggest a venous etiology.[7]

The function of the nose is to warm, filter, and humidify airflow. Inspired air also carries odorants that interact with the olfactory neuroepithelium at the roof of the nasal vault and contribute to the sense of smell. The nose also is a first-line immunologic defense against airborne pathogens, as the epithelial mucosa secretes IgA.[8]

## ETIOLOGY

Epistaxis may be due to factors ranging from local to systemic and can also be subdivided into anterior and posterior causes. The majority of cases are idiopathic.

### Local Causes

Local causes include trauma, structural/anatomical abnormalities, mucosal irritation, and tumors.[5,9,10]

- Trauma
  - Nose-picking — "Digital" trauma is common in children. Bleeding is usually anterior from the vessels of Kiesselbach's plexus.
  - Facial/head trauma — Blunt trauma, such as due to contact sports, can cause nasal fracture that may include injury to the septum, as well as injury to the orbit and lamina paprycea. Subsequent bleeding can be from laceration of vessels or from damaged mucosal surfaces. Massive epistaxis after head or face trauma can be from carotid pseudoaneurysm.
  - Foreign body — Unilateral epistaxis accompanied by foul-smelling nasal discharge suggests a nasal foreign body. The foreign body causes local trauma through mucosal irritation and ulceration. Epistaxis can be exacerbated by attempted removal of the foreign body. Disc battery nasal foreign bodies are particularly dangerous, and urgent surgery for

removal is indicated. A septal perforation may result from such retained caustic nasal foreign bodies.

- o Nasal intubation — Nasal intubation can cause bleeding at the time of insertion or may abrade mucosa and thereby promote epistaxis. Dilation of the nasal airway with a lubricated soft nasopharyngeal airway after decongestion with oxymetazoline may help reduce the mucosal trauma of nasal intubation, as may rigid or flexible fiberoptic endoscopic guidance of a nasal tube to avoid septal spurs and adenoid tissue.
- o Surgery — Adenoidectomy, endoscopic sinus surgery, turbinate reduction, etc. all can result in postoperative epistaxis.

— *Structural/anatomical abnormalities*

- o Septal perforation/deviation — These intranasal abnormalities can disrupt nasal airflow with resultant desiccation of adjacent tissues, leading to epistaxis. Chronic septal perforations may be rimmed with delicate granulation tissue that can be friable and easily bleed. "Eddy currents" of airflow may be created by septal deviations that exacerbate drying of mucosa and promote vascular breakdown and subsequent epistaxis.

— *Mucosal irritation* may result from changes in humidity, seasonal or allergic changes, infection (bacterial or viral), chronic rhinitis, use of nasal sprays, use of systemic drying medications, and exposure to inhalants such as cigarette spoke and cocaine, as well as airborne pollutants.

— *Tumors* are a rare cause of epistaxis, presenting usually with unilateral epistaxis with nasal discharge, obstruction, and dysosmia or anosmia.[11] Benign tumors (such as juvenile nasopharyngeal angiofibroma, hemangiomas, pyogenic granulomas, and inverting papillomas) and malignant tumors (such as rhabdomyosarcoma and nasopharyngeal carcinoma) may be seen in children. Nasopharyngeal extension may impair eustachian tube patency and result in serous otitis media. Juvenile nasopharyngeal angiofibroma most commonly occurs in adolescent males and are very vascular, fed generally from the internal maxillary artery. These tumors arise from the lateral nasopharyngeal wall and bulge into the nasal cavity. Pyogenic granulomas can form after trauma and are associated with capillary proliferation. Inverting papillomas generally arise from the lateral nasal wall, septum, or turbinates. They are benign but cause local destruction and have an approximately 10% potential for malignant transformation.[12]

### Systemic Causes

Systemic causes include bleeding diatheses, disorders of blood vessels, medications, neoplasms, inflammatory disorders, and hypertension.[5,9,10]

- *Bleeding disorders* include hereditary and acquired disorders of coagulation and platelet dysfunction.
- *Hereditary hemorrhagic telangiectasia* (HHT; Osler-Weber-Rendu syndrome) is an autosomal dominant condition that commonly presents with epistaxis. The telangiectasias are mucocutaneous vascular formations that are widespread over the body. Episodes of epistaxis may worsen over time, and bleeding can be severe during treatment.
- *Medications* — Children taking systemic medications such as anti-inflammatory/antiplatelet and anticoagulant medications are at increased risk for epistaxis.
- *Inflammatory disorders* such as Wegener's granulomatosis may present with bloody nasal discharge. Wegener's is also characterized by oral and nasal ulcers, persistent rhinorrhea, and myalgias or polyarthralgias. Renal and pulmonary anomalies are seen.
- *Hypertension* — Although much less common than in adults, children can suffer from hypertension. Secondary hypertension may result from renal disease or systemic corticosteroid use.

## EVALUATION

Evaluation of epistaxis should begin with attention to respiratory and hemodynamic stability. An expedient assessment of general appearance, mental status, and vital signs should be conducted.

## History

Important information to gather includes the following.[5,9]

- *Age of the child* — The younger the child, the more consideration should be given to trauma or serious illness.
- *Onset and duration of bleeding* — Prolonged bleeding suggests a bleeding disorder.
- Whether the *bleeding is unilateral or bilateral* — Unilateral bleeding suggests obstruction related to tumor or foreign body or isolated trauma.
- Whether there is *blood in the mouth or vomitus* — Bleeding from the mouth or with vomit may suggest a source beyond the nose or nasopharynx, or may indicate a posterior nasal bleeding source.
- *Prior measures* used to stop bleeding — Bleeding that does not stop spontaneously or with minimal interventions such as nasal pressure suggests a more serious etiology or posterior location of bleeding.
- An *estimation of the quantity* of blood loss.
- *Trauma*, nasal fracture history, insertion of a foreign body or nose-picking.
- *Nasal congestion, runny nose, or obstruction* may suggest allergic or infectious rhinitis or a tumor.
- *Recent history of oral or nasal surgery.*
- *Prolonged bleeding at other sites, easy bruising, and previous treatment for epistaxis.*
- *Family history* of easy bruising or bleeding problems.
- *Medications or drugs of abuse* such as inhaled cocaine.
- *Associated symptoms* such as headaches, facial pain, dysosmia or anosmia, hearing loss, otalgia.

## Physical

Evaluation and management is facilitated by seating the child, for younger children, usually in the caregiver's lap, with protection of parent, child, and staff clothing with drapes and gowns, eye protection and masks for staff, and a basin and suction for the child so that she can clear her mouth of bloody secretions. Application of a topical vasoconstrictor such as 0.05% oxymetazoline with or without 4% lidocaine via nasal spray or on a cotton pledget may facilitate examination and management.[5,9] Caution due to adrenergic effects of these medications is warranted.

After obtaining vital signs, physical exam should proceed systematically beginning with a general inspection with a focus on signs of hemodynamic or respiratory instability, such as decreased responsiveness or lethargy, cutaneous pallor, and coughing. Exam should next proceed to a full head and neck exam. Visual acuity and extraocular motility should be tested in this setting as well. Otoscopy may reveal hemotympanum from trauma or from reflux of blood from the nasal cavity. Oral cavity and oropharyngeal exam may reveal a source for the bleeding, bleeding onto the posterior pharyngeal wall suggestive of a posterior nasal bleed, mucosal lesions, petechiae, telangectasias, hemangiomas, etc. Exam of the skin may reveal stigmata of liver disease such as jaundice, which may cause a coagulopathy, as well as bruises, telangectasias, or petechiae suggestive of a bleeding disorder.[5,9]

Nasal exam should focus on identifying the source of bleeding. This may be difficult depending of the extent of the epistaxis. If bleeding precludes a thorough exam, then the bleeding should be controlled first with a pack and/or cautery as detailed below. Clots in the nose or temporary packing placed previously may need to be removed to allow for adequate visualization. Instruments such as an otoscope and a nasal speculum are indispensable for exam. The examiner should begin by using a thumb or finger to elevate the nasal tip to permit better anterior nasal vault exposure, including the nasal vestibule, the anterior septum (the location of Kiesselbach's plexus), and the anterior aspect of the inferior turbinate. An otoscope with or without the nasal speculum can then be used to perform anterior rhinoscopy, which generally allows for inspection of more posterior structures such as the rest of the septum, inferior turbinates, and anterior middle turbinates. Failure to identify a source of bleeding using these methods may indicate a posterior bleeding source. Exam by rigid or flexible endoscopy allows for further visualization of the nasal cavity, as well as the nasopharynx. A magnifying and illuminating headlight may be helpful as well.[5,9]

During exam, attention should be paid to the mucosa of the nasal cavity for signs of dryness, color, irritation, ulceration, laceration, vascular hypertrophy or anomalies, edema, erythema, and/or drainage. Masses or foreign bodies may be identified.[5,9]

### Labs

Generally, because most cases of epistaxis are benign, self-limited, and caused by local factors, laboratory evaluation is usually not necessary. However, if a systemic cause is indicated by history or physical exam then a complete blood count with differential, peripheral blood smear, partial thromboplastin time, prothrombin time, international normalized ratio, and blood type and screen may be helpful. In addition, specialized hematologic labs to detect clotting factor deficiencies, von Willebrand's disease, hemophilia, may be needed.[5]

### Imaging

If concern exists for a mass or vascular malformation, computed tomography (CT) or magnetic resonance imaging/angiography (MRI/A) may be indicated. The CT scan should be performed with and without contrast. A CT scan may also be needed for image guidance for certain endoscopic surgical procedures (see below).[5]

## TREATMENT

Patients with epistaxis are seen in a variety of settings including the ED, inpatient units, or outpatient offices. The goal of management in any setting is to control the bleeding. There are many different treatment approaches, both surgical and non-surgical, that may be used depending on the clinical situation. Non-surgical treatment is effective in the majority of cases.[13] Immediate "field" management is accomplished by anterior compression of the nares, contrary to the common misconception that pinching the bridge of the nose is effective for stopping nosebleeds.[14,15]

## Non-Surgical Emergency Department Management

If the patient is unstable, as determined by vital signs and rapid general assessment, then the patient should be placed on a cardiorespiratory monitor and an intravenous (IV) line should be placed to initiate rehydration or for transfusion if necessary. Pressure should be applied if the patient is bleeding and stable. Pressure is applied by compressing the nasal alae together for five to ten minutes while sitting up with head and body slightly forward to prevent bleeding from draining into the mouth and throat. Most cases of epistaxis resolve with simple pressure or compression.[16]

During this time, the provider can prepare for the exam and treatment by assembling the necessary equipment. A nasal speculum, a bayonet forceps, tongue depressor, a suction catheter, and/or Frazier and Yankauer tip suctions, cotton pledgets, a topical anesthetic and decongestant/vasoconstricting agent (e.g. 0.05% oxymetazoline with 4% gel or topical lidocaine), topical antibiotic ointment, and packing materials should be readily available. The child may need to be secured, such as in a parent's or providers lap and arms, or in a papoose.[9]

The anesthetic/vasoconstricting agent can be sprayed into the nose bilaterally or used to soak cotton pledgets. A nasal speculum is inserted into the nasal vestibule to gently spread open the anterior nasal cavity and pledgets are placed with bayonet forceps along the nasal floor or angled slightly superior towards the middle turbinate. Appropriate time should be allowed for the effect of the medication (approximately seven to ten minutes for oxymetazoline). The pledgets are then removed and the bleeding source is identified. In up to 65% of patients, this intervention alone has been found to successfully stop epistaxis.[17]

### *Chemical cautery*

If pressure fails to stop the bleeding, then control should next be attempted using cautery. Topical application of local anesthetic with vasoconstriction is recommended. Suction to remove clot and allow effective and efficient cauterization may be held in the same hand as the cautery stick (Fig. 2a).

In the awake patient, this is generally done with silver nitrate sticks (GF Health, Atlanta, GA), which provide chemical cautery (Fig. 2b). Coagulation should begin at the periphery of the active vessel, and then, with one hand holding the nasal speculum and the other hand holding both the suction and the silver nitrate sticks.

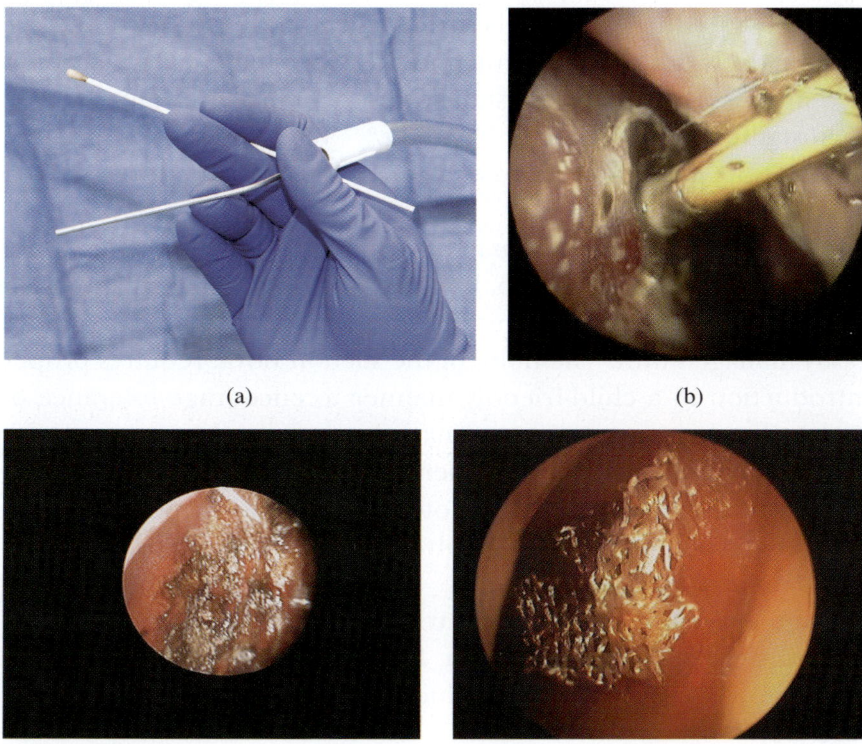

(a) (b) (c) (d)

**Fig. 2.** Control of epistaxis.

**(a)** Holding cautery (top) and suction (below) in one hand.

**(b)** Silver nitrate cautery. *Permission requested from K. Cavanaugh, MD (entusa.com).*

**(c)** Post-cautery.

**(d)** Surgicel over cauterized area.

Silver nitrate sticks have an applicator tip that is applied with a gentle rolling motion at the site of bleeding for several seconds until a grey-black eschar forms (Fig. 2c). Moist gauze may be used to remove debris from cautery on the lips and skin to prevent chemical injury to these to these tissues. Care must be taken to avoid using too much pressure, avoid keeping the tip on the spot longer then necessary, and to avoid deeply cauterizing corresponding locations on the contralateral nasal septum, as this can cause necrosis of nasal mucosa and lead to septal perforation. Additionally, cautery may predispose to rhinorrhea and crusting. Silver nitrate is most effective in a relatively dry environment, and therefore the area to be cauterized must be relatively hemostatic prior to application. This method is most effective for anterior bleeding.[5,10] When used appropriately, silver nitrate cautery has a greater than 90% success rate at controlling epistaxis.[18]

Suction electrocautery may be applied in selected cases using the suction Bovie (Valley Lab, Boulder, CO) in a similar manner, on a spray setting, thereby permitting suction and cautery with a more easily managed unit. The noise of the suction Bovie requires proper introduction in a child-friendly manner to encourage tolerance of this technology for epistaxis management in the awake child. Adequate anesthesia and a cooperative child are absolutely critical for use in this population.[19] Of note, a small study demonstrated no difference in effectiveness of silver nitrate or electrocautery for mild, anterior nasal bleeding.[20]

Antibacterial ointment over trimmed absorbable packing such as SurgiCel (Johnson & Johnson, New Jersey, USA) may be placed over the cauterized area to reduce airflow and promote healing (Fig. 2d).

### *Anterior nasal packing*

Whether or not chemical cautery is effective, anterior nasal packing may be used. There are many materials that can be used for packing, both non-resorbable and resorbable. In the former category, Vaseline gauze (Covidien, Mansfield, MA), compressed sponges (e.g. Merocel sponges; Medtronic, Jacksonville, FL), or nasal balloons (e.g. RapidRhino; (ArthroCare, Austin, TX) are used. In general, non-resorbable packing materials should be amply coated with a topical antibiotic such as bacitracin prior to insertion to avoid the development of infection including sinusitis and toxic shock syndrome. Packing should fill the nasal cavity, bearing in mind that the superior and middle aspects are frequently overlooked and inadequately packed to sustain enough pressure to maintain hemostasis. A nasal endoscope is helpful to guide placement of packing. A small otologic alligator forceps or thin pediatric endoscopic sinus instruments are also useful.[5,9,15]

Vaseline gauze comes as a long, continuous ribbon. Gauze packing may effectively compress bleeding sites while being insinuated into the crevices of the lateral nasal wall and medially against the septum by grasping several centimeters from the end so that when placed the most inferior gauze layer is exiting the nose just at the ala: this permits easy removal. A nasal speculum may be placed in the nose so that the blade secures the ribbon against the lower aspect of the nasal vestibule. The packing is then regrasped several centimeters from the point at which it enters the nose and is placed into the nose over the initial layer. This process is repeated until the nasal vault is completely packed. When complete, two free ends of the ribbon should protrude from the nose.[5,9]

Compressed sponges are generally firm and flat but come in many shapes and sizes. Most have an attached string that facilitates removal. Sponges may need to be trimmed and shaped, especially in the pediatric population. After coating generously with topical antibiotic ointment or a sterile lubricant, they are gently inserted into the nasal cavity until the proximal edge can be seen just inside the nasal vestibule. Care must be taken to avoid the tendency to insert the sponge in a superior direction, and rather to direct the sponge along the path of the nasal floor. The sponge should not protrude past the vestibule as that would put pressure on the skin of the ala, increasing the risk of alar necrosis or ulceration. Once in place, the sponges should be soaked by a spray of saline or the mixture of anesthetic/vasoconstrictor to cause expansion.[5,9] Oral antibiotics are recommended when packing the nose to prevent toxic shock syndrome, discussed below.

Anterior epistaxis balloons come in different lengths but work similarly to a Foley catheter. They are coated with ointment inserted into the nose. Saline is injected to inflate the balloon until the bleeding stops. Saline is used as air has the tendency to leak out of the balloon over time, compromising hemostasis. Care should be taken to avoid overfilling the balloon, as this can lead to complications associated with pressure injury. Several studies suggest that balloons are superior to sponges in terms of ease of insertion and patient comfort, but equal in effectiveness.[21,22]

The most common absorbable packing materials include solids such as Gelfoam (Baxter, Deerfield, IL) and Surgicel (Ethicon, Somerville, NJ), and paste-like substances including Surgifoam (Ethicon, Somerville, NJ) and Floseal (Baxter, Deerfield, IL). These products have pro-thrombotic effects. Surgicel comes as rectangular sheets is placed into the nasal cavity in a layered fashion with bayonet forceps, similar to placement of Vaseline gauze, or in small pieces directly over bleeding points. Surgifoam comes as a dry, flaky material that is mixed with 5 to 6 ml of saline immediately prior to use. The resulting paste-like substance is placed into a 10 ml syringe affixed with a large-bore angiocather and injected into the nasal cavity. The foam can be injected in a directed fashion or used to fill most of the cavity.[5] Non-absorbable packing, especially the paste-like substances, have been shown to be easier to use, more effective, and less uncomfortable to patients compared to non-resorbable packing.[23]

Regardless of the material, once the packing is placed, inspection of the nasal cavity (including the contralateral side) and the oral cavity/oropharynx should be performed to assure the bleeding has stopped. Further oozing from the ipsilateral side indicates that packing is inadequate in amount or position, and adjustments should be made. If bleeding is noted on the contralateral side or in the oropharynx, it may also indicate that the anterior packing is inadequate, or that the bleeding is from a posterior source.[5]

*Posterior nasal packing*

If the bleeding source is known or suspected to be posterior, then a posterior pack may need to be placed. Careful consideration must be made of the need for a posterior pack, as it is associated with increased morbidity and potential risks. In most cases, posterior packs are combined with anterior packs. Once the packing is placed, inspection of the nasal cavity (including the contralateral side) and the oral cavity/oropharynx should be performed to assure the bleeding as stopped. Overall, posterior packing has a 70% success rate in controlling epistaxis.[5,24]

As with anterior packs, there is a variety from which to choose. Several companies produce packs composed of anterior and posterior balloons (e.g. Epistat; Medtronic, Jacksonville, FL), which can be quickly and easily placed. The pack is inserted through the nose to the nasopharynx. The posterior balloon is filled with saline and pulled forward to fit snugly in the choana. The anterior balloon is then filled. Besides being easier to use, the newer commercially available posterior or anterior/posterior packs have a nasal airway built in so that nasal obstruction can be avoided, which decreases potential complications. The potential drawbacks of these preformed packs are a tendency to migrate anteriorly (which can place pressure on the nasal ala) and to put severe pressure on the nasal septum, or posteriorly and be asprirated. Taping ties attached to the packs or tying these across the columella may prevent such movement. Padding to protect the columella against erosion from the strings of the ties may be necessary.[5,24]

A traditional anterior/posterior pack typically consists of a combination of a 12 French Foley catheter (Bard, Covington, GA) and either Vaseline gauze or a compressed sponge. After decongestion, anesthesia, and evacuation of blood and clots, the Foley is advanced into the nose along the nasal floor until the tip is just visible in the posterior oropharynx when the patient opens their mouth. The catheter is then withdrawn approximately 2 cm and the balloon is inflated with enough saline so that it fits in the choana and resists movement with gentle backward traction. Then anterior pack is then placed as described above. Once both packs are placed, the Foley is secured with a clamp.[5]

Recently, hot water irrigation has been used as a non-surgical method for controlling intractable posterior epistaxis. In this method, a balloon catheter (e.g. a Foley catheter) is introduced into the nasal cavity as described above after topical anesthesia/vasoconstriction. The nasal cavity is then continuously irrigated using 500 ml of 50°C hot water. The balloon is then removed. Studies have found this method to be at least as effective as conventional non-surgical methods while avoiding packing, hospitalizations, or immediate surgery, and allowing the patient to breathe normally through unobstructed nasal cavities. The mechanism of action may be due to increased tissue edema with vessel compression and activation of the clotting process.[25]

*Follow-up*

If hemostasis is achieved without the use of anterior or posterior packing, the patient can typically be discharged safely from the ED. They should be given instructions to avoid nose blowing, to sneeze through the mouth, and avoid strenuous activity or exertion for several days. They should use nasal saline irrigation liberally (generally four times a day) and topical antibiotic ointment applied to the nasal vestibule and anterior septum (generally twice a day). Oral antibiotics are not indicated. Patients are instructed to use pressure and/or spray a topical vasoconstrictor into the nose if rebleeding occurs, and to go to the ED if bleeding does not remit. Finally, the bleeding is suspected to be the result of a systemic disorder or mass, appropriate and prompt follow-up should be arranged.[5]

If an anterior pack is placed, the patient can also often be discharged. They are given the same instructions as above in regards to nasal saline and activity restrictions. In addition, patients may be given prescriptions for analgesics (as packing may be very uncomfortable) and should be prescribed oral antibiotics effective against sino-nasal pathogens (such as clindamycin, or amoxicillin-clavulanic acid). They are given instructions to return to the ED or to an outpatient office in three to five days for removal of the packing (or to check the status of absorbable packing). Finally, they should be counseled on the warning signs of infection such as increased pain, fever, and purulent rhinorrhea.[5]

If a posterior pack is placed, the patient must be admitted to the hospital, usually to a monitored bed or intensive care unit depending on age and medical comorbidities. Patients should receive supplemental oxygen as needed, as posterior packs are associated with systemic hypoxemia. They may be given analgesics and antibiotics and instructed to use nasal saline several times a day. The packs are removed three to five days after placement, either at bedside or in the operating room.[5]

## Non-Surgical Inpatient and Outpatient Management

Epistaxis management for patients who are seen as inpatient consultations or who present to an outpatient offices are managed similarly to the above description for emergency department management. Outpatients who have posterior packs placed or who will require surgical management must be transferred to a local hospital. In addition, patients treated effectively in the office or inpatient setting can be set up for elective, more definitive management in the operating room at a later date.[16]

## Surgical Management

In some cases of epistaxis, management in the operating room is required. Indications for surgical management include: refractory epistaxis, recurrent epistaxis, the need for transfusion, a nasal anomaly precluding packing, patient refusal or intolerance of packing, or the need for posterior packing.[5,26] Because of the potential difficulties in managing pediatric patients, who may be uncooperative and in great emotional distress, it is occasionally necessary to take children to the operating room to attempt non-surgical management such as packing. They can then be monitored under sedation or general anesthesia. If there is concern for airway protection, management in the operating room can be the safest, most controlled setting with an experienced airway management team.

Anesthesia in epistaxis cases has potential risks and pitfalls. Depending on the severity of bleeding and how much is present in the oral cavity and oropharynx, views on direct laryngoscopy may be suboptimal for intubation. A rapidly placed, temporary pack may need to be placed prior to intubation attempts. Careful suctioning of the upper airway from the oral cavity to the larynx must be done prior to intubation as clots could inadvertently be pushed down in the airways as the endotracheal tube or laryngeal mask is placed. Often, these cases are taken to the operating room emergently, without regard to the child's NPO status. Also, depending on the severity of bleeding, the child is likely to have swallowed some of the blood. These factors increased the risk of reflux and aspiration during anesthesia induction mandating cricoid pressure (the "Sellick" maneuver). Finally, the patient may be hemodynamically unstable secondary to blood loss, which may or may not be immediately reflected on lab values such as hemoglobin and hematocrit, as well as on vital signs.

As with conservative management, there are a variety of surgical techniques and procedures that can be employed to manage epistaxis in the operating room. Often these techniques are used in combination.

### *Endoscopic nasal cautery*

The use of endoscopy can greatly facilitate identification and treatment of bleeding sites. The necessary equipment includes zero and 30-degree rigid endoscopes, a standard nasal tray which includes a variety of nasal specula and a Cottle elevator, silver nitrate sticks, and a suction cautery device.

After the child is anesthetized, the rigid endoscopes are used to carefully search the nasal cavity and nasopharynx for bleeding sources. If possible, this should be done prior to the administration of topical decongestants via pledgets or injection of local anesthesia because of the ability to identify active bleeding sites. Adequate attention should be paid to all areas, but especially to sites associated with prominent vasculature including the nasal septum, the anterior and posterior superior nasal cavity, the middle meatus, the posterior aspect of the middle turbinate, and the sphenoethmoid recess. If views are limited by anatomy, then procedures such as turbinate medialization or lateralization by in- or out-fracturing, medialization of the middle turbinate, or septoplasty may need to be preformed. In addition to active bleeding sites, the surgeon should inspect for lesions or masses, sites of recent bleeding (sites with mucosal injury, ulceration, clots, prominent vasculature), and sites of trauma caused by previous attempts at control.[5,10]

If not already completed, the nasal cavity is then decongested and anesthetized with a topical agent on pledgets as described above, as well as with injection of a local agent, typically lidocaine with 1:100,000 epinephrine. Cauterization then proceeds under direct visualization with the endoscope. If bleeding points are small and not severe, chemical cauterization with silver nitrate can be performed. If not, the suction cautery is used to cauterize bleeding points. The device is typically set at eight to 20 Watts of power on a spray setting of coagulation. Care should be taken to minimize cauterization of surrounding normal mucosa and when cauterizing the septum. After the bleeding is controlled, the nasal cavity and oral cavity/oropharynx should be carefully inspected. Packing may or may not be placed depending on the comfort level of the surgeon and the severity of initial bleeding. All materials should be kept ready in the operating room in case of rebleeding during emergence from anesthesia.[5,10] Endoscopic nasal cautery has been reported to have a greater than 90% success rate at controlling epistaxis.[13]

*Septal dermoplasty*

Septal dermoplasty may be used surgically as another option in epistaxis refractory to other treatment methods.

*Young's procedure*

Surgical closure of the nasal vestibule has been recommended for refractory epistaxis and may require "reversal" once the mucosa and nasal vault have had time to heal. This is rarely performed today.[27,28]

*Arterial ligation*

In extreme cases of refractory epistaxis, attempts at control include surgical ligation of primary vessels supplying blood to the nasal cavity and nasopharynx. The vessels typically ligated are the anterior ethmoid, the internal maxillary, and the external carotid arteries.[10,14]

Ligation of the anterior ethmoid artery is performed either by trans-nasal endoscopic technique or through an external ethmoidectomy approach beginning with a Lynch incision. After dissection through the soft tissues and periosteum, the periosteum is elevated and the lacrimal fossa and frontoethmoid suture line are identified. The anterior ethmoid artery is approximately 15 to 20 mm posterior to the anterior lacrimal crest. The artery is clipped, ligated, or cauterized with a bipolar device. If the posterior ethmoid artery needs to be addressed, it can be identified approximately 10 mm posterior to the anterior ethmoid artery. Care must be taken to avoid injury to the nearby optic nerve.[5,29]

In the endoscopic approach, an anterior ethmoidectomy is performed to expose nasofrontal recess. The artery is generally visible beneath the surface of mucosa, or identifiable in a prominent ridge or septation. The artery is then exposed and clipped or cauterized. A preoperative CT scan for use with image guidance may be necessary.[29] Success rates of greater than 80% have been reported in the literature for ethmoid artery ligation.[30]

Ligation of the internal maxillary artery is performed either through a transantral or, less commonly, a transoral approach. The transantral approach is relatively contraindicated in pediatric patients, depending on age and development, because of potential damage to maxillary tooth roots. It is contraindicated in maxillary sinus trauma and hypoplasia. The transantral approach begins with a Caldwell-Luc incision. After the periosteum has been elevated off of the anterior face of the maxillary sinus and infraorbital nerve identified, the maxillary sinus is exposed using a mallet and osteotome, and a ronguer. The mucosa is elevated off the posterior maxillary wall, and an approximately 1–2 cm square of bone is removed closer to the medial aspect of this posterior wall, below the orbit, to expose the pterygomaxillary space. Blunt dissection is used to isolate the internal maxillary tissue from the investing fat of this space. The artery, along the sphenopalantine and descending palantine distal branches, is clipped or ligated. Care must be taken to identify and avoid the maxillary division of the trigeminal nerve.[5] Image guidance may be useful in such cases.

The transoral approach to internal maxillary artery ligation begins with a posterior gingivobuccal incision beginning at the second molar which is carried through the buccinator muscle. The buccal fat pad is removed, to be replaced later at closure. The maxillary artery is then identified prior to the pterygomaxillary space, relative to the temporalis muscle medially and the ramus of the mandible. The artery is then clipped.[31] This technique is useful in epistaxis associated with maxillary sinus trauma and children, but it is generally less effective and more difficult than the transantral approach.[5]

More recently, the technique of transnasal endoscopic sphenopalantine artery ligation (TESPAL) has been described, which avoids the extensive dissection outlined above. TESPAL begins with the identification of the posterior attachment of the middle turbinate. The mucosa is elevated of the lateral nasal wall at this point. The sphenopalantine artery is identified as it exits the sphenopalantine foramen and is clipped and cauterized distally. The mucosal flap is replaced and the nasal cavity is packed with resorbable material. This technique has an approximately 90% success rate.[29,32,33]

Finally, external carotid artery ligation may be necessary as a last resort measure if refractory bleeding cannot be controlled by ligation of distal branches. This technique begins with an incision along the medial border of the sternocleidomastoid muscle. The common carotid artery is identified in relation to the jugular vein and followed to the bifurcation of the internal and external branches. The external carotid is identified by locating at least two of its branches; the internal carotid will have no branches. The external carotid artery is then ligated. This technique has a high long-term failure rate due to collateral contributions from the contralateral external carotid system.[5,10]

*Arterial embolization*

Management of epistaxis by interventional radiology may be a good option for bleeding that is refractory to surgical management; for poor surgical candidates; and for children with vascular anomalies, blood dyscrasias, or tumors. This technique can generally address bleeding from the internal maxillary artery and its branches only and is usually recommended for bleeding rates of at least 0.5 ml/min. It should not be performed if diagnostic angiography indicates anomalous anastomoses of the internal and external carotid systems or if the child has a contrast dye allergy.[10,34,35]

Diagnostic angiography of both the external and internal carotid systems bilaterally is performed first. The internal maxillary artery is then embolized, usually with Gelfoam, alcohol, or platinum coils, at the most distal site possibly permitting for precise, selective embolization with low risk. Recent studies have shown this technique to have a high success rate of approximately 90%.[10,35]

*Lasers*

Lasers have been used for managing epistaxis, often for patients with HHT. Several types of lasers have been used, including the pulsed dye laser and the Nd:YAG laser. Often, multiple treatments are needed, and surgical and non-surgical techniques to control epistaxis may be needed in conjunction.[36,37]

## COMPLICATIONS

### Non-Surgical Management

Complications of anterior nasal packing include pressure necrosis of the nasal mucosa internally and of the nasal ala. Intranasal mucosal necrosis can lead to ulceration, synechiae formation, septal perforation, and future bleeding. Anterior packs can lead into intranasal and sinus infections due to disruption of normal mucociliary outflow and secondary bacterial overgrowth. Such infections mandate antibiotic use with packing. Although more common with posterior packing, toxic shock syndrome can occur (see below).[16,26]

Complications of posterior nasal packing are more extensive and potentially more serious. Combined use of anterior and posterior nasal packing is associated with a complication rate ranging from 2% to 69%, with an average of 17%.[26] As with anterior packing, posterior packing can cause injuries associated with pressure necrosis, as well as intranasal and sinus infections. Infections are caused by pathogens such as *Hemophilus influenzae, Streptococcus pneumoniae, Moraxella catarrhalis,* and *Staphylococcus aureus. Staphylococcus aureus* infection can lead to toxic shock syndrome through the release of a preformed endotoxin. This endotoxin attacks multiple sites in the body, causing multiorgan failure, systemic shock, and death. Signs and symptoms include fever, malaise, nausea, vomiting, diarrhea, hypotension and signs of hypoperfusion, desquamation, and mucosal hyperemia.[24] Finally posterior packing can initiate the nasopulmonary reflex, in which irritation of the nasal mucosa by packing results in bronchoconstriction, leading to hypoxemia and hypercarbia. The use of narcotic analgesics to treat the significant discomfort experienced by patients with posterior nasal packing can exacerbate this effect by causing hypoventilation. This impact on respiration can lead to cardiac dysrhythmias and exacerbate other medical comorbidities.[26]

## Surgical Management

All techniques performed in the operating room carry the risks associated with general anesthesia, as well as those involving potentially difficult airways, particularly when brisk bleeding puts children at greater risk of aspiration during intubation.

### *Endoscopic nasal cautery*

Complications of nasal cautery include mucosal injury and subsequent necrosis and ulceration. Excessive bilateral cauterization of the septum can lead to perforation. Endonasal scarring can result, which can lead to rebleeding, synechiae formation, chronic rhinorrhea, and sinusitis.

Patients may experience transient or permanent palatal numbness or pain. Finally, any of the risks associated with endoscopic sinus surgery may result, including damage to the orbit and skull base.[5,9]

*Arterial ligation*

Complications associated with ligation of the anterior and/or posterior ethmoid arteries via the external approach include cosmetic deformity, wound infection, ecchymosis, hypesthesias/paresthesias, injury to the lacrimal duct, diplopia, enophthalmos, and blindness. Complications via the endoscopic approach include those associated with endoscopic sinus surgery and frontal sinus obstruction.[29]

Complications associated with ligation of the internal maxillary artery occur in approximately 25–30% of cases, and include intraoperative and/or postoperative bleeding, damage to tooth roots, wound infection, oroantral fistula, sinusitis, hypesthesias/paresthesias, and damage to the orbit.[34,38]

The complication rate of TESPAL has been reported as less than 10%, and includes those associated with endoscopic sinus surgery including damage to orbital contents and cerebrospinal fluid leak, as well as intraoperative and/or postoperative bleeding, scar formation, epiphora, palate hypoesthesias/paresthesias, sinusitis, and mucocele formation.[32,33,39]

Complications external carotid artery ligation include injury to the hypoglossal, vagus, and superior laryngeal nerves with associated sequlae, as well as injury to the internal jugular vein and common carotid arteries and can cause significant intraoperative bleeding. Finally, wound infections can occur.[5]

*Arterial embolization*

The complication rate of arterial embolization has been reported at 27%. The most significant risk of catheterization of the carotid artery is the risk of precipitating a cerebrovascular accident, resulting in permanent neurologic deficits. Other complications include recurrence of bleeding, facial pain and paraesthesia, trismus, and skin necrosis.[34,35]

## SUMMARY

Epistaxis is a common and potentially serious condition affecting the pediatric population. The range of presentation can range from minor and self-limiting to severe and life-threatening. It can be caused by a host of factors, both local and systemic, and can be symptomatic of a more serious underlying problem. A wide variety of approaches may be used to manage epistaxis. Awareness and consideration of potential complications associated with each intervention is necessary. Treatment should be determined on an individual basis for each patient. Providers are therefore urged to appreciate the breadth and skills required for effective management of pediatric epistaxis, including knowledge of referral sites for the less common but potentially useful procedures such as TESPAL and interventional radiographic approaches.

## REFERENCES

1. McIntosh N, Mok JY, Margerison A. Epidemiology of oronasal hemorrhage in the first 2 years of life: implications for child protection. *Pediatrics* 2007;120:1074–1078.
2. Bray D, Monnery P, Toma AG. Airborne environmental pollutant concentration and hospital epistaxis presentation: a 5-year review. *Clin Otolaryngol Allied Sci* 2004;29:655–658.
3. Danielides V, Kontogiannis N, Bartzokas A, Lolis CJ, Skevas A. The influence of meteorological factors on the frequency of epistaxis. *Clin Otolaryngol Allied Sci* 2002;27:84–88.
4. Petruson B. Epistaxis in childhood. *Rhinology* 1979:17:83–90.
5. Massick D, Tobin EJ. Epistaxis. In: Cummings CW, Flint PW, Harker LA, Haughey BH, Richardson MA, Robbins KT, Schuller DE, Thomas JR, eds. *Otolaryngology Head and Neck Surgery*, 4th Ed. Philadelphia: Elsevier Mosby, 2005, pp. 942–961.
6. Ballenger HC. Diseases of the nasal septum. In: Jackson C, Jackson CL, eds. *Diseases of the Nose, Throat, and Ear.* Philadelphia: WB Saunders, 1959, pp. 38–43.
7. Chiu TW, Shaw-Dunn J, McGarry GW. Woodruff's plexus. *J Laryngol Otol* 2008;122:1074–1077.

8. Levinson W. Humoral immunity. In: Weitz M, Naglieri C, eds. *Review of Medical Microbiology and Immunology*, 10th Ed. New York: McGraw-Hill, 2008, pp. 436–437.
9. Alvi A, Joyner-Triplett N. Acute epistaxis. How to spot the source and stop the flow. *Postgrad Med* 1996;99:83–90.
10. Pope LE, Hobbs CG. Epistaxis: an update on current management. *Postgrad Med J* 2005;81:309–314.
11. Shah UK, Potsic WP. Tumors and polyps of the nose. In: Burg FD, Ingelfinger JR, Polin RA, Gershon AA, eds. *Gellis and Kagan's Current Pediatric Therapy*, 17th Ed. Philadelphia: WB Saunders, 2002, pp. 918–920.
12. Mackle T, Chambon G, Garrel R, Meieff M, Crampette L. Endoscopic treatment of sinonasal papilloma: a 12-year review. *Acta Otolaryngol* 2008;128:670–674.
13. Pollice PA, Yoder MG. Epistaxis: a retrospective review of hospitalized patients. *Otolaryngol Head Neck Surg* 1997;117:49–53.
14. Douglas R, Wormald PJ. Update on epistaxis. *Curr Opin Otolaryngol Head Neck Surg* 2007;15:180–183.
15. Frazee TA, Hauser MS. Nonsurgical management of epistaxis. *J Oral Maxillofac Surg* 2000;58:419–424.
16. Kucik CJ, Clenney T. Management of epistaxis. *Am Fam Physician* 2005;71:305–311.
17. Krempl GA, Noorily ND. Use of oxymetazoline in the management of epistaxis. *Ann Otol Rhinol Laryngol* 1995;104:704–706.
18. Link TR, Conley SF, Flanary V, Kerschner JE. Bilateral epistaxis in children: efficacy of bilateral septal cauterization with silver nitrate. *Int J Pediatr Otorhinolaryngol* 2006;70:1439–1442.
19. Ahmed A, Woolford TJ. Endoscopic bipolar diathermy in the management of epistaxis: an effective and cost-efficient treatment. *Clin Otolaryngol Allied Sci* 2003;28:273–275.
20. Toner JG, Walby AP. Comparison of electro and chemical cautery in the treatment of anterior epistaxis. *J Laryngol Otol* 1990;104:617–618.
21. Badran K, Malik TH, Belloso A, Timms MS. Randomized controlled trial comparing Merocel and RapidRhino packing in the management of anterior epistaxis. *Clin Otolaryngol* 2005;30:333–337.

22. Singer AJ, Blanda M, Cronin K, LoGuidice-Khwaja M, Gulla J, Bradshaw J, Katz A. Comparison of nasal tampons for the treatment of epistaxis in the emergency department: a randomized controlled trial. *Ann Emerg Med* 2005;45:134–139.
23. Mathiasen RA, Cruz RM. Prospective, randomized, controlled clinical trial of a novel matrix hemostatic sealant in patients with acute anterior epistaxis. *Laryngoscope* 2005;115:899–902.
24. Viducich RA, Blanda MP, Gerson LW. Posterior epistaxis: clinical features and acute complications. *Ann Emerg Med* 1995;25:592–596.
25. Schlegel-Wagner C, Siekmann U, Linder T. Non-invasive treatment of intractable posterior epistaxis with hot-water irrigation. *Rhinology* 2006;44:90–93.
26. Johnson J. New approaches to the management of epistaxis. In: Johnson J, ed. *Maintenance Manual for Lifelong Learning,* 2nd Ed. Dubuque: Kendall-Hunt, 2002, pp. 254–258.
27. Brooker DS, Cinnamond MJ. Young's procedure in the treatment of epistaxis. *J Laryng Otol* 1991;105:847–848.
28. Lund VJ, Howard DJ. Closure of the nasal cavities in the treatment of refractory hereditary haemorrhagic telangiectasia. *J Laryngol Otol* 1997;111:30–33.
29. Snyderman CH, Carrau RL. Epistaxis. In: Myers EN, Carrau RL, Eibling DE, Ferguson BJ, Ferris RL, Gillman GS, Golla S, Grandis JR, Hirsch BE, Johnson JT, Raz Y, Rosen CA, Schaitkin VM, Snyderman CH, Toh EA, eds. *Operative Otolaryngology: Head and Neck Surgery,* 2nd Ed. Philadelphia: WB Saunders, 2008, pp. 7–16.
30. Klotz DA, Winkle MR, Richmon J, Hengerer AS. Surgical management of posterior epistaxis: a changing paradigm. *Laryngoscope* 2002; 112: 1577–1582.
31. Maceri DR, Makielski KH. Intraoral ligation of the maxillary artery for posterior epistaxis. *Laryngoscope* 1984;94:737–741.
32. Abdelkader M, Leong SC, White PS. Endoscopic control of the sphenopalatine artery for epistaxis: long-term results. *J Laryngol Otol* 2007;121:759–762.
33. Voegels RL, Thome DC, Iturralde PP, Butugan O. Endoscopic ligature of the sphenopalantine artery for severe posterior epistaxis. *Otolaryngol Head Neck Surg* 2001;124:464–467.

34. Cullen MM, Tami TA. Comparison of internal maxillary artery ligation versus embolization for refractory posterior epistaxis. *Otolaryngol Head Neck Surg* 1998;118:636–642.
35. Tseng EY, Narducci CA, Willing SJ, Sillers MJ. Angiographic embolization for epistaxis: a review of 114 cases. *Laryngoscope* 1998;108:615–619.
36. Mahoney EJ, Shapshay SM. Nd-YAG laser photocoagulation for epistaxis associated with hereditary hemorrhagic telangiectasia. *Laryngoscope* 2005;115:373–375.
37. Shah RK, Dhingra JK, Shapshay SM. Hereditary hemorrhagic telangiectasia: a review of 76 cases. *Laryngoscope* 2002;112:767–773.
38. Strong EB, Bell DA, Johnson LP, Jacobs JM. Intractable epistaxis: transantral ligation vs. embolization: efficacy, review, and cost analysis. *Otolaryngol Head Neck Surg* 1995;113:674–678.
39. Snyderman CH, Goldman SA, Carrau RL, Ferguson BJ, Grandis JR. Endoscopic sphenopalantine artery ligation is an effective method of treatment for posterior epistaxis. *Am J Rhinol* 1999;13:137–140.

# AIRWAY AND SWALLOWING

7

# Airway Obstruction in the Newborn*

*Matthew T. Brigger and Christopher J. Hartnick*

## INTRODUCTION

The first several months of life are a time of great change and adaptation for the newborn. In the vast majority of births, this time is characterized by few difficulties and rapid growth. However, for an unfortunate few children, this period is characterized by a turbulent course with potentially deadly complications. The newborn airway is not only smaller in physical size, but more dynamic than the adult airway due to the immaturity of the tissues, musculature and nervous system. As such, the newborn airway is acutely susceptible to a variety of insults, both congenital and acquired. Symptoms of airway obstruction in the newborn are the clinical manifestations of a wide spectrum of conditions. The range of presentations can vary from simply noisy breathing to that of severe distress requiring emergent intervention. As such, the evaluation and management of individual conditions is often predicated by the presentation of the specific etiology of obstruction. The goal of this chapter is to review

* The views expressed in this article are those of the authors and do not necessarily reflect the official policy or position of the Department of the Navy, the Department of Defense, nor the U.S. Government.

pertinent anatomic and physiologic issues and then to highlight evaluation and treatment strategies for conditions that compromise the newborn airway.

## Anatomy

The coordination of respiration and feeding is the evolutionary goal of newborn airway. The crossroads of this coordination occurs at the level of the larynx. However, this intricate interaction requires a certain level of anatomic development and neurologic integrity from the nasal cavity to the lungs. Our discussion will focus on the airway as part of the complex aerodigestive tract.

The respiratory mechanics of the first months of life are critically important to the evaluation of neonates. At birth, the neonatal epiglottis extends to a point superior to the soft palate while the tongue remains in contact with both the hard and soft palate.[1] This configuration provides for respiration during suckling. Although efficient during feeding, the configuration requires the neonate to be an obligate nasal breather. Crying is the only time when the normally developed neonate breathes orally. Mouth breathing is learned over the first four to six weeks of life.[1] As such, in the critical first month of life, any cause of nasal obstruction can result in respiratory distress to the non-crying infant.

Development of the aerodigestive tract derives from the primitive foregut through a series of outpouching, obliteration and recanalization that begins at 25 days gestation and is nearly complete by 27 weeks gestation.[2] During this time a variety of errors can occur including failure to fuse the tracheoesophageal septum, failure to recanalize the larynx or abnormal cartilaginous development. As part of the aerodigestive tract, nasal and midface development begins *in utero* by the fourth gestational month and continues through adolescence. Errors of midfacial differentiation can result in obstruction of the nasal passages and thus result in distress at birth.

As stated above, the larynx serves as the junction between the airway and the digestive tract and serves to provide ventilation, prevention of aspiration and vocalization. Neurologic and structural integrity are necessary for an infant's well-being and survival. Neurologic abnormalities or injuries that manifest as respiratory distress can occur both centrally and peripherally. Central manifestations resulting from anoxic insults, intracerebral hemorrhage or structural anomalies such as a Chiari malformation can result in vocal fold paralysis or loss of airway coordination. Peripherally, the course of the recurrent laryngeal nerves which descend from the vagus nerve and loop posteriorly around the subclavian artery on the right or the aorta on the left become of particular importance in infants requiring cardiac surgery.

At birth, the larynx is located high in the neck where the cricoid cartilage aligns with the fourth cervical vertebra. During childhood and adolescence, the cricoid cartilage will descend to the adulthood location of the seventh cervical vertebra. Furthermore, a relatively short thyrohyoid membrane results in the hyoid bone telescoping over the thyroid cartilage and obscuring the thyroid notch when palpated transcervically. Internally, the laryngeal inlet of an infant communicates with the trachea with the narrowest fixed portion at the subglottis. This region is at the level of the cricoid cartilage, which represents the only part of the airway that is circumferentially surrounded by cartilage. Therefore, from an anatomic standpoint, the subglottis with its narrow lumen and inability to expand secondary to the cricoid ring is at particular risk for instrumentation injury. Throughout the neonatal airway, soft tissue and cartilage are more supple when compared to adults thus resulting in a susceptibility to dynamic collapse, swelling and clinically significant intraluminal changes.

## Physiology

Two laws of fluid dynamics are of critical importance regarding the physiology of airflow in the infant. Using a fluid dynamics model, the airway can be thought of as a tube with flow through it. Poiseuille's law states that resistance within such a system is inversely proportional to the radius of the tube raised to the fourth power. In this model, if one considers an infant with a subglottic diameter of 4 mm who sustains 1 mm of swelling, the resistance to flow can be expected to increase by 16-fold and the cross-sectional area decrease by 75% while an adult with a 12 mm subglottis would experience only a twofold increase in resistance and 30% reduction in cross-sectional area. This law explains why infants, particularly those with subglottic stenosis, are susceptible to what might appear as relatively minor insults.[3]

Bernuolli's law states that as velocity increases in a tube with a constant diameter, the wall pressure decreases. Thus when air moves through a region of constriction at a high velocity, the drop in wall pressure may further contribute to dynamic collapse. The dynamic collapse is often manifested as stridor and is frequently generated from the supraglottic tissues or from the trachea.[3]

## Evaluation

As in any case of respiratory distress, evaluation always begins with structured Pediatric Advanced Life Support (PALS) algorithms including an assessment in the well-known *ABC* format. Initial assessment of a patent *airway* followed by an assessment of the child's *breathing* status and ultimately whether *circulation* is occurring ensures that the immediate needs of the newborn are met. Once the infant is confirmed to be stable, a further structured evaluation can occur. Regardless of whether the evaluation occurs in an inpatient or outpatient setting, attention must be directed to the functions of the upper aerodigestive tract. Specifically, the balance between airway patency, control of swallowing and the ability to vocalize must be considered jointly when investigating the potential etiology of airway obstruction. Further-more, this balance becomes particularly important in consideration of therapy as specific therapeutic interventions may improve airway patency at the expense of swallowing or vocalization.

Evaluation of infants with symptoms of airway obstruction is best accomplished in a multidisciplinary fashion. Dependent on the birth history, the type of obstructive symptoms, other comorbidities and urgency required many different practitioners might serve as part of a team-based approach to managing such children. Commonly involved specialties include otolaryngology, general pediatrics, neonatology, pulmonology, speech pathology, gastroenterology, anesthesiology, pediatric critical care, general or thoracic surgery and emergency medicine. An open stream dialogue is requisite between the specialties to ensure a comprehensive evaluation of these children.

## Outpatient Management

The variety of etiologies as well as the spectrum of severity associated with neonatal airway obstruction dictates the urgency and location of management. Stable children with an uncomplicated birth history and a mild degree of symptoms can safely be evaluated in the outpatient setting. Furthermore, some newborns only begin to manifest symptoms after discharge and will often present for evaluation in the outpatient setting. The absence of potentially worrisome symptoms such as cyanosis, apneic episodes, respiratory distress associated with retractions, frank aspiration symptoms or failure to thrive suggests that an outpatient strategy may be feasible. A diagnostic flexible fiberoptic laryngoscopy in an office setting gives important information regarding the neonatal airway above the level of the glottis and can help guide decision making regarding the need for admission. Radiography of the chest can serve to rule out the presence of an undiagnosed distal tracheal stenosis in children who warrant a diagnostic bronchoscopy under anesthesia.

## Inpatient Management

Inpatient management is required for all newborns demonstrating evidence of oxygen desaturations including cyanotic episodes. Furthermore children who present with any of the above described worrisome symptoms are often best evaluated initially as an inpatient. Children with associated anatomic or structural anomalies such as craniofacial dysmorphisms or cardiac malformations often benefit from initial evaluation in a controlled inpatient setting with appropriate multidisciplinary services available.

## Emergency Evaluation and Treatment

Emergent life threatening neonatal airway obstruction is one of the most feared and stress invoking situations in medicine. Clear thinking, calm decision-making and well-trained personnel can make the difference between life and death for a newborn in distress. As described above, appropriate PALS protocols should always be followed. Of critical importance is to realize the low functional reserve of newborns, particularly those with concurrent morbidities, as related to the rapid clinical decline that can occur in what appears to be a stable situation. As such, all members of the care team need to be well versed in emergency protocols and be able to function within their predefined roles. Furthermore, the goal of all centers that provide newborn care is to minimize the occurrence of emergent situations by actively assessing and identifying potentially dangerous situations. Adequate preparation and dialogue among the team members can significantly decrease the tension and improve the outcome of such situations. A discussion regarding various methods to secure a child's airway as well as the proper use of necessary equipment must be common knowledge among all practitioners.

Emergent situations can occur in any setting. Stabilizing maneuvers may provide valuable time to allow transfer of the child to a more appropriate setting such as an operating room for definitive management. A variety of adjunctive measures ranging from simple oral or nasal airway devices to the laryngeal mask airway and video based intubating devices or even Heliox can be invaluable to aid in securing a newborn's airway. In the setting of an uncontrolled airway that cannot be secured transorally or transnasally, a needle cricoidotomy can be a life saving procedure (Table 1). Of paramount importance is the strict avoidance of neuromuscular paralysis in the setting of a tenuous airway when the airway configuration is unknown.

## Complications and Their Management

Complications related to neonatal airway obstruction can be devastating. Failure to secure an adequate airway in an emergent situation

**Table 1. Needle cricoidotomy procedure.**

*Equipment needed*: 3 cc syringe, 14 gauge angiocatheter, size 8 endotracheal tube (ETT), bag-valve mask (BMV).

*Procedure*:
1. Fill syringe with 1.5 cc saline and connect angiocatheter.
2. Locate cricothyroid membrane, rapid cervical skin prep.
3. Transcutaneously pass needle through cricothyroid membrane.
4. Confirm placement in airway by withdrawing plunger to see bubbles.
5. Remove needle, maintain catheter in neck, empty syringe, remove plunger and reconnect to angiocatheter.
6. Connect standard 15 mm endotracheal tube adaptor from size 8 ETT to open end of syringe (with plunger removed).
7. Attach BMV or jet ventilator.
8. Proceed to tracheostomy in a controlled fashion.

can result in severe hypoxic neurologic injury or death. Additional complications can occur as a result of maneuvers used to secure an emergent airway. Immediate concerns after a difficult emergent intubation or obtaining a surgical airway include the development of a pneumothorax or pneumomediastinum potentially requiring further intervention. Traumatic intubation and high tracheostomy placement can result in future subglottic stenosis or worsening of a pre-existing airway lesion. Individual management is tailored to the specific complication, time course of development and severity. The thoughtful use of cuffed endotracheal or tracheostomy tubes to bypass areas of air escape into the mediastinum may prove useful.

## Operative Interventions

Operative interventions are tailored to the specific etiology of the child's airway obstruction. Depending on the urgency, careful evaluation of risks and benefits is necessary. Potential long-term effects versus immediate benefits must be considered. An important consideration must be given to the value of a short-term tracheostomy in children with potentially tenuous airways. Certainly, the decision to proceed must not be taken lightly. However, such a bridging measure, despite the well-known morbidity of tracheostomies, may ultimately improve the child's overall course. When the luxury of time exists, such decisions are made in conjunction with a frank discussion between the caretakers and other involved providers.

## ETIOLOGIES OF AIRWAY OBSTRUCTION

### Pyriform Aperture Stenosis

Pyriform aperture stenosis is characterized by excessive bony growth at the pyriform aperture resulting in anterior nasal obstruction. Clinically symptomatic cases are rare as there have been less than 100 reported.[4] However, there has been suggestion that the condition is underdiagnosed.[5] Presentation in the neonatal period is consistent with obligate nasal breathing and demonstrates cyclic respiratory distress relieved by crying. A spectrum of manifestations from mild to severe are possible. Diagnosis is made by anterior rhinoscopy or the inability to pass a small endoscope and confirmed with computed tomography.

An association with a single maxillary incisor as well as the spectrum of holoprosencephaly has been described.[6] The developmental defect associated with holoprosencepahly may include midline defects including dysfunction of the hypothalamic and pituitary axis which may suggest that a endocrine evaluation may be prudent in children with pyriform aperture stenosis.[7–10]

If a newborn with pyriform aperture stenosis were to demonstrate marked obstruction requiring an airway intervention, oral intubation may be necessary. However, the more common scenario is persistent cyclic nasal obstruction as described above. Thus treatment of pyriform aperture stenosis is dependent upon severity. Mild cases may be managed expectantly with nasal steroid drops while awaiting adequate growth. More severe cases are treated surgically by removing the stenotic bone of the anterior midface with a powered drill via a sublabial approach followed by stenting for several weeks.[11]

**Choanal Atresia**

Neonatal airway obstruction secondary to bilateral posterior choanal atresia presents as marked cyanosis that is relieved with crying. The prevalence is estimated to be approximately one in 5000 to 8000 live births with a female predominance in a ratio of 2:1.[12,13] Embryologically, persistence of the nasobuccal membrane occurs during the fourth gestational week.[12] The classic teaching is that unilateral atresia is present twice as often as bilateral atresia and more commonly affects the right nasal passage.[14–16] Historically, it has been reported that 90% of atretic plates are osseous and 10% are membranous. However, improvement in imaging techniques has demonstrated that most atresias are mixed.[17] Choanal atresia has been associated with a number of additional congenital anomalies and syndromes, particularly when the atresia is bilateral. The most common anomalies are those within the CHARGE (*c*olobomas, *h*eart defects, choanal *a*tresia, growth or mental *r*etardation, *g*enitourinary anomalies and *e*ar anaomalies) association. Other associated anomalies include Treacher Collins syndrome, Crouzon's syndrome, craniosynostosis, polydactyly, palate dysmorphism, tracheoesophageal fistula and meningoceles.[1,13] Diagnosis is generally made by a failure to pass #6 French nasal catheters and confirmed endoscopically or with a CT scan. A CT scan is essential in planning treatment to best determine the quality and degree of the atretic plate as well as potentially hazardous surgical anatomy.

At birth, children with complete bilateral choanal atresia may present in florid respiratory distress. As such, PALS algorithms are followed and some children may require oral intubation dependent upon severity. In some children, a McGovern nipple may be useful to relieve cyanosis.[12] Rapid accumulation of thick secretions occurs due to the inability to drain posteriorly.

Definitive management requires surgical opening of the obstructed choanae. Surgical approaches include the transnasal (both endoscopic or with an operating microscope), transpalatal, transseptal and transantral methods. All result in surgically removing the atretic plate to relieve the obstruction. Nasal stenting postoperatively has been advocated, however current trends have decreased the duration of stenting or avoided stenting altogether.[1,11,18] Some authors have advocated mitomycin-C or instillation of nasal steroid drops to prevent restenosis, but overall there is a lack of supporting data.[19–22] Outcomes are generally good, with an endoscopic restenosis rate of 12% that can be salvaged with additional procedures. However, it is generally accepted that the children with the CHARGE association represent a more challenging patient population and may have a lower primary success rate.[12]

Regarding timing of repair, in cases of bilateral atresia early repair is advocated unless contraindications such as extreme prematurity or multiple congenital anomalies are present.[23] In such cases, a tracheostomy may be placed and the repair planned approximately a year after adequate growth. Several authors have advocated the waiting approach particularly in children with the CHARGE association.[12,24,25]

## Nasolacrimal Duct Cysts

Nasolacrimal duct cysts represent a rare cause of airway obstruction in the neonate. At birth, approximately 30% of neonates have a patent nasolacrimal duct.[26] The remainder have a thin membrane that spontaneously ruptures within the first month of life.[27] Failure to rupture can result in recurrent dacrocystitis and resultant epiphora. If the cyst attains sufficient size, nasal obstruction can occur at the level of the inferior meatus. There has been a report of a child with bilateral nasolacrimal duct obstruction in a child with CHARGE association, however there is no clear genetic or associated anomalies.[28] In the appropriate clinical picture, CT scan confirms the diagnosis.

Few children with nasolacrimal duct cysts present in airway distress requiring PALS algorithms. However, in such a child, oral intubation would alleviate the airway distress and allow for further management. Most authors propose endoscopic marsupialization of the cyst wall with or without nasolacrimal duct cannulation as therapy.[27]

## Congenital Nasal Masses

Any congenital nasal or nasopharyngeal mass present at birth can manifest as airway obstruction similar to other forms of nasal obstruction. Such masses include nasal dermoids, gliomas, encepahalocele, teratomas, Thornwaldt cysts, craniopharyngiomas. The vast majority of such lesions do not present in neonates, but should be included in a differential diagnosis. Therapy is surgical excision, reduction or decompression.

## Nasal Malformations

Any malformation of facial development including cleft palate, cleft lip or the less common facial clefts can result in nasal obstruction. Treatment is often directed at reconstructive efforts of the primary malformation.

## Neonatal Rhinitis

As demonstrated above, given that neonates are obligate nasal breathers, any cause of nasal obstruction can result in airway obstruction. As such, non-structural mucosal edema can also result in airway obstructive symptoms. Neonatal rhinitis is the presence of mucosal edema in the absence of active infection or any structural abnormalities.[29] Such children often respond to topical decongestants or steroids with aggressive suctioning. Some authors have reported the success of nasal stents in refractory cases.[30]

## Laryngomalacia

Laryngomalacia is the most frequent cause of stridor in children.[31,32] However, the condition rarely causes symptoms in the immediate newborn period. Generally, symptoms develop over the first two weeks to two months of life. The symptoms are a manifestation of excessive soft tissue, hypermobility and decreased sensation of the supraglottic laryngeal structures, primarily the epiglottis and arytenoid cartilages. The pathophysiology has not been completely elucidated but gastroesophageal reflux, neurologic underdevelopment and structural anomalies have been suggested.[33] Of key importance is that laryngomalacia is a dynamic problem and as such the degree of obstruction is intermittent and frequently associated with feeding and crying.

Diagnosis is based on clinical suspicion and awake fiberoptic laryngoscopy to assess the dynamic function of the supraglottic larynx. Findings include redundant arytenoid mucosa which is dynamically drawn anteriorly into the airway (floppers), excessive curling of the epiglottis (curlers) or a combination. In children with severe symptoms resulting in cyanosis, apparent life threatening events or failure to thrive, an operative endoscopy is performed to rule out synchronous lesions and possibly allow a surgical intervention. Preoperatively, it is prudent to obtain airway and chest radiography.

Treatment is expectant observation in the majority of children. Few children require emergent intervention for laryngomalacia. However, if a child were to present in life threatening respiratory distress, oral intubation may be necessary to secure the child's airway. Surgical therapy is indicated in severely affected children with progressive desaturations, obstructive sleep apnea or failure to thrive. The procedure of choice is a supraglottoplasty. The procedure is tailored to the specific findings on the child's dynamic laryngeal exam and primarily involves removing excess tissue from the arytenoids and/or releasing tight aryepiglottic folds to allow the epiglottis to displace anteriorly. Instrumentation includes traditional laryngeal knife and scissors, $CO_2$ lasers or more recently powered microdebriders. A key tenant of surgery is to minimize tissue excision to prevent the development of supraglottic scarring.

### Vocal Fold Immobility

Vocal fold immobility (VFI) has been reported to be the second most common etiology of stridor in infants and accounts for 5% to

10% of pediatric tracheostomies.[34–36] Although, bilateral VFI is more commonly associated with airway obstruction and the need for a tracheostomy, children with unilateral VFI present with some degree of stridor, primarily inspiratory, as high as 77% of the time.[37] Etiologies are generally attributed to one of several classifications: neurogenic, birth trauma, cardiovascular, iatrogenic or idiopathic causes. The type of immobility generally depends on where the injury or lesion has occurred in relation to recurrent laryngeal nerve. Central causes generally result in bilateral immobility, while peripheral causes are generally unilateral in nature. Iatrogenic causes include surgical injury, compression injuries secondary to cuffed endotracheal tubes as well as trauma to the laryngeal cartilage complex.

Appropriate evaluation always requires imaging of the brain with a MRI when no clear etiology, such as history of surgically damaging the nerve, is present to rule out the presence of a central lesion or malformation.

Children presenting with marked distress at birth require oral intubation and stabilization. Ultimately, treatment is directed by the degree of symptoms and etiology of VFI. Traditional management of bilateral VFI in a neonate with airway obstruction is placement of a tracheostomy and observation for a period of 12 months. The prolonged observation period is prudent because high rates of spontaneous recovery (52%–100%) have been reported particularly when the etiology is idiopathic or secondary to neurological dysfunction.[38,39] Procedures designed to open the glottis and allow decannulation include removal of a unilateral portion of the posterior vocal fold with or without a partial arytenoidectomy, arytenoidopexy procedures or performing a posterior cricoid split and placing a cartilage graft. Any attempt to open the glottis in this fashion reflects the precarious airway, swallowing and voice balance that exists in such children. As such, potential complications that must be considered include aspiration and poor voice outcomes in the future. In general, most children with unilateral VFI do not require intervention for obstructive symptoms.

## Congenital Structural Anomalies of the Airway

A wide variety of congenital airway anomalies can result in various degrees of neonatal airway obstruction. These anomalies represent a spectrum of developmental derangements ranging from small laryngeal webs to complete laryngeal atresia. Some anomalies represent mild shape disturbances of normal structures, such as an elliptical as opposed to a circular cricoid ring as in congenital subglottic stenosis, that manifest clinically due to the small caliber of the infant airway. Other anomalies including laryngeal clefts and tracheoesophageal fistulae result in direct communication to the digestive tract. As such, presentation in the newborn can range from mild stridor when crying to life threatening obstruction immediately at birth. The extreme case is complete atresia which requires the presence of another anomaly such as a tracheoesophageal fistula to be compatible with life. Such children require an immediate tracheostomy at birth.

At the level of the larynx, a specific anomaly secondary to congenital obstruction of the laryngeal saccule can lead to formation of a saccular cyst. The saccule is an extension of the anterior portion of the laryngeal ventricle and is rich in mucous secreting glands that provide lubrication to the larynx. Obstruction of the orifice leads to accumulation of secretions and thus a mass effect. This is in distinction to a laryngocele which occurs when air fills the saccule, but rarely causes airway obstruction.

A commonly discussed term referred to as congenital high airway obstruction syndrome (CHAOS) has been used to describe a variety of situations presenting as airway obstruction at birth. The term generally connotes airway obstruction in a neonate that requires a surgical airway within one hour of birth.[40] Etiologies include laryngeal atresia or near complete obstruction within the proximal trachea or subglottis. Prenatal diagnosis is possible with ultrasound demonstrating evidence of the inability for fluid to egress from the fetal lungs. Ultrasonically this failure to clear fluid is reflected as large lung volumes, flattened or inverted diaphragms, dilated airways distal to the obstruction as well as late fetal ascites and/or hydrops.[41]

Children born with abnormalities involving the separation of the trachea from the esophagus are at risk of developing airway obstructive symptoms at birth dependent upon severity. Mild cases may go unrecognized into childhood, but major anomalies frequently present immediately after birth with choking and aspiration.

As in other etiologies of neonatal airway obstruction, management is based on the precise cause and urgency of intervention required. All children must be stabilized with PALS protocols if necessary. The delicate balance of airway, swallowing and vocalization becomes integral to the long-term management of these conditions. Treatment for simple thin webs requires little more than endoscopic excision. However, as the complexity of the lesion increases, more advance procedures including open layngotracheoplasty are frequently required. Saccular cysts generally require surgical excision. A stepwise approach of needle aspiration followed by endoscopic $CO_2$ laser excision and ultimately open excision of such saccular cysts has been advocated.[42] In the case of prenatally diagnosed CHAOS, the *ex utero* intrapartum treatment (EXIT) procedure allows a neonate's airway to be secured by initially delivering the child while pharmacogically maintaining placental circulation. After the airway is secured, the conversion from *in utero* to *ex utero* circulation is allowed to proceed.

Children requiring emergent airway interventions at birth frequently have a variety of concurrent medical and surgical issues. As such, the group tends to be at a higher risk of complications. The complexity of many of these conditions or proximity to the larynx often results in the need for further swallowing therapy, voice therapy or surgical therapy after the primary procedure.

## Tracheomalacia

Tracheomalacia represents a subset of congenital airway anomalies that are present in approximately half of all children with stridor.[32] Two primary forms exist. Intrinsic tracheomalacia refers to the setting where the primary defect is within the tracheal walls. These children have excessively pliant airways that easily collapse and compress under dynamic loads. In a child with a normal caliber airway, the anterior cartilaginous to posterior membranous trachea ratio is approximately four to one when viewed in cross-section. Children with intrinsic tracheomalacia frequently demonstrate ratios as low as three or even two to one.[43] In such children, the trachea takes on a much flatter, hyperdynamic state that is subject to marked collapse. Intrinsic tracheomalacia is commonly seen in premature infants.

Extrinsic tracheomalacia occurs when the tracheal cartilage has normal structural integrity, but an external compression occurs from within the mediastinum. When symptoms manifest during infancy, any compression of the trachea can result in airway obstruction, however great vessel anomalies are the most frequently discussed. Much has been written about the configuration, diagnosis and repair of such anomalies. Presentation depends on the severity of compression and whether the trachea is simply compressed as in the case of an aberrant innominate artery versus encircled as in the case of a double aortic arch.

Suspected tracheomalacia can be diagnosed radiographically prior to endoscopic confirmation. Airway fluoroscopy frequently demonstrates an anterior posterior compression on lateral view. Endoscopic assessment is used to further quantify the degree of severity, the length of the trachea involved and clues about causes of extrinsic compression. Contrasting views of rigid endoscopy versus flexible endoscopy are often complementary. If extrinsic compression is suspected, high resolution computed tomography with simulated angiography can provide invaluable evidence regarding the intrathoracic abnormality causing compression.

Therapy is generally conservative as most children with intrinsic tracheomalacia improve over time. Children with life threatening airway collapse require a tracheostomy or even the placement of an airway stent to provide palliation while giving a child time to further develop. Clear cases of great vessel abnormalities, particularly in the setting of tracheal encasement such as the ring of a double aortic arch must be surgically repaired. There has been recent anecdotal interest in the use of ipratropium to medically treat tracheomalacia.

## Subglottic Hemangioma

Subglottic hemangiomas represent a rare cause of neonatal airway obstruction with progressive airway obstruction manifesting over the first several months of life as the lesion proliferates. As the lesion expands, stridor and symptoms of persistent croup ensue. Misdiagnosis is common prior to the child undergoing endoscopy. At endoscopy a characteristic firm, but compressible red lesion in the posterior subglottis is seen. Deep submucosal lesions may not exhibit the red hue of superficial lesions. Confirmatory biopsy may be necessary in some cases, but is not requisite. If necessary, bleeding is easily controlled with topical vasoconstrictor agents. Associations with cutaneous hemangiomas have been reported of which the "beard" distribution was reportedly associated with subglottic lesions in 63% of children in one study.[44]

Preoperative airway radiography may demonstrate classic signs of subglottic narrowing, which in distinction to viral croup may be asymmetric in nature. In children diagnosed by endoscopy, further evaluation with neck and chest imaging is indicated to rule out mediastinal and intrathoracic extension prior to initiating therapy.

As described above, children with subglottic hemangiomas generally present with progressive respiratory distress. However if a young child with an enlarging hemangioma contracts a viral infection or has subglottic edema for any reason, frank distress can occur. PALS algorithms will dictate securing the child's airway immediately. In general, these children can be intubated with a small endotracheal tube. If unsuccessful, a surgical airway may be required. As the natural course of hemangiomas is a gradual involution, the goal of treatment is to provide the child with a secure airway with the least amount of morbidity. Surgical methods including bypassing the obstruction with a tracheostomy, laser ablation, intralesional steroid therapy and open excision are recommended based of the extent of the lesion and the desires of the family. Pharmacologic interventions include systemic corticosteroids, interferon and more recently vincristine or propanolol.[45–47] Each individual therapy must be considered with regard to success rates, number of procedures required and potential complications. Surgical therapies often demonstrate high success rates, but may potentially lead to scarring or development of voice or swallowing difficulties. Medical therapies may be limited by incomplete control or systemic side effects.

## Iatrogenic Causes

As neonatal care has progressed and the limits of fetal viability have been extended over the past four decades, an increasing number of neonates experience complications associated with such life giving care. Acquired subglottic stenosis secondary to intubation injury is far more common than congenital narrowing and should be suspected in any child with symptoms of airway obstruction after extubation. The incidence appears to have reached a plateau in recent years secondary to heightened awareness, meticulous NICU care and improved materials used in endotracheal tube construction.

In addition to acquired subglottic stenosis, acute injuries can occur during instrumentation of a child's airway. Children with extreme prematurity or other congenital anomalies are particularly at risk. Injuries such as intubation granulomas or a displaced arytenoid cartilage can result in life threatening airway obstruction. Acute tracheal tears can additionally result in mediastinal complications.

Management of iatrogenic injuries follows the same protocols and procedures as other causes of airway obstruction. In general, PALS algorithms dominate the acute phase of such injuries. After stabilization, a thoughtful identification of the injury as well as the development of a team based treatment plan based on the principles of balancing the child's airway needs while maximizing swallowing ability and long-term vocalization is necessary.

Table 2. Etiologies of neonatal airway obstruction.

| Etiology | Pyriform aperture stenosis | Choanal atresia | Nasolacrimal duct cyst | Neonatal rhinitis |
|---|---|---|---|---|
| **Above the Larynx** | | | | |
| Symptoms | Cyclic obstruction relieved by crying | Cyclic obstruction relieved by crying | Nasal obstruction and epiphora or dacrocystitis | Mild to moderate nasal congestion |
| Diagnosis | Exam/CT | Exam/CT | Endoscopic exam/CT | Exam |
| Medical | Steroid drops | None | Antibiotics for infection | Topical decongestants |
| Surgical | Sublabial resection | Transnasal or transoral resection | Marsupialization | None |

| Etiology | Laryngomalacia | Bilateral vocal fold immobility | Saccular cyst |
|---|---|---|---|
| **At the larynx** | | | |
| Symptoms | Choking, stridor | Stridor, abnormal cry | Stridor |
| Diagnosis | Flexible laryngoscopy | Flexible laryngoscopy | Operative laryngoscopy/CT |
| Medical | Thickened feeds | Observation tracheostomy, cordotomy or lateralization | None |
| Surgical | Supraglottoplasty | | Excision |

(*Continued*)

**Table 2.** (*Continued*)

| Etiology | Subglottic or tracheal stenosis | Tracheoesophageal fistula | Congenital high airway obstruction syndrome (CHAOS) | Tracheomalacia | Subglottic hemangioma |
|---|---|---|---|---|---|
| **Below the Larynx** | | | | | |
| Symptoms | Stridor | Stridor, aspiration, failure to thrive | Emergent airway at birth | Stridor worse with exertion | Progressive stridor |
| Diagnosis | Operative bronchoscopy | Operative bronchoscopy, barium swallow | Prenatal ultrasound, clinically at birth | Operative bronchoscopy, fluoroscopy | Operative bronchoscopy |
| Medical | None | None | None | Ipratropium | Propanalol, steroids, vincristine |
| Surgical | Tracheostomy, airway reconstruction | Transthoracic repair | Tracheostomy/EXIT procedure | Tracheostomy, repair of extrinsic causes | Excision |

CT: Computed tomography.
EXIT: *Ex utero* intrapartum treatment procedure.

## CONCLUSION

Airway obstruction in the infant has a wide variety of etiologies and presentations. Table 2 serves as a summary of many of the etiologies of neonatal airway obstruction. A comprehensive assessment from the level of the nasal cavity to the bronchi with a broad awareness of potential etiologies is requisite to managing infants suffering from airway obstruction. Facility with a variety of airway maintenance techniques and cooperation among an interdisciplinary team of providers, nurses and staff serves as a framework for successful evaluation and management of such children.

## REFERENCES

1. Keller JL, Kacker A. Choanal atresia, CHARGE association, and congenital nasal stenosis. *Otolaryngol Clin North Am* 2000 Dec;33(6):1343–1351, viii.
2. Isaacson G. Developmental anatomy and physiology of the larynx, trachea and esophagus. In: Bluestone CD, Stool SE, Alpert CM *et al.*, eds. *Pediatric Otolaryngology*, Vol. 2. Philadelphia: Saunders, 2003, pp. 1361–1370.
3. Hartnick CJ, Cotton RT. Stridor and airway obstruction. In: Bluestone CD, Stool SE, Alpert CM, *et al.*, eds. *Pediatric Otolaryngology*, Vol. 2. Philadelphia: Saunders, 2003, pp. 1437–1447.
4. Brown OE, Myer CM, 3rd, Manning SC. Congenital nasal pyriform aperture stenosis. *Laryngoscope* 1989 Jan;99(1):86–91.
5. Van Den Abbeele T, Triglia JM, Francois M, Narcy P. Congenital nasal pyriform aperture stenosis: diagnosis and management of 20 cases. *Ann Otol Rhinol Laryngol* 2001 Jan;110(1):70–75.
6. Arlis H, Ward RF. Congenital nasal pyriform aperture stenosis. Isolated abnormality vs developmental field defect. *Arch Otolaryngol Head Neck Surg* 1992 Sep;118(9):989–991.
7. Royal SA, Hedlund GL, Wiatrak BJ. Single central maxillary incisor with nasal pyriform aperture stenosis — CT diagnosis prior to tooth eruption. *Pediatr Radiol* 1999 May;29(5):357–359.

8. Tavin E, Stecker E, Marion R. Nasal pyriform aperture stenosis and the holoprosencephaly spectrum. *Int J Pediatr Otorhinolaryngol* 1994 Jan;28(2–3):199–204.
9. Artman HG, Boyden E. Microphthalmia with single central incisor and hypopituitarism. *J Med Genet* 1990 Mar;27(3):192–193.
10. Liberfarb RM, Abdo OP, Pruett RC. Ocular coloboma associated with a solitary maxillary central incisor and growth failure: manifestations of holoprosencephaly. *Ann Ophthalmol* 1987 Jun;19(6):226–227.
11. Rutter MJ. Evaluation and management of upper airway disorders in children. *Semin Pediatr Surg* 2006 May;15(2):116–123.
12. Hengerer AS, Brickman TM, Jeyakumar A. Choanal atresia: embryologic analysis and evolution of treatment, a 30-year experience. *Laryngoscope* 2008 May;118(5):862–866.
13. Myer CM, 3rd, Cotton RT. Nasal obstruction in the pediatric patient. *Pediatrics* 1983 Dec;72(6):766–777.
14. Deutsch E, Kaufman M, Eilon A. Transnasal endoscopic management of choanal atresia. *Int J Pediatr Otorhinolaryngol* 1997 4 May;40(1): 19–26.
15. Poswillo D. The pathogenesis of the treacher collins syndrome (mandibulofacial dysostosis). *Br J Oral Surg* 1975 Jul;13(1):1–26.
16. Josephson GD, Vickery CL, Giles WC, Gross CW. Transnasal endoscopic repair of congenital choanal atresia: long-term results. *Arch Otolaryngol Head Neck Surg* 1998 May;124(5):537–540.
17. Brown OE, Pownell P, Manning SC. Choanal atresia: a new anatomic classification and clinical management applications. *Laryngoscope* 1996 Jan;106(1 Pt 1):97–101.
18. Schoem SR. Transnasal endoscopic repair of choanal atresia: why stent? *Otolaryngol Head Neck Surg* 2004 Oct;131(4):362–366.
19. Kubba H, Bennett A, Bailey CM. An update on choanal atresia surgery at Great Ormond Street Hospital for Children: preliminary results with Mitomycin C and the KTP laser. *Int J Pediatr Otorhinolaryngol* 2004 Jul;68(7):939–945.
20. McLeod IK, Brooks DB, Mair EA. Revision choanal atresia repair. *Int J Pediatr Otorhinolaryngol* 2003 May;67(5):517–524.
21. Prasad M, Ward RF, April MM, Bent JP, Froehlich P. Topical mitomycin as an adjunct to choanal atresia repair. *Arch Otolaryngol Head Neck Surg* 2002 Apr;128(4):398–400.

22. Holland BW, McGuirt WF, Jr. Surgical management of choanal atresia: improved outcome using mitomycin. *Arch Otolaryngol Head Neck Surg* 2001 Nov;127(11):1375–1380.
23. Samadi DS, Shah UK, Handler SD. Choanal atresia: a twenty-year review of medical comorbidities and surgical outcomes. *Laryngoscope* 2003 Feb;113(2):254–258.
24. Coniglio JU, Manzione JV, Hengerer AS. Anatomic findings and management of choanal atresia and the CHARGE association. *Ann Otol Rhinol Laryngol* 1988 Sep-Oct;97(5 Pt 1):448–453.
25. Freng A. Subperiosteal early resection of the mid-palatal suture. A morphological study in twelve patients operated for choanal atresia. *Scand J Plast Reconstr Surg* 1979;13(2):289–293.
26. Shott SR, Myer CM, 3rd, Willis R, Cotton RT. Nasal obstruction in the neonate. *Rhinology* 1989 Jun;27(2):91–96.
27. Paoli C, Francois M, Triglia JM, Frydman E, Polonovski JM, Narcy P. Nasal obstruction in the neonate secondary to nasolacrimal duct cysts. *Laryngoscope* 1995 Jan;105(1):86–89.
28. Bowling BS, Chandna A. Superior lacrimal canalicular atresia and nasolacrimal duct obstruction in the CHARGE association. *J Pediatr Ophthalmol Strabismus* 1994 Sep-Oct;31(5):336–337.
29. Nathan CO, Seid AB. Neonatal rhinitis. *Int J Pediatr Otorhinolaryngol* 1997 14 Feb;39(1):59–65.
30. Tolley NS, Ford G, Commins D. The management of neonatal rhinitis. *Int J Pediatr Otorhinolaryngol* 1992 Nov;24(3):253–260.
31. Zoumalan R, Maddalozzo J, Holinger LD. Etiology of stridor in infants. *Ann Otol Rhinol Laryngol.* 2007 May;116(5):329–334.
32. Holinger LD. Etiology of stridor in the neonate, infant and child. *Ann Otol Rhinol Laryngol* 1980 Sep-Oct;89(5 Pt 1):397–400.
33. Thompson DM. Abnormal sensorimotor integrative function of the larynx in congenital laryngomalacia: a new theory of etiology. *Laryngoscope* 2007 Jun;117(6 Pt 2 Suppl 114):1–33.
34. Corbett HJ, Mann KS, Mitra I, Jesudason EC, Losty PD, Clarke RW. Tracheostomy — a 10-year experience from a UK pediatric surgical center. *J Pediatr Surg* 2007 Jul;42(7):1251–1254.
35. Hadfield PJ, Lloyd-Faulconbridge RV, Almeyda J, Albert DM, Bailey CM. The changing indications for paediatric tracheostomy. *Int J Pediatr Otorhinolaryngol* 2003 Jan;67(1):7–10.

36. Grundfast KM, Harley E. Vocal cord paralysis. *Otolaryngol Clin North Am.* 1989 Jun;22(3):569–597.
37. Daya H, Hosni A, Bejar-Solar I, Evans JN, Bailey CM. Pediatric vocal fold paralysis: a long-term retrospective study. *Arch Otolaryngol Head Neck Surg* 2000 Jan;126(1):21–25.
38. de Gaudemar I, Roudaire M, Francois M, Narcy P. Outcome of laryngeal paralysis in neonates: a long term retrospective study of 113 cases. *Int J Pediatr Otorhinolaryngol* 1996 Jan;34(1–2):101–110.
39. Zbar RI, Smith RJ. Vocal fold paralysis in infants twelve months of age and younger. *Otolaryngol Head Neck Surg* 1996 Jan;114(1):18–21.
40. Hartnick CJ, Rutter M, Lang F, Willging JP, Cotton RT. Congenital high airway obstruction syndrome and airway reconstruction: an evolving paradigm. *Arch Otolaryngol Head Neck Surg* 2002 May;128(5):567–570.
41. Hedrick MH, Ferro MM, Filly RA, Flake AW, Harrison MR, Adzick NS. Congenital high airway obstruction syndrome (CHAOS): a potential for perinatal intervention. *J Pediatr Surg* 1994 Feb;29(2):271–274.
42. Holinger LD. Congenital laryngeal anomalies. In: Holinger LD, Lusk RP, Green CG, eds. *Pediatric Laryngology and Bronchoesophagology*. Philadelphia: Lippincott-Raven, 1997, p. 146.
43. Holinger LD, Green CG, Benjamin B, Sharp JK. Tracheobronchial tree. In: Holinger LD, Lusk RP, Green CG, eds. *Pediaric Laryngology and Bronchoesophagology*. Philadelphia: Lippincott-Raven, 1997, p. 189.
44. Orlow SJ, Isakoff MS, Blei F. Increased risk of symptomatic hemangiomas of the airway in association with cutaneous hemangiomas in a "beard" distribution. *J Pediatr* 1997 Oct;131(4):643–646.
45. Kubba H, Murphy D. Subglottic haemangioma in children: experience with open surgical excision. *J Laryngol Otol* 2007 Dec;121(12):1215; author reply 1215–1216.
46. Fawcett SL, Grant I, Hall PN, Kelsall AW, Nicholson JC. Vincristine as a treatment for a large haemangioma threatening vital functions. *Br J Plast Surg* 2004 Mar;57(2):168–171.
47. Denoyelle F, Leboulanger N, Enjolras O, Harris R, Roger G, Garabedian EN. Role of Propranolol in the therapeutic strategy of infantile laryngotracheal hemangioma. *Int J Pediatr Otorhinolaryngol* 2009 Aug;73(8):1168–1172.

8

# Clinical Evaluation of Stridor

*Seth M. Pransky and Lawrence M. Simon*

## DEFINITION OF STRIDOR

Stridor is a harsh, vibratory sound caused by turbulent air flow. Its occurrence is explained by the Bernoulli principle, which states that the velocity of fluid travelling in a column is inversely proportional to the diameter of the column. Additionally, the pressure of the fluid against the walls of the column is inversely proportional to the velocity. In this case, the fluid is air, and the column is the upper tracheobronchial tree. As the airway narrows, the velocity of air increases. This phenomenon decreases the pressure of air stenting the airway open, allowing collapse. The collapse produces turbulent flow, which we hear as stridor.

## DIFFERENTIAL DIAGNOSIS

*Congenital*

Laryngomalacia — various types
Tracheomalacia
Laryngeal cleft
Vocal cord paralysis
Vascular ring/sling
Glottic stenosis
Subglottic stenosis
Subglottic cyst

*Idiopathic/Iatrogenic*

Vocal cord paralysis
Subglottic stenosis
Intubation trauma

*Inflammatory*

GERD
Eosinophilic esophagitis

*Neoplastic*

Subglottic hemangioma

*Trauma/Toxic*

Foreign body — tracheal or esophageal
Caustic ingestion
Laryngo-tracheal trauma

*Infectious*

Recurrent respiratory papillomatosis
Croup (laryngotracheitis)
Epiglottitis
Tracheitis
"Croup Masquerade"

## ASSESSMENT OF THE STRIDULOUS PATIENT

### Initial Assessment

Several factors need to be considered in the initial assessment of children with stridor. First is the age of the patient. For example, a seven-week-old infant with stridor is more likely to have a congenital etiology; whereas a seven-month-old child is more likely to have an acquired etiology. Second are the characteristics of the stridor. Inspiratory stridor suggests a supraglottic or glottic etiology; expiratory stridor suggests an intrathoracic tracheal etiology; and biphasic stridor suggests a glottic/subglottic or extrathoracic tracheal etiology.

### History

As with most conditions, an accurate diagnosis for stridor can usually be obtained through taking a thorough history. History taking is unique for the pediatric patient because the information is often second hand. Additionally, while parents generally provide very accurate information, they cannot tell us how a patient "feels." Bearing this in mind, the key elements of the otolaryngologic history for stridor include:

- Onset: acute, chronic, progressive
- Age of onset
- Prior respiratory problems
  - Recurrent croup
  - Aspiration

  - Pneumonia
  - "Reactive airways disease"
- Birth history
  - Ex-preemie
  - NICU stay
- Prior intubation
- GERD symptoms
- Sleep disordered breathing
  - Snoring
  - Nocturnal cough
  - Witnessed apneas
- Wheezing episodes
- Feeding problems
  - FTT, weight gain
- Choking episodes
- Acute changes in clinical status
  - Fever
  - Respiratory distress
  - Cough
  - Drooling
  - Change in voice or cry
  - Decrease in oral intake
  - Body position

**Physical Examination**

Pediatric otolaryngologists must have a very astute sense of observation when examining stridulous children. Key points to bear in mind are:

- Assess urgency
  Is the child in acute distress?
  - Nasal flaring
  - Tachypnea
  - Cyanosis
  - Retractions
  - Tripod position
- Let the parent hold the child
  Allowing the parent to hold the child can help to keep him/her calm.
- Use a mirror to examine for nasal airflow
  Allows assessment of nasal patency and distinction between stridor and stertor.
- Use a "headless" stethoscope

To accomplish this, remove the diaphragm and head from the stethoscope tubing. Then, auscultate the child's nostrils and neck with only the tubing.

- Observe for positional changes
  Certain conditions (such as laryngomalacia) improve when prone.

**Flexible Laryngoscopy**

This is the gold standard for office evaluation of stridor. The technique allows excellent assessment of the supraglottic and glottic larynx and is easy to perform in the clinic setting. In neonates and small infants, endoscopy can often be performed transorally. Older children typically require topical decongestion and local analgesia for transnasal laryngoscopy. However, as valuable as this technique is, there are several limitations. These are:

- VC mobility may be difficult to assess
  - Especially neonates
- Excess secretions
- Poor view of subglottis
  - Easily misinterpreted
- Interpretation of erythema difficult
- Overhanging epiglottis
- Must be careful with local anesthesia in neurologically impaired child

**Operative Direct Laryngoscopy and Bronchoscopy**

Operative endoscopy is not indicated for every child with stridor. It requires a general anesthetic and is the only way to accurately assess the subglottis. The key indications are:

- To establish a diagnosis (when other measures fail)
- To evaluate for synchronous lesions (usually suspected when the clinical picture is not fully explained by the diagnosis provided by other measures)

- Concern for subglottic lesion
- Severe or progressive stridor
- Cyanosis or apnea concerns
- Radiologic abnormalities
- Concern for foreign body
- Parental or physician anxiety

The key limitation of rigid operative endoscopy is that it does not assess the larynx in its native state. This can make evaluation of dynamic changes, such as vocal fold movement or tracheomalacia, difficult. For this reason, it is crucial to communicate with the anesthesiologist. The anesthesiologist must be:

- Comfortable with spontaneous ventilation anesthesia. This technique facilitates assessment of dynamic pathology
- Comfortable with sharing the airway
- Fully aware of suspected pathology — so that a joint plan can be formulated for dealing with anticipated problems

When considering airway surgery, specific risks must be discussed and certain complications must be anticipated. These include:

- Postoperative edema and infection
- Possible need for long term treatment with steroids
- Extended hospitalization with possible need for mechanical ventilation
- Airway injury
- Voice abnormalities[1–3]

## SPECIFIC PATHOLOGY

### Laryngomalacia

Laryngomalacia is the most common cause of stridor in infants. It occurs in varying degrees of severity and is characterized by staccato inspiratory stridor that is typically worse with exertion, feeding or crying and supine position. The stridor usually begins around four to six weeks of life and worsens during the first six months before

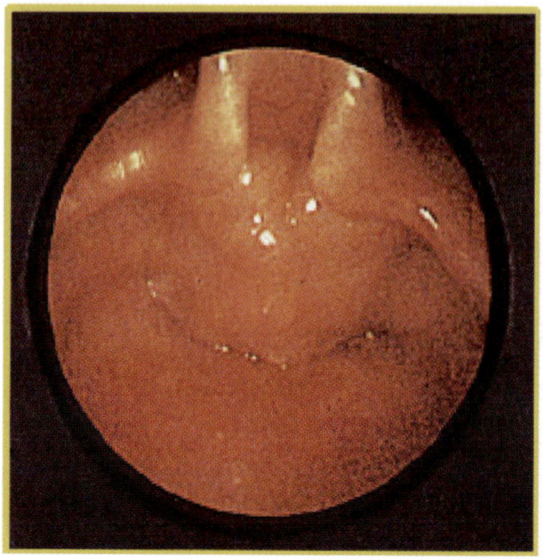

**Fig. 1.** Laryngomalacia — note omega shaped epiglottis; edematous, overhanging arytenoids; and shortened aryepiglottic folds.

gradually resolving spontaneously. The condition is usually diagnosed by history and office flexible laryngoscopy. The key findings are demonstrated in Fig. 1. These include:

(a) omega shaped epiglottis
(b) over-hanging arytenoids
(c) short aryepiglottic folds

There are multiple theories regarding the pathophysiology of laryngomalacia; however the underlying result is collapse of the cartilaginous laryngeal framework. Obstruction can arise from epiglottic prolapse, inward collapse of the arytenoid cartilages, overall narrowing of the supraglottic introitus from short aryepiglottic folds, or all of the above.[4–7] There is an approximately 80% correlation between laryngomalacia and GERD. The relationship is not well understood, but all of these patients should be screened for GERD, and many require empiric treatment.[8]

Laryngomalacia has varying degrees of severity. Some children are barely affected by it all, whereas others experience failure to thrive. Moreover, the severity of stridor often has little to do with the severity of the laryngomalacia. It is important to explain this fact to parents, as they are often preoccupied with the stridor.

The treatment of laryngomalacia must be tailored to the patient. Most patients with this condition do not have respiratory difficulty. However, many of them have feeding problems, and failure to thrive is the most common indication for treatment. About 80% of these patients will do well with reflux medications, close monitoring of weight, and reassurance. However, the remaining 20% will require surgery. The primary surgical therapy for laryngomalacia is aryepiglottoplasty, in which the aryepiglottic folds are divided, releasing the tethering of the epiglottis and arytenoids. Other therapies include reduction of the arytenoids and epiglottopexy.

Fifteen to twenty percent of patients with laryngomalacia will have a synchronous airway lesion, and this should be suspected in patients with severe respiratory distress and/or failure to thrive. These patients must be evaluated with rigid direct laryngoscopy and bronchoscopy.

Lastly, patients with severe laryngomalacia may have underlying CNS pathology, resulting in hypotonia. It is important to identify this because aryepiglottoplasty is contraindicated in these patients — it may worsen the condition.[4,9–11]

**Discoordinate Pharyngolaryngomalacia**

This is a condition characterized by stridor in the absence of classic laryngomalacia findings. It is caused by prolapse of pharyngolaryngeal tissues due to hypotonia and dysfunction. Frequently, these children will have associated neurologic or myogenic conditions, such as mitochondrial disease, and will be grossly hypotonic. It is important to keep this diagnosis in mind because their treatment is very different than that for laryngomalacia. These children do not respond to reflux medications and aryepiglottic fold division. In fact, as this is primarily a disease of poor pharyngolaryngeal tone, aryepiglottic fold division can actually worsen the condition and lead to aspiration. Instead, these children need to have their airway stented open. Therefore, the mainstay of therapy is Bi-PAP. If Bi-PAP is unsuccessful, then tracheostomy must be considered.[12]

**Tracheomalacia**

Tracheomalacia is often confused with laryngomalacia, and otolaryngologists are frequently consulted for children with "laryngotracheomalacia." However, these two conditions have very different pathophysiologies and natural histories. Laryngomalacia is a typically benign condition that produces inspiratory stridor and resolves spontaneously with growth. Tracheomalacia is rarely benign; children with this condition often manifest significant respiratory distress and failure to thrive. The most common etiology is external tracheal compression associated with congenital heart disease; however, it may be idiopathic and/or due to an anatomic defect of the trachea. The characteristic presentation is biphasic or expiratory stridor and a very characteristic cough. Therefore, it is important to distinguish between laryngomalacia and tracheomalacia and to educate patients and practitioners about their differences. Key features of tracheomalacia are:

(1) Tracheal wheeze — an expiratory wheeze that typically begins around four to eight weeks of age. It does not respond to, and may even worsen with, bronchodilator therapy. It will worsen with exertion and infection, and, unlike the wheeze of asthma or cystic fibrosis, does not cause distress or oxygen desaturations.
(2) "Brassy" cough. This cough is almost pathognomonic and has a characteristic harsh expiratory sound.
(3) Failure to thrive. Unlike children with laryngomalacia, many children with tracheomalacia have difficulty with weight gain.
(4) Increasing respiratory distress with growth.

The diagnosis of tracheomalacia is made with bronchoscopy. Rigid direct laryngoscopy and bronchoscopy in the operating room is preferable because it provides more control of the airway and more accurate assessment of the location and extent of the compression/collapse. If rigid endoscopy is used, it must be performed with spontaneous ventilation and no muscle relaxation. Paralysis or positive pressure ventilation may mask the true extent of the malacia. Congenital vascular anomalies causing tracheal compression are the most common causes of tracheomalacia. Therefore, these children must also receive a thorough cardiovascular examination, including a CT angiogram of the thorax.

The mainstay of treatment is positive pressure ventilation to stent the airway open. Frequently, these children will present in the NICU as children who are difficult to ventilate. This problem occurs because the tracheal collapse is occurring distal to the end of the endotracheal tube. In some cases, it may be necessary to use flexible bronchoscopy to titrate the PEEP. In extubated children, BiPAP/CPAP may be used.

Refractory cases may require tracheostomy with custom length tubes to bypass the collapse. Stents can be used for endobronchial collapse, although they are primarily palliative and rarely successful. Lastly, cardiothoracic surgery may be consulted for vascular decompression.[13–15]

## Croup (Laryngotracheobronchitis)

Croup is a viral infection of the upper airway caused by the *parainfluenza* virus. It produces edema of the subglottis resulting in a characteristic biphasic stridor and "seal-like" barking cough. Unless there is concomitant airway or cardiovascular pathology, infections usually resolve with conservative treatment.

It is important to note that children younger than six months do not contract croup as often as children older than six months. Congenital obstruction is more common than croup in this young age range, and therefore, these children are more likely to need diagnostic endoscopy in the operating room.

The diagnosis of croup is primarily clinical with children presenting with fever and biphasic stridor that responds to humidified air and steroids. Other tests that may prove useful include:

(1) High KV AP of neck: symmetric subglottic narrowing ("steeple sign") (Fig. 2)
(2) Endoscopy: two "sets" of vocal cords (Fig. 3)
(3) Airway fluoroscopy

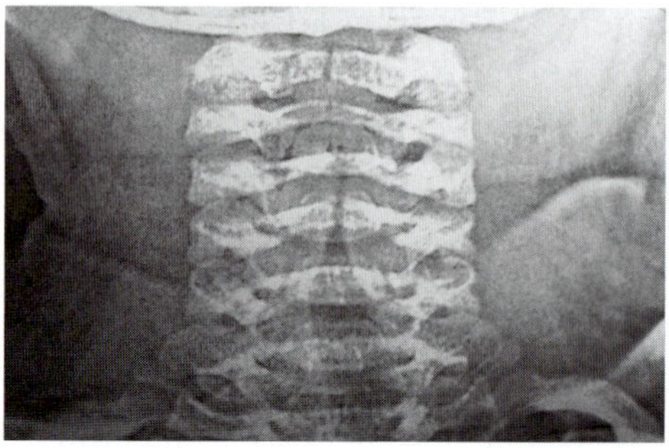

**Fig. 2.** Classic "steeple sign" of croup.

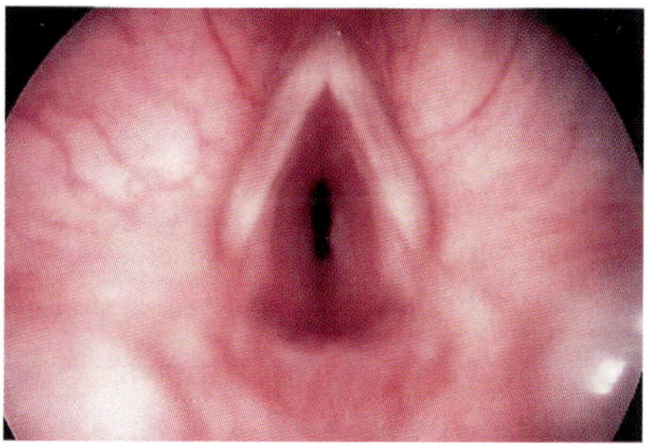

**Fig. 3.** Classic endoscopic appearance of croup with two "sets" of vocal folds.

While useful in diagnosis, endoscopy is rarely done in the acute setting, as these children represent a high anesthetic risk and airway manipulation may exacerbate the condition.

Treatment is primarily conservative and consists of steroids, nebulizer treatments and humidified air (placing children in a warm shower for 20 minutes every few hours can help tremendously.) However, clinicians should maintain a low threshold for admission in children exhibiting significant distress. While in the hospital, children can be monitored and treated with IV steroids, racemic epinephrine, supplemental oxygen, heliox and cool mist tent. Children with recurrent croup (three or more infections per year) or with an atypical course deserve airway endoscopy once the acute infection has resolved.[16–18]

## Epiglottitis

In the age of the *Haemophilus Influenza Type B* vaccine, epiglottitis is fortunately extremely rare. The majority of cases are now caused by Group A *Streptococcus* and *Staphylococcus aureus.* Additionally, traumatic epiglottitis may be caused by foreign body aspiration, thermal ingestion or an overly aggressive finger sweep. The presentation is characterized by the sudden onset and rapid progression of high fever (when infections), drooling, throat pain and respiratory distress. Children often assume a "tripod" position in an effort to stent their airway open. Diagnosis is clinical. Lateral neck X-ray shows a stereotypical "thumb print sign," representing an enlarged epiglottis, but children are often too unstable. Treatment should consist of immediate intubation in the operating room with culture of the epiglottis followed by aggressive, broad-spectrum antibiotic therapy. Steroids may also help with inflammation. It is important that the intubation occur in the operating room and that the airway not be manipulated in the emergency department. Flexible laryngoscopy could potentiate an airway crisis and should be avoided. Lastly, given the rarity of the condition, immunocompromise should be considered in all children with confirmed epiglottitis.[19–21]

## Tracheitis

Acute bacterial infection of trachea/main bronchi. This condition often develops as bacterial super-infection of viral URI, such as influenza or croup. Diagnosis is clinical, and is characterized by the sudden onset of acute airway obstruction, high fever, biphasic or expiratory stridor and deep, sometimes painful cough with extremely thick secretions. In fact, the secretions are so thick, that they sometimes cannot be expectorated and must be suctioned. Symptoms typically begin approximately two to three days after the onset of a viral illness. If this diagnosis is suspected, airway endoscopy is indicated for both pulmonary toilet and tracheal aspirate for culture.

*Staphylococcus aureus* and *Pseudomonas* are the most common causative organisms. Infections with *Pseudomonas* can be particularly concerning and may be associated with a necrotizing laryngotracheitis.

Endoscopically, acute tracheitis appears as erythematous tracheal mucosa coated with thickened secretions. Treatment consists of pulmonary toilet, monitoring, humidified air/oxygen, and culture directed antibiotics. Intubation may be necessary, and some patients require serial bronchoscopy to clear the secretions. Tracheostomy may be indicated for the most severe cases. Lastly, after resolution of the acute infection, patients should be monitored closely for signs of tracheal scarring and stenosis with a low threshold for post-treatment endoscopy.[22–24]

## Subglottic Hemangioma

These rare congenital airway lesions produce biphasic stridor beginning at about six to eight weeks of age. Unfortunately, the mean age of diagnosis is four months. This delay is due to frequent misdiagnosis early in the disease course as asthma or croup.

The classic presentation is the onset of "croup" symptoms beginning at six to eight weeks of age. This condition is one of the key reasons to do endoscopy when children have "croup" before six months of age. Unlike croup, children with subglottic hemangioma (SGH) have a good cry and no fever. Additionally, the respiratory distress and stridor often respond to typical asthma/croup therapy — humidified air, nebulizers and steroids. This response confounds diagnosis; however, suspicion is raised when the croup recurs several weeks later.

These hemangiomas follow the same clinical course as other hemangiomas, including a proliferative phase that lasts two to 12 months followed by spontaneous involution. They must be taken very seriously because the airway can be threatened during the proliferative phase.

Work up of SGH includes first assessing the degree of respiratory distress and performing a through physical exam. Approximately 50% of these children will have other hemangiomas. The classically associated lesion is a facial hemangioma in a "Beard distribution." These children must also be screened for PHACES syndrome. Comprehensive airway endoscopy is always indicated for both diagnosis and treatment. The classic endoscopic appearance is that of a smooth submucosal mass. They tend to favor the left posterolateral airway, and bilateral lesions may be mistaken for a "soft" subglottic stenosis. Biopsy is not essential, and CT/MRI may be considered to evaluate for extraluminal extension.

Management of SGH is classically both medical and surgical. Standard medical therapy includes GERD medications and steroids — both long term maintenance therapy and high dose pulses for acute distress, frequently in the setting of an upper respiratory tract infection. Both interferon and vincristine have been tried, but were abandoned due to unacceptable toxicity.

Recently, the treatment of SGH has been revolutionized by an observation published by Labrèze *et al.* in *The New England Journal of Medicine* in 2008. These physicians observed that children on propanolol for other indications experienced near total resolution of their hemangiomas. Since this publication, propanolol has become widely used for subglottic hemangioma with reportedly excellent success.

Surgical treatment for SGH is becoming more and more rare with the success of propanolol. However, having a basic knowledge and understanding of these modalities is important, as not all lesions respond to medical therapy. Tracheostomy remains a viable option in an emergent setting for clinicians who do not have extensive experience with treating SGH. Decannulation is almost always possible after involution. Open surgical excision with or without anterior cartilage grafting also remains a viable option, but requires considerable expertise and is rarely used given the plethora of medical and endoscopic treatment options. From an endoscopic standpoint, these lesions can be managed with any combination of lasers ($CO_2$, KTP, pulsed dye laser) and/or the microdebrider. Additionally, endoscopic intralesional steroid injections are frequently helpful, but must be repeated in six to eight weeks. Ultimately, these children usually do very well. Care must be taken in securing a reliable airway, but remember that this is a self-limited condition. The lesions will spontaneously involute with time.[25–28]

**Post-Intubation Injuries**

Post-intubation injuries are fairly common. Usually, they are not very serious, but they can occasionally cause significant morbidity. Also, it is important to note that these injuries can occur with as little as a few hours of intubation. The classic history includes the following:

- Intubation — even transient (hours)
- NICU Graduate
- Stridor and/or distress with even mild upper respiratory infections
- History of recurrent or prolonged croup or asthma
- Poor response to standard therapy

Specific injuries include the following:

(1) *Anterior commissure web*: These can be either congenital or acquired after intubation. Children present with a weak, hoarse cry and typically mild respiratory distress. Treatment involves endoscopic division with or without topical application of Mitomycin-C. An open approach is rarely necessary, but occasionally a laryngeal keel may be required for refractory cases. If intubation is required post-operatively, steroids should be used, and the patient should be extubated as soon as possible. All children with congenital anterior glottis webs should be screened for 22q11 deletion syndrome.[29–31]

(2) *Posterior glottic injury*: These can be more serious than anterior injuries. They fall into a spectrum of problems that begin with simple granulation tissue and progress to ulceration, furrow and finally, in the most severe cases, interarytenoid scarring. Interarytenoid scarring is a serious problem. It causes bilateral true vocal fold immobility and is extremely difficult to treat.

As with all post-intubation injuries, the primary method of treatment is prevention. However, once injury has occurred, management begins with reflux medications and steroids. Surgical intervention may be needed for persistent granuloma, severe furrow or interarytenoid scarring.

(3) *Interarytenoid web*: This condition is similar to interarytenoid scarring and causes bilateral vocal fold immobility. It can easily be mistaken for vocal fold paralysis. Diagnosis requires suspension laryngoscopy with palpation of the arytenoid.

Minimally invasive techniques, such as endoscopic division with or without Mitimycin C and mucosal interposition flaps, are often unsuccessful for interarytenoid webbing/banding/scarring. Effective repair usually involves open or endoscopic laryngotracheoplasty with division and posterior grafting.[32,33]

(4) *Subglottic cysts* (Fig. 4): This process is along the spectrum of traumatic endotracheal tube injuries. The typical progression of injury is: edema→granulation tissue→cysts→ulceration→scarring→stenosis. Cysts typically occur along the posterior lateral subglottic wall and are often multiple. They present with stridor and airway obstruction. They can be removed using a variety of techniques, including the microdebrider, blunt forceps, and various lasers. Recurrence is common, and serial endoscopy must be performed until the airway has fully healed.[34,35]

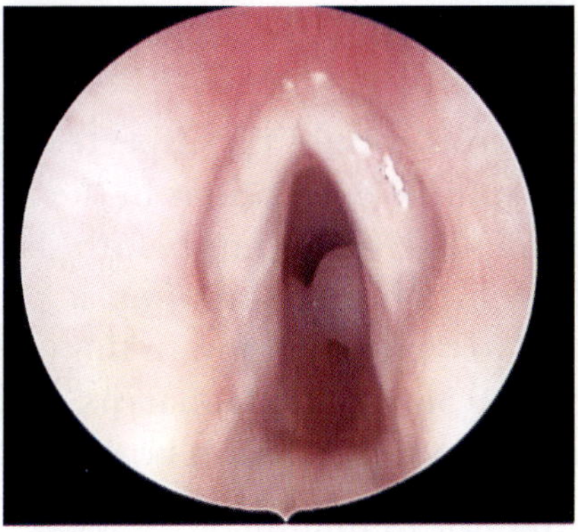

**Fig. 4.** Subglottic cysts.

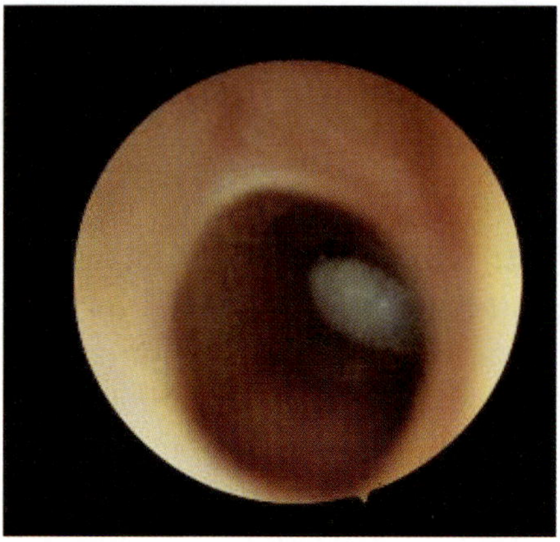

**Fig. 5.** Subglottic stenosis with tracheostomy tube in place.

(5) *Subglottic stenosis* (Fig. 5): This is the classic disease that was part of the foundation of pediatric otolaryngology. The problem has tremendous variation in both its presentation and level of severity. The classic history is failed extubation in a premature infant with prolonged ventilation. However, presentations also include dyspnea with exertion, recurrent stridor and recurrent croup. Fortunately, the incidence of this disease is decreasing with improved NICU ventilation techniques. Subglottic stenosis can be either congenital or acquired. Congenital stenosis is caused by an abnormally narrow, oval shaped cricoid ring in the absence of scar. Acquired stenosis is caused by scar that results from airway manipulation.

Subglottic stenosis should be suspected whenever a premature infant fails multiple extubations in the NICU, when a child presents with croup-like symptoms before six months of age (as with subglottic hemangioma) or when a presumed asthmatic does not respond to typical therapy. In this case, complete upper airway endoscopy from the nasopharynx to the carina is indicated. If stenosis is found, it should be reported as such:

(a) Length of stenosis in millimeters
(b) Location of stenosis (glottic, subglottic or tracheal)

(c) Character of stenosis — soft or firm. This helps determine the age/maturity of the stenosis. Early stenosis consisting primarily of granulation tissue will be managed differently than mature scar.

(d) Size and grade stenosis
Grade I (0%–50% occlusion)
Grade II (50%–70% occlusion)
Grade III (70%–99% occlusion)
Grade IV (No visible lumen)

Treatment of subglottic stenosis is complex and is guided by the endoscopic findings as well as by the overall clinical picture. First and foremost is to ensure an adequate airway, which means tracheostomy if there is uncertainty or if the child is in distress. In milder cases, children will often respond to steroids and nebulized breathing treatments. Additionally, caretakers should maintain a low threshold for admission for routine upper respiratory infections, as these children have decreased airway reserve. Next, all airway irritants should be controlled. To this end, these children are frequently on allergy/asthma regimens and long term proton pump inhibitor (PPI) therapy. Once the airway is secure and all irritants are controlled, correction of the stenosis can be considered. Grade I and asymptomatic grade II stenoses can frequently be managed with observation and serial endoscopy. Symptomatic grade II and mild grade III stenoses are amenable to multiple modalities. Serial endoscopic dilatation with or without kenalog injection is becoming the standard for managing these mild to moderate cases. Both endotracheal tubes and balloons are useful tools for dilation. Sharp instrumentation or LASER with or without Mitomycin C may also be used to weaken or lyse these scar bands either alone or as an adjunct to dilatation, depending on the clinical picture.

Severe grade III and grade IV stenosis, as well as stenoses that fail to respond to endoscopic treatments are candidates for open surgical therapy. When considering open airway surgery, many variables must be considered, and these primarily center around whether or not the patient is a good surgical candidate. Children with acquired subglottic stenosis frequently have cardiac and/or pulmonary comorbidities as well as other sequelae of prematurity. These must be fully addressed before successful airway surgery can occur.

When planning airway reconstruction, there are three primary grafting choices: anterior, posterior and both. The choice is based on where the tension needs to be released. Two examples will illustrate this concept. Congenital stenosis is characterized with an oval shaped cricoid. Surgery to fix this must convert an oval to a circle. To do this, you simply need to release the tension at the anterior curve of the oval and the force from the posterior bend will often draw the ring into a circle. In fact, these children may often be treated by simply performing an anterior cricoid split with no graft, but cartilage grafts are usually used for other anterior releases.

The opposite of this situation is posterior stenosis with interarytenoid scarring. In this case, movement of the vocal folds is typically limited, and a posterior scar release with posterior grafting is necessary. Placing an anterior graft with the scar band along the posterior airway will accomplish very little. Lastly, severe grade III and grade IV stenoses will often require both anterior and posterior grafting.

A few final notes on airway reconstruction: This operation should not be undertaken lightly. It is high risk and highly specialized and requires a comprehensive, multidisciplinary approach. The recovery is complex, and the care of these children should include a multidisciplinary airway team consisting of: pediatric otolaryngology, pediatric surgery, speech pathology, occupational therapy, critical care, pulmonology, anesthesiology and sometimes cardiology and gastroenterology. Preoperative pulmonary function tests and PPI therapy are mandatory. A great deal is also made about single versus multiple stage reconstructions. This decision is surgeon and institution dependent and based on the clinical situation. The overall principle to remember is that earlier extubation is preferable when possible.[36–48]

## Vocal Cord Paralysis

Vocal cord (TVC) paralysis in children is classified along two major lines: congenital versus acquired and unilateral versus bilateral. Congenital is usually present at birth and should be suspected in cases of stridor at birth and/or a history of difficult/forceps delivery. Acquired is most often seen after intubation, cardiac surgery or thyroid surgery.

Understanding the differences between unilateral and bilateral is critical to the treatment of these patients. Unilateral paralysis rarely causes airway obstruction, as the paralyzed cord is frequently located at a paramedian position. The children have a coarse stridor that is worse with crying and a weak voice. In infancy, their problems center around feeding and airway protection; they are at high risk for aspiration, and must be followed closely by speech pathology. Additionally, the inability to cough results in pooling of secretions and can cause airway obstruction. As these children grow, speech production becomes more of an issue from both a psychological and functional standpoint. Common etiologies include intubation and surgical trauma.

In contrast to unilateral paralysis, bilateral TVC paralysis causes problems with airway obstruction instead of feeding and aspiration. These children usually swallow well and have a good voice and cry. The vocal folds are frequently fixed in a partially adducted position, and acute airway distress can occur. In fact, tracheostomy is sometimes needed. Common causes include Arnold Chiari malformation, posterior fossa central nervous system insults (tumor, hemorrhage, surgery) and interarytenoid scarring (glottic stenosis).

The work up of children with vocal fold paralysis should assess the entire course of the recurrent laryngeal nerves. This should include:

- Chest X-ray
- Complete neurologic exam
- Flexible laryngoscopy

Direct laryngoscopy and bronchoscopy should be considered if there is suspicion of an anatomic abnormality, such as glottic/subglottic stenosis. Additional studies particular to unilateral or bilateral paralysis include:

- Unilateral:
  - Video fluoroscopic or endoscopic swallowing study to look for aspiration
  - CT scan of skull base to thoracic inlet

- Bilateral: Airway issues, Aspiration issues
  - Video fluoroscopic swallowing study
  - Closely monitor oxygen saturation, weight gain and sleep patterns — watch for apnea
  - MRI of brain and skull base to look for Chiari malformation and CNS abnormalities

Management is dictated by both the nature of the paralysis and the clinical picture. Unilateral paralysis can be managed with observation if the patient is asymptomatic. Children frequently compensate well and spontaneous recovery may occur. However, if the child is having difficulties with either speech or swallowing, injection of the paralyzed cord with either temporary or semi-permanent material can be successful. Open thyroplasty is rarely indicated in children and should only be considered in cases of known permanent vocal fold paralysis.

Management of bilateral TVC paralysis is focused on securing the airway. As with unilateral paralysis, bilateral paralysis can be managed expectantly if the patient is stable. However, surgical management is often needed to stabilize these patients. There are a multitude of options, including:

- Tracheotomy — Gold standard
- BOTOX injection
- Posterior laryngeal expansion
- Cordotomy/Cordectomy
- Arytenoidectomy
- Re-innervation procedures

Each of these treatments has their own unique indications, risks and benefits. However, the key point of each is to create a patent and stable airway.[49–52]

### Congenital Airway Anomalies

There are several common congenital airway anomalies that must be discussed.

(1) *Glottic webs*
These tend to occur on the anterior glottis between the anterior 1/3 of the TVC. They also tend to be thick and extend to the subglottis. All children with webs should be screened for 22q11 deletion, and rare variants are associated with laryngeal atresia. They typically require surgical treatment, which can be done either endoscopic or open, and keel placement is controversial.[53]

(2) *Laryngeal clefts*
Larygeal clefts (also called laryngotracheoesophageal clefts) are a midline defect representing a failure of formation of the posterior laryngeal wall and the common wall separating the trachea and esophageal introitus. These children present with stridor, but their primary issues center around aspiration and inability to handle their secretions.

A cleft should be suspected whenever a child develops stridor and recurrent aspiration pneumonia early in life, and these children should be assessed with suspension microlaryngoscopy. This technique allows for bimanual manipulation of the larynx and two-handed distraction to fully inspect the interarytenoid region. Clefts are classified as types I to IV based on the extent of laryngeal involvement. Type I clefts are isolated to the supraglottic posterior laryngeal wall; type II clefts extend into the subglottis but do not involve the entire cricoid; type III clefts involve the entire cricoid cartilage and extend into the cervical trachea; and type IV clefts extend deep into the thoracic trachea and are often fatal. The differential diagnosis for this condition includes tracheoesophageal fistula, choanal atresia and esophageal atresia. These children should also be screened for cardiovascular defects.

All cleft patients require treatment with proton pump inhibitor therapy. Additionally, speech pathology or occupational therapy should be involved to determine the safety of swallowing. If oral feeding is unsafe, then a feeding tube can be placed. Once these steps are completed, treatment is then based on the type of cleft. Type I clefts are rarely problematic and can often be observed. Type II and some type III clefts may be amenable to endoscopic repair with. Many type III clefts require a laryngofissure with posterior buttressing, and type IV clefts require open repair via thoracotomy.[54–56]

(3) *Vascular rings/slings*

Children with cardiovascular anomalies often manifest stridor and some degree of airway obstruction related to their abnormal mediastinal vasculature. Three predominate abnormalities seen are:

(a) Aberrant course of innominate artery — most common
(b) Right sided/double aortic arch
(c) Aberrant right subclavian artery — the artery may course posterior to the esophagus, producing obstruction and the characteristic "dysphagia lusoria"

The classic presentation of vascular rings is tracheomalacia. These children have a harsh expiratory stridor, characteristic cough and "dying spells." Evaluation should include an esophogram and imaging of the thoracic vasculature. Tracheobronchoscopy is also indicated and typically reveals a "fish mouth" appearance of the airway with pulsatile compression. Symptomatic children require open vascular decompression. As with laryngeal webs, all children with vascular rings must be screened for 22q11.[57–59]

## Recurrent Respiratory Papillomatosis (RRP)

RRP occurs in two forms: juvenile onset and adult onset (Fig. 6). This chapter will deal exclusively with juvenile onset recurrent respiratory papillomatosis. This is one of the hallmark diseases of pediatric otolaryngology and should be ruled out in all children with stridor or hoarseness. Children with RRP are often diagnosed around three years of age, and correct diagnosis may be delayed for years with children being initially treated for asthma or recurrent croup. RRP can cause airway obstruction, especially in non-compliant patients. Also, a child's initial presentation may be in extremis, requiring urgent surgical intervention. Lastly, sexual abuse should always be considered in preadolescent cases. Diagnosis is made with

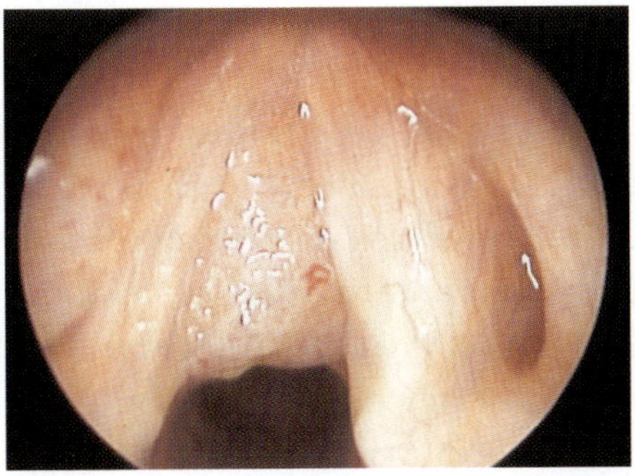

**Fig. 6.** Recurrent respiratory papillomatosis.

office flexible laryngoscopy. Bronchoscopy to screen for pulmonary lesions should be performed at the time of initial direct laryngoscopy as well as at least on an annual basis.

The incidence of RRP is 4.3 per 100,000 children in the United States and key risk factors are young mother, first-born child, vaginal delivery and vaginal lesions present at birth. There is a great deal of controversy regarding the utility of cesarean section in the children of mothers with vaginal papillomas; however, most authorities agree that cesarean section is indicated in the setting of active disease at the time of delivery.

The natural history of RRP is varied and unpredictable. The two most common serotypes of HPV found in children are HPV-6 and HPV-11, and much published and anecdotal evidence suggests that type 11 follows a more aggressive clinical course. Fortunately, HPV-16 and HPV-18, which carry a much higher risk of malignant transformation, are rarely found in laryngeal papilloma. Sadly, children with RRP are challenging patients. Their course is characterized by frequent recurrence and a devastating physical, logistical and psychological impact. Their weak voice can limit social interaction, and bulky disease can cause obstruction that limits physical activity. Additionally, distant travel, such as for vacation, is rarely feasible, as the child needs to remain close to a major medical center at all times.

Spread of the disease beyond the confines of the larynx occurs to the distal airways in 6%–13% of cases and to the lungs in 2%–7%

of cases. Malignant transformation is extremely rare, occurring in 1%–4% of patients.

Therapy for RRP can be frustrating, and no predictive therapeutic intervention is available. Surgical extirpation is rarely curative, and must be aimed at controlling disease burden. Medical adjuvants are available for severe disease.

When planning surgery for RRP, preoperative preparation is critical. The parents must be counseled about the need for multiple surgeries and of the inherent risks of airway surgery. Also, a detailed anesthesia plan must be formulated. These cases must often be performed under spontaneous ventilation to afford access to the larynx and decrease the risk of spreading disease distally. Multiple instruments can be used, including forceps, the microdebrider and a variety of LASERs. No matter which modality is chosen, the basic principles remain the same:

(1) Reduce tumor burden
(2) Avoid tracheostomy
(3) Decrease spread of disease
(4) Create a safe and patent airway
(5) Preserve voice quality
(6) Increase interval between surgical procedures

Usually, these objectives can be met by adhering to two overriding principles: protect the anterior commissure (damage here is extremely difficult to reconstruct) and to "first do no harm." RRP is essentially a benign disease that will recur regardless of the extent of surgery.

Therefore, it is preferable to leave disease in the larynx rather than damage the larynx to achieve a complete resection.

For the most severe cases of RRP, medical adjuvant therapy is available. These therapies should only be considered when patients are still experiencing either airway obstruction or great psychological distress despite full surgical therapy. The more commonly used medical adjuvants are:

- MMR vaccine
- Interferon — rarely used due to side effect profile
- Cidofovir

Intralesional cidofovir is currently the most widely used adjuvant. Approximately 80% of cases respond to cidofovir, and there is usually a dramatic initial improvement. Typically, the medication is injected directly into the lesions — often at two- to four-week intervals — for ten or more doses per course. Once the course is complete, the persistent disease is often less extensive than before the injections were given, and some rare cases may even progress to a lasting remission. Additionally, it is important to understand that patient selection is critical for cidofovir. This therapy is not designed to facilitate a cure or to help patients whose disease is already well controlled with surgery. Its main impact is to increase the surgical interval for patients with the most severe disease. For example, it can help a patient who requires endoscopy every six weeks to need it only every four months. Lastly, systemic cidofovir is known to have liver and kidney toxicity, and intralesional cidofovir may carry an increased risk of malignant transformation. Therefore, liver and kidney tests and biopsies should be sent at least every three months while on cidofovir.

The last therapy to discuss with regards to RRP is Gardisil®. There is no direct data regarding Gardisil® and RRP, but the FUTURE I and FUTURE II studies have shown 98%–100% efficacy at prevention of HPV-6 and HPV-11. Therefore, there is the possibility that Gardisil® could drastically decrease the incidence of RRP, and future studies will need to investigate this relationship.[60–66]

## Foreign Body-Airway

Foreign bodies are a ubiquitous problem in pediatric otolaryngology and can range from nearly asymptomatic to immediately life threatening. History is the most important component of the diagnosis, and can help distinguish airway from esophageal foreign bodies. Importantly, a witnessed aspiration or ingestion is not necessary for this diagnosis.

Airway foreign bodies usually present as a coughing spell while eating or playing, and post-tussive emesis is not uncommon.

Sunflower seeds, peanuts and popcorn kernels are among the most commonly aspirated foods, and hot dogs carry the highest mortality.[67] Children may also have cyanotic ("blue") spells, but many aspirations do not have cyanosis. A critical component in the history for airway foreign bodies is the quiescent interval. Frequently, objects that do not cause total or subtotal tracheal obstruction will progress from an intense coughing spell to a nearly asymptomatic period as the coughing reflex fades. Then, days to weeks later, the patient will develop a subacute pneumonia and become severely ill with atelectasis, pneumothorax (secondary to erosion of the bronchial wall), empyema, respiratory failure and sepsis.

Physical findings in patients with aspiration include stridor, tachypnea, tachycardia, diaphoresis and poor oxygen saturation. There is often a characteristic barky cough with hoarseness and intermittent dyspnea. Auscultation of the chest may reveal a unilateral wheeze or decreased aeration, which can help determine the side of the obstruction. Imaging with chest X-ray — including inspiration, expiration and decubitus films — and airway fluoroscopy can help secure the diagnosis in uncertain cases. The affected side may either be atelectatic or may not deflate appropriately due to the ball-valve effect that some foreign bodies can create.

Bronchoscopy with removal is the mainstay of treatment. Ideally, the patient should first be stabilized with fluids and oxygen, but this is not always possible in cases of total or subtotal obstruction. Sometimes, if the parents know what the child aspirated, it may be helpful to practice on a similar object. Additionally, it is critical to communicate closely with anesthesia. These patients are usually able to maintain their airway while upright and awake. However, they rarely tolerate laying supine, are often difficult to mask and can quickly decompensate when given even mild relaxants. Therefore, it is important that everything be in place before the first anesthetic is given. Lastly, one should always consider perioperative antibiotics and admission to ensure complete recovery.[68–73]

### Foreign Body — Esophageal

Esophageal foreign bodies can also present with stridor due to either laryngeal inflammation or extrinsic posterior compression of the trachea from the esophagus. Their history is distinct from airway foreign bodies. As opposed to an intense coughing episode, children who ingest foreign objects present with a gagging episode (which may be interpreted as "choking" by many parents) that then progresses to drooling and intolerance of oral intake. Frequently, the parents may try to help the child by giving them something to drink, which then produces emesis. It is important to remember that emesis does not rule out esophageal foreign bodies. Many objects that children ingest are large and will remain lodged in the esophagus in spite of prolonged heaving and vomiting. Lastly, when assessing a child with a suspected esophageal foreign body, it is critical to ask about possible button (disk) battery ingestion. As opposed to coins and many other inert objects, button batteries are an absolute surgical emergency and must be removed immediately. When lodged in the esophagus, the batteries conduct a current through the esophagus that produces sodium hydroxide and can result in erosion and perforation within hours of ingestion.

When assessing these children in the clinic or emergency department, one must first assess the degree of respiratory distress. Many esophageal foreign bodies are benign and can wait in line until operating room time is available on the regular schedule. However, in some circumstances, posterior compression of the trachea and drooling can create airway compromise — necessitating urgent surgical removal. If the patient is stable, a routine foreign body X-ray series should be ordered. This will detect most metallic foreign bodies and can help distinguish a button battery from other objects. On AP or PA views, there is frequently a double density with an inner circle corresponding to the back-side of the battery. On lateral views, there is a characteristic step-off corresponding to the profile of the battery.

If a fishbone impaction is suspected and the X-ray series is negative, CT scan of the neck and chest may have a higher sensitivity.

However, the risk of radiation must be compared against the risk of esophagoscopy and discussed with the family.

Management of these patients is typically surgical with rigid esophagoscopy and removal of the foreign object. Button batteries should be removed urgently, but other objects can wait for operating room space to become available. If several hours pass between initial diagnosis and surgical intervention, a repeat X-ray should be considered to ensure that the object did not pass spontaneously. Parents should also be counseled that the object may pass with induction of anesthesia. Additionally, one should remain suspicious of a second foreign object, and the esophagus must be cleared with repeat endoscopy after the object is removed. Many children can then be discharged home from the recover room if they pass an oral challenge. However, some children require admission and observation to ensure an adequate recovery.

Children who ingest button batteries should be admitted for observation and inpatient gastroenterology consultation. Perioperative antibiotics and steroids should be considered, especially in the case of perforation. An esophogram should be obtained prior to discharge. If the study is negative, then the child may be discharged after passing an oral challenge. These children should then be followed closely to ensure that they do not develop long term strictures.[74–81]

## Gastroesophageal Reflux Disease (GERD)

The final cause of stridor to discuss is GERD — manifesting as laryngopharyngeal reflux disease (LPRD). Diagnosing this condition requires a high index of suspicion, as laryngeal reflux may have no classic GERD symptoms (sometimes called "silent GERD"). In fact, stridor or hoarseness may be the only symptom. Other symptoms of LPRD include:

- Emesis
- Dysphagia
- Burping
- Choking

- Gagging
- Sleep disturbance
- Irritability
- Apnea/breath holding spells
- Arching
- Nocturnal cough
- Stertor
- Hoarseness
- Halitosis
- Laryngospasm
- Rumination

In addition to the above symptoms, LPRD is related to multiple pediatric otolaryngologic problems. These include:

- Rhinitis of infancy
- Recurrent otitis
- Chronic sinusitis
- Hoarseness
- Chronic cough
- Halitosis
- Severe laryngomalacia
- Recurrent croup
- Subglottic stenosis exacerbation
- Recurrent bronchitis
- Asthma exacerbation

The assessment of children with suspected GERD/LPRD is both non-operative and operative. The diagnosis is usually empiric and a successful therapeutic response to proton pump inhibitors will suffice. However, both a barium swallow/upper GI series and double lumen pH probes (with a pharyngeal probe) can be helpful in equivocal cases. Should the child not respond to medical therapy or exhibits symptoms of airway compromise, assessment in the operating room is indicated. These children should receive a combined assessment by both otolaryngology and gastroenterology with direct laryngoscopy, bronchoscopy and esophagogastroduodenoscopy (EGD) with esophageal biopsies. The endoscopy must focus on subtle mucosal changes such as pseudosulcus vocalis, thickened secretions, erythema/edema (especially of arytenoids), nodules and tracheal inflammation. Esophageal biopsies should be sent to look for inflammation and eosinophilic esophagitis, and tracheal aspirate may be sent for lipid laden macrophages.[82–87]

Lastly, eosinophilic esophagitis (EE) deserves special mention. EE is essentially an esophageal mucosal allergy to certain foods and should be suspected whenever there is an inadequate response to reflux therapy in a child with symptoms suggestive of GERD. Boys predominate 3:1 over girls in cases of EE, and the disease tends to present in the preadolescent years. The diagnosis is made by a distal esophageal biopsy showing >15–20 eosinophils per high power field. Each child suspected of EE should also receive a food allergy work up. Treatment focuses on dietary manipulation, reflux medications and inhaled or swallowed steroids.[88–95]

## REFERENCES

1. Cotton RT, Reilly JS. Stridor and airway obstruction. In: Bluestone C, Stool S, Kenna M, eds. *Pediatric Otolaryngology*, 3rd Ed. Philadelphia, PA: WB Saunders Co, 1995; pp. 1275–1286.
2. Bent J. Pediatric laryngotracheal obstruction: current perspectives on stridor. *Laryngoscope* Jul 2006;116(7):1059–1070.
3. Holinger LD. Etiology of stridor in neonate, infant and child. *Ann Otol Rhinol Laryngol* 1980;89:397–400.
4. Olney DR, Greinwald JH, Smith RJ, Bauman NM. Laryngomalacia and its treatment. *Laryngoscope* 1999;109:1770–1775.
5. Awan S, Saleheen D, Zafar A. Laryngomalacia: an atypical case and review of the literature. *Ear Nose Throat J* 2004;83:334–338.
6. Baxter MRN. Congenital laryngomalacia. *Can J Anaesth* 1994;41: 332–339.
7. Belmont JR, Grundfast K. Congential laryngeal stridor (laryngomalacia): etiologic factors and associated disorders. *Ann Otol Rhinol Laryngol* 1984;93:430–437.

8. Giannoni C, Sulek M, Friedman EM, Duncan NO 3rd. Gastroesophageal reflux association with laryngomalacia: a prospective study. *Int J Pediatr Otorhinolaryngol* 1998;43:11–20.
9. Mancuso RF, Choi SS, Zalzal GH, Grundfast KM. Laryngomalacia: the search for a second lesion. *Arch Otolaryngol Head Neck Surg* 1996; 122:302–306.
10. O'Donell S, Murphy J, Bew S, Knight LC. Aryepiglottoplasty for laryngomalacia: results and recommendations following a case series of 84. *Int J Pediatr Otorhinolaryngol* 2007;71:1271–1275.
11. Pereira Valera FC, Tamashiro E, de Araujo MM, Sander HH, Kupper DS. Evaluation of the efficacy of supraglottoplasty in obstructive sleep apnea syndrome associated with severe laryngomalacia. *Arch Otolaryngol Head Neck Surg* 2006;132:489–493.
12. Froehlich P, Seid AB, Denoyelle F, Pransky SM, Kearns DB, Garabedian EN, Morgon A. Discoordinate pharyngolaryngomalacia. *Int J Pediatr Otorhinolaryngol* 1997 14 Feb;39(1):9–18.
13. Carden KA, Boiselle PM, Waltz DA, Ernst A. Tracheomalacia and trachea-bronchomalacia in children and adults: an in-depth review. *Chest* 2005 Mar;127(3):984–1005.
14. Jaquiss RD. Management of pediatric tracheal stenosis and tracheomalacia. *Semin Thorac Cardiovasc Surg* 2004 Fall;16(3):220–224.
15. Benjamin B. Tracheomalacia in infants and children. *Ann Otol Rhinol Laryngol* 1984;93:438–442.
16. Johnson D. Croup. *Clin Evid (Online).* 10 Mar 2009.
17. Ausejo M, Saenz A, Pham B, Kellner JD, *et al.* The effectiveness of glucocorticoids in treating croup: meta-analysis. *BMJ* 1999 4 Sep; 319(7210):595–600.
18. Bjornson CL, Johnson DW. Croup. *Lancet* 2008 26 Jan;371(9609): 329–339.
19. Cressman WR, Myer CM 3rd. Diagnosis and management of croup and epiglottitis. *Pediatr Clin North Am* 1994 Apr;41(2):265–276.
20. Guldfred LA, Lyhne D, Becker BC. Acute epiglottitis: epidemiology, clinical presentation, management and outcome. *J Laryngol Otol* 2008 Aug;122(8):818–823
21. Kavanagh KR, Batti JS. Traumatic epiglottitis after foreign body ingestion. *Int J Pediatr Otorhinolaryngol* 2008 Jun;72(6):901–903.

22. Eckel HE, Widemann B, Damm M, Roth B. Airway endoscopy in the diagnosis and treatment of bacterial tracheitis in children. *Int J Pediatr Otorhinolaryngol* 1993 Aug;27(2):147–157.
23. Huang YL, Peng CC, Chiu NC, *et al.* Bacterial tracheitis in pediatrics: 12 year experience at a medical center in Taiwan. *Pediatr Int* 2009 Feb;51(1):110–113.
24. Salamone FN, Bobbitt DB, Myer CM, Rutter MJ, Greinwald JH Jr. Bacterial tracheitis reexamined: is there a less severe manifestation?. *Otolaryngol Head Neck Surg* 2004 Dec;131(6):871–876.
25. Pransky SM, Canto C. Management of subglottic hemangioma. *Curr Opin Otolaryngol Head Neck Surg* 2004 Dec;12(6):509–512.
26. Léauté-Labrèze C, Dumas de la Roque E, Hubiche T, Boralevi F, Thambo JB, Taïeb A. Propranolol for severe hemangiomas of infancy. *N Engl J Med* 2008 12 Jun;358(24):2649–2651.
27. Siegfried EC, Keenan WJ, Al-Jureidini S. More on propranolol for hemangiomas of infancy. *N Engl J Med* 2008 25 Dec;359(26):2846; author reply 2846–2847.
28. Denoyelle F, Leboulanger N, Enjolras O, Harris R, Roger G, Garabedian EN. Role of Propranolol in the therapeutic strategy of infantile laryngotracheal hemangioma. *Int J Pediatr Otorhinolaryngol* 2009 Aug;73(8):1168–1172. Epub May 2009.
29. Miyamoto RC, Cotton RT, Rope AF, Hopkin RJ, Cohen AP, Shott SR, Rutter MJ. Association of anterior glottic webs with velocardiofacial syndrome (chromosome 22q11.2 deletion). *Otolaryngol Head Neck Surg* 2004 Apr;130(4):415–417.
30. Vivero RJ, Roy S. Anterior glottic web. *Ear Nose Throat J* 2008 Jul;87(7):372–375.
31. Milczuk HA, Smith JD, Everts EC. Congenital laryngeal webs: surgical management and clinical embryology. *Int J Pediatr Otorhinolaryngol* 2000;52(1):1–9.
32. Inglis AF Jr, Perkins JA, Manning SC, Mouzakes J. Endoscopic posterior cricoid split and rib grafting in 10 children. *Laryngoscope* 2003 Nov;113(11):2004–2009.
33. Zalzal GH. Posterior glottic stenosis. *Int J Pediatr Otorhinolaryngol* 1999;49(Suppl 1):S279–S282.

34. Freed GL, Derkay CS. Subglottic cysts: a cause of pediatric stridor. *Ear Nose Throat J* 2007 Jul;86(7):386–387.
35. Jaryszak EM, Collins WO. Microdebrider resection of bilateral subglottic cysts in a pre-term infant: a novel approach. *Int J Pediatr Otorhinolaryngol* 2009 Jan;73(1):139–142.
36. Fearon B, Cotton R. Surgical correction of subglottic stenosis of the larynx in infants and children. Progress report. *Ann Otol Rhinol Laryngol* 1974 Jul–Aug;83(4):428–431.
37. Seid AB, Pransky SM, Kearns DB. One-stage laryngotracheoplasty. *Arch Otolaryngol Head Neck Surg* 1991 Apr;117(4):408–410.
38. Cotton RT, O'Connor DM. Evaluation of the airway for laryngotracheal reconstruction. *Int Anesthesiol Clin* 1992 Fall;30(4):93–98.
39. Zalzal GH. Treatment of laryngotracheal stenosis with anterior and posterior cartilage grafts. A report of 41 children. *Arch Otolaryngol Head Neck Surg* 1993 Jan;119(1):82–86.
40. Rothschild MA, Cotcamp D, Cotton RT. Postoperative medical management in single-stage laryngotracheoplasty. *Arch Otolaryngol Head Neck Surg* 1995 Oct;121(10):1175–1179.
41. Zalzal GH, Choi SS, Patel KM. Ideal timing of pediatric laryngotracheal reconstruction. *Arch Otolaryngol Head Neck Surg* 1997 Feb;123(2): 206–208.
42. Cotton RT. Management of subglottic stenosis. *Otolaryngol Clin North Am* 2000 Feb;33(1):111–130.
43. Lee KH, Rutter MJ. Role of balloon dilation in the management of adult idiopathic subglottic stenosis. *Ann Otol Rhinol Laryngol* 2008 Feb;117(2):81–84.
44. Myer CM 3rd, O'Connor DM, Cotton RT. Proposed grading system for subglottic stenosis based on endotracheal tube sizes. *Ann Otol Rhinol Laryngol* 1994 Apr;103(4 Pt 1):319–323.
45. Seid AB, Canty TG. The anterior cricoid split procedure for the management of subglottic stenosis in infants and children. *J Pediatr Surg* 1985 Aug;20(4):388–390.
46. Stern Y, Gerber ME, Walner DL, *et al.* Partial cricotracheal resection with primary anastomosis in the pediatric age group. *Ann Otol Rhinol Laryngol* 1997 Nov;106(11):891–896.

47. Boardman SJ, Albert DM. Single-stage and multistage pediatric laryngotracheal reconstruction. *Otolaryngol Clin North Am* 2008 Oct;41(5): 947–958.
48. Lando T, April MM, Ward RF. Minimally invasive techniques in laryngotracheal reconstruction. *Otolaryngol Clin North Am* 2008 Oct;41(5): 935–946.
49. King EF, Blumin JH. Vocal cord paralysis in children. *Curr Opin Otolaryngol Head Neck Surg* 2009 Dec;17(6):483–487.
50. Kwon TK, Buckmire R. Injection laryngoplasty for management of unilateral vocal fold paralysis. *Curr Opin Otolaryngol Head Neck Surg* 2004 Dec;12(6):538–542.
51. Miller S. Voice therapy for vocal fold paralysis. *Otolaryngol Clin North Am* 2004 Feb;37(1):105–119.
52. Chen EY, Inglis Jr AF. Bilateral vocal cord paralysis in children. *Otolaryngol Clin North Am* 2008 Oct;41(5):889–901.
53. Nicollas R, Triglia JM. The anterior laryngeal webs. *Otolaryngol Clin North Am* 2008 Oct;41(5):877–888.
54. Moungthong G, Holinger LD. Laryngotracheoesophageal clefts. *Ann Otol Rhinol Laryngol* 1997;106(12):1002–1011.
55. Eriksen C, Zwillenberg D, Robinson N. Diagnosis and management of cleft larynx: literature review and case report. *Ann Otol Rhinol Laryngol* 1990;99(9 Pt 1):703–708.
56. Pezzettigotta SM, Leboulanger N, Roger G, Denoyelle F, Garabédian E-N. Laryngeal cleft. *Otolaryngol Clin North Am* 2008 Oct;41(5):913–933.
57. Backer CL, Mavroudis C. Surgical approach to vascular rings. *Adv Card Surg* 1997;9:29–64.
58. Castaneda AR, Jonas RA, Mayer JE. Vascular rings, slings, and tracheal anomalies. In: *Cardiac Surgery of the Neonate and Infant.* Philadelphia, PA: WB Saunders, 1994; pp. 397–408.
59. Momma K, Matsuoka R, Takao A. Aortic arch anomalies associated with chromosome 22q11 deletion (CATCH 22). *Pediatr Cardiol* 1999;20: 97–102.
60. Derkay CS, Wiatrak B. Recurrent respiratory papillomatosis: a review. *Laryngoscope* 2008 Jul;118(7):1236–1247.
61. Zacharisen MC, Conley SF. Recurrent respiratory papillomatosis in children: masquerader of common respiratory diseases. *Pediatrics* 2006 Nov;118(5):1925–1931.

62. Hartnick CJ, Boseley ME, Franco RA Jr, Cunningham MJ, Pransky S. Efficacy of treating children with anterior commissure and true vocal fold respiratory papilloma with the 585-nm pulsed-dye laser. *Arch Otolaryngol Head Neck Surg* 2007 Feb;133(2):127–130.
63. Pransky SM, Albright JT, Magit AE. Long-term follow-up of pediatric recurrent respiratory papillomatosis managed with intralesional cidofovir. *Laryngoscope* 2003 Sep;113(9):1583–1587.
64. Pransky SM, Brewster DF, Magit AE, Kearns DB. Clinical update on 10 children treated with intralesional cidofovir injections for severe recurrent respiratory papillomatosis. *Arch Otolaryngol Head Neck Surg* 2000 Oct;126(10):1239–1243.
65. Pransky SM, Magit AE, Kearns DB, Kang DR, Duncan NO. Intralesional cidofovir for recurrent respiratory papillomatosis in children. *Arch Otolaryngol Head Neck Surg* 1999 Oct;125(10):1143–1148.
66. FUTURE II Study Group. Quadrivalent vaccine against human papillomavirus to prevent high-grade cervical lesions. *N Engl J Med* 2007 10 May;356(19):1915–1927.
67. Altkorn R, Chen X, Milkovich S, Stool D, Rider G, Bailey CM, Haas A, Riding KH, Pransky SM, Reilly JS. Fatal and non-fatal food injuries among children (aged 0–14 years). *Int J Pediatr Otorhinolaryngol* 2008 Jul;72(7):1041–1046. Epub 2 May 2008.
68. Pak MW, van Hasselt CA. Foreign bodies in children's airways: a challenge to clinicians and regulators. *Hong Kong Med J* 2009 Feb; 15(1):4–5.
69. Eren S, Balci AE, Dikici B, *et al.* Foreign body aspiration in children: experience of 1160 cases. *Ann Trop Paediatr* 2003 Mar;23(1):31–37.
70. CDC. Nonfatal choking-related episodes among children — United States, 2001. *MMWR Morb Mortal Wkly Rep* 25 Oct 2002;51(42):945–948.
71. Zaupa P, Saxena AK, Barounig A, Hollwarth ME. Management strategies in foreign-body aspiration. *Indian J Pediatr* 2009 Feb;76(2): 157–161.
72. Chung MK, Jeong HS, Ahn KM, *et al.* Pulmonary recovery after rigid bronchoscopic retrieval of airway foreign body. *Laryngoscope* 2007 Feb;117(2):303–307.
73. Bloom DC, Christenson TE, Manning SC, *et al.* Plastic laryngeal foreign bodies in children: a diagnostic challenge. *Int J Pediatr Otorhinolaryngol* 2005 May;69(5): 657–662.

74. Stack LB, Munter DW. Foreign bodies in the gastrointestinal tract. *Emerg Med Clin North Am* Aug 1996;14(3):493–521.
75. Balci AE, Eren S, Eren MN. Esophageal foreign bodies under cricopharyngeal level in children: an analysis of 1116 cases. *Interact Cardiovasc Thorac Surg* 2004 Mar;3(1):14–18.
76. Cheng W, Tam PK. Foreign-body ingestion in children: experience with 1,265 cases. *J Pediatr Surg* 1999 Oct;34(10):1472–1476.
77. Little DC, Shah SR, St Peter SD, Calkins CM, Morrow SE, Murphy JP, *et al.* Esophageal foreign bodies in the pediatric population: our first 500 cases. *J Pediatr Surg* 2006 May;41(5):914–918.
78. Miller RS, Willging JP, Rutter MJ, Rookkapan K. Chronic esophageal foreign bodies in pediatric patients: a retrospective review. *Int J Pediatr Otorhinolaryngol* 2004 Mar;68(3):265–272.
79. Litovitz T, Schmitz BF. Ingestion of cylindrical and button batteries: an analysis of 2382 cases. *Pediatrics* 1992 Apr;89(4 Pt 2):747–757.
80. Bronstein AC, Spyker DA, Cantilena LR Jr, Green J, Rumack BH, Heard SE. 2006 Annual Report of the American Association of Poison Control Centers' National Poison Data System (NPDS). *Clin Toxicol (Phila)* 2007 Dec;45(8):815–917.
81. Chan YL, Chang SS, Kao KL, Liao HC, Liaw SJ, Chiu TF, *et al.* Button battery ingestion: an analysis of 25 cases. *Chang Gung Med J* 2002 Mar;25(3):169–174.
82. Bhatia J, Parish A. GERD or not GERD: the fussy infant. *J Perinatol* 2009 May;29(Suppl 2):S7–S11.
83. Rudolph CD. Supraesophageal complications of gastroesophageal reflux in children: challenges in diagnosis and treatment. *Am J Med* 2003 18 Aug;115(Suppl 3A):150S–156S.
84. Mousa H, Woodley FW, Metheney M, Hayes J. Testing the association between gastroesophageal reflux and apnea in infants. *J Pediatr Gastroenterol Nutr* 2005;41:169–177.
85. Gold BD. Gastroesophageal reflux disease: could intervention in childhood reduce the risk of later complications?. *Am J Med* 2004 6 Sep; 117(Suppl 5A):23S–29S.
86. Diaz DM, Gibbons TE, Heiss K, *et al.* Antireflux surgery outcomes in pediatric gastroesophageal reflux disease. *Am J Gastroenterol* 2005;100: 1844–1852.

87. Orenstein SR. Management of supraesophageal complications of gastroesophageal reflux disease in infants and children. *Am J Med* 2000; 108(4A):139S–143S.
88. Dellon ES, Gibbs WB, Fritchie KJ, Rubinas TC, Wilson LA, Woosley JT, *et al.* Clinical, endoscopic, and histologic findings distinguish eosinophilic esophagitis from gastroesophageal reflux disease. *Clin Gastroenterol Hepatol* 2009 Dec;7(12):1305–1313; quiz 1261.
89. Rothenberg ME. Biology and treatment of eosinophilic esophagitis. *Gastroenterology* 2009 Oct;137(4):1238–1249.
90. Ramakrishnan JB. The role of food allergy in otolaryngology disorders. *Curr Opin Otolaryngol Head Neck Surg* 2010 Jun;18(3):195–199.
91. Furuta GT, Liacouras CA, Collins MH, *et al.* Eosinophilic esophagitis in children and adults: a systematic review and consensus recommendations for diagnosis and treatment. *Gastroenterology* 2007 Oct;133(4): 1342–1363.
92. Spergel JM. Eosinophilic esophagitis in adults and children: evidence for a food allergy component in many patients. *Curr Opin Allergy Clin Immunol* 2007 June;7(3):274–278.
93. Liacouras CA, Wenner WJ, Brown K, Ruchelli E. Primary eosinophilic esophagitis in children: successful treatment with oral corticosteroids. *J Pediatr Gastroenterol Nutr* 1998 Apr;26(4):380–385.
94. Noel RJ, Rothenberg ME. Eosinophilic esophagitis. *Curr Opin Pediatr* 2005 Dec;17(6):690–694.
95. Chan SK, Mahmoudi M. Eosinophilic esophagitis. *Compr Ther* 2009 Fall-Winter;35(3–4):160–166.

# 9

# Pediatric Laryngeal Disorders

*N. Scott Howard and Gerald Berke*

## INTRODUCTION

The pediatric voice is influenced by laryngeal development. From the infant's first cry to her first vocal expression and words, and later, during pubertal growth changes, the voice is in a continual state of flux. It is, therefore, not uncommon for children to develop voice abnormalities that follow the anatomical changes and physiological differences in the larynx. These changes can cause significant anxiety for the patient and may result in improper adaptations resulting in abnormal voice changes. Early identification and treatment of these disorders is important for the emotional and social development of the child.

Although accurate prevalence and incidence is not known for many pediatric voice disorders, the frequency of occurrence overall is estimated to range from 6% to 11%.[1,2] The high variability in incidence is partly due to the diversity of voice patterns in children and the inability for even trained professionals to correctly diagnose the problem in pediatric patients.[3] Many of these voice changes are thought to be transient, but surprisingly, in a longitudinal study of rural school aged children, nearly 40% of patients with voice disorders had persistent voice abnormalities at one and five years without treatment.[4] "Voice disorders" can be placed within categories of disordered laryngeal movement/phonation, vocal tract/resonance abnormalities, or decreased respiratory functioning as well as classified as either congenital or acquired.

Examples of congenital pediatric disorders that cause voice abnormalities include vocal fold immobility, laryngeal stenosis, laryngomalacia, laryngocele, webbing, and anterior laryngeal clefts. Several of these etiologies including bilateral abductor paralysis are more thoroughly discussed in other chapters.

Examples of acquired voice disorders include chronic laryngitis caused by vocal fold fibrovascular lesions (nodules, ulcers, granulomas and scar), laryngeal polyposis, reflux and microvascular lesions as well as laryngeal hyperfunction, paradoxical vocal fold motion, velopharyngeal incompetence or hypernasality, and laryngeal trauma.

## Anatomy

The pediatric larynx is smaller than the adult larynx. As seen in Table 1, in newborns, the length of the vocal folds is 2.5–3.0 mm and increases over the subsequent 20 years. Adult vocal fold length is approximately 11–15 mm in females and 17–21 mm in males.[5] In addition to a substantial increase in length of the folds, the

**Table 1. Changes in the structure of the vocal folds and influence on fundamental frequency.**

| Age | Membranous cord | Posterior cord | Total length | Pitch ($F_0$) |
|---|---|---|---|---|
| Newborn | 1.25–1.5 mm (50%) | 1.25–1.5 mm | 2.5–3.0 mm | 500 Hz |
| Ten years old | 6–8 mm (variable) | 2–3 mm | Variable | Decr. by 50% ~250 Hz |
| Adult female | 8.5–12 mm (77%–80%) | Incr. 1.5 to 4 mm | 11–15 mm | 150–250 Hz |
| Adult male | 14.5–18 mm (85%) | Incr. 4 to 11 mm | 17–21 mm | 80–150 Hz Drops additional 50 Hz at puberty. |

composition of the vocal folds also changes over time. At birth, the membranous portion of the fold (the distance from the anterior commisure to the vocal process) accounts for 50% of the total fold length. As the child matures, the membranous portion of the cord lengthens relative to the arytenoids. Initially, this lengthening is equal in boys and girls until age 10 where a significant increase in growth occurs for the male. As the child enters puberty and adulthood, the relative length of the membranous cord to the posterior glottis ranges from 77%–85% of the total vocal fold length.

The composition of the vocal cord also changes significantly over time.[6] The vocalis muscle of an infant inserts anteriorly into the vocal process and the mucosa is thinner with a high percentage of collagen and no discernable difference between the layers of lamina propria. Newborns have no vocal ligament. It slowly develops over the first one to four years of life. In adults, the vocalis muscle is thicker with three specific layers of lamina propria with variable composition.[7]

Other notable features of the developing vocal tract include a high laryngeal position, a high and pliant epiglottis that is omega shaped in over 50% of normal infants, a narrow conical shaped glottal and subglottal spaces, and anteriorly flexed airway. In the newborn, the subglottal space is the narrowest part of the airway with normal full term diameter of 4 mm. The cricoid ring is the least pliable portion of the airway and is the most likely site of laryngeal trauma and stenosis. The infant larynx is less susceptible to blunt trauma due to its high position protected by the mandible and its cartilaginous flexibility.[8] The newborn larynx lies between the first and third cervical spaces while in the adult it lies between the sixth and seventh cervical levels.[9] With growth, the vocal tract elongates into a more cylindrical shape with expansion of the cricoid and widening of the thyroid ala causing changes in vocal tract resonance.

As the male child enters puberty between the ages of ten and 14 years of age, the laryngeal structures grow rapidly — lengthening and widening the vocal tract. Increased bulk of the thyroaryenoid muscle causes vertical thickening of the vocal fold. As the cricoid expands, the vocal folds lengthen and these forces narrow the

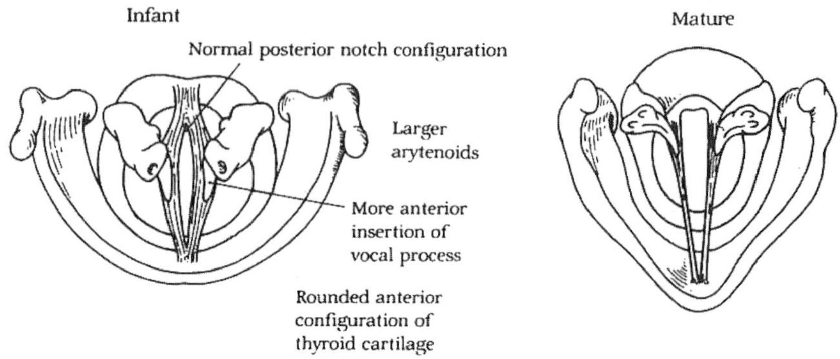


**Fig. 1.** Superior view of vocal folds demonstrates the relative large size of the pediatric arytenoids and short length of the membranous cord. From Bent JP, Alexander RE, Eavey RD. The pediatric larynx. In: Fried MP, Ferlito A, eds. *The Larynx,* 3rd Ed., Vol. 1, p. 78. Copyright © 2009 Plural Publishing, Inc. All rights reserved. Used with permission.

thyroid cartilage creating an angle of 90–110 degrees compared to the infant (130 degrees) and female adult angle of 120 degrees.[10] The size of the vocal tract and pharynx relative to the oral cavity increases significantly in the adolescent male resulting in a decrease in the fundamental frequency.

Figure 1 shows an endoscopic view perspective of the pediatric and adult larynx. Figure 2 shows the posterior view demonstrating the large relative size of the arytenoids.

## Physiology

The voice is a result of the complex coordination of multiple motor systems controlling the respiratory, laryngeal, and articulation movements required for creating the voice. The lungs provide a driving force for the vocal cords. Due to the small relative size of the pediatric membranous fold, the subglottic pressures required for phonation exceeds adult levels. For phonation to occur, this increased pressure is developed despite a lung volume less than half that of adults. The elevated pressure is primarily exerted via increased accessory muscle use with rib cage excursion of an eight-year-old nearly double that

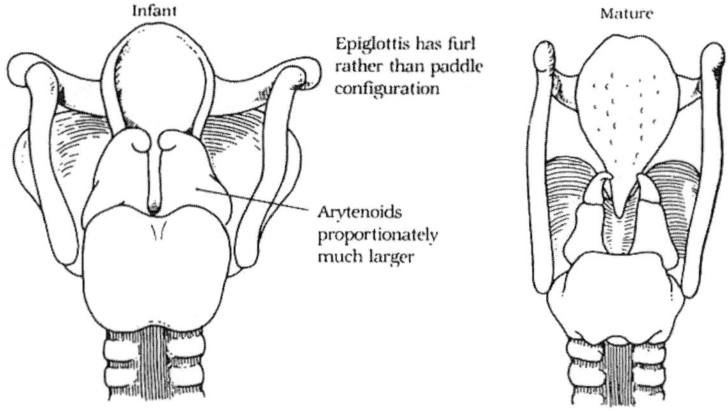


**Fig. 2.** Posterior view demonstrates the omega shaped epiglottis, overlapped thyroid cartilage and hyoid bone, and prominent cricoid cartilage. From Bent JP, Alexander RE, Eavey RD. The pediatric larynx. In: Fried MP, Ferlito A, eds. *The Larynx*, 3rd Ed., Vol. 1, p. 78. Copyright © 2009 Plural Publishing, Inc. All rights reserved. Used with permission.

of an adult. It is no coincidence that hyperfunction and overuse injury is very common in this age group.[11]

The acoustic output of the larynx is produced from vibrations of the membranous cord during periodic puffs of air release during cord movement. The vibratory movements of the vocal fold occur in both an inferior-superior direction and an anterior-posterior direction. The oscillation of the vocal folds is secondary to the innate elastic recoil of the vocal fold mucosa and the subglottic pressures that open and close the mucosal margin. Interruptions in the uniformity of the vibratory mucosal wave due to imperfections of the surface or alteration of the elastic properties of the vocal cord cause harshness or breathiness.

The acoustic output from the vocal cords is further modified at the level of the oropharynx, oral cavity, velopharynx, and lips. The human ability to create intelligible speech is primarily due to the phenomenal coordination of the musculature of the pharynx, velopharynx, and tongue. Abnormalities in these areas result in articulation and resonance disorders. Of particular importance in pediatric patients is the action of the velopharynx. The velopharynx acts as a valve for deglutition, respiration, and speech. Paired muscular slings — palatopharyngeus, palatoglossis, levator veli palatine, superior constrictor, and uvulae musculature — enable us to elevate, depress, constrict, or relax the palate. In the English language, the valve is open with nasal consonant sounds /m/, /n/, /ng/ and closed in all others.

## Evaluation

Pediatric voice abnormalities can usually be categorized into alterations of quality, pitch, loudness, articulation or resonance. Frequently, parents or teachers initiate the evaluation by noting changes in voice or an inability to match peer improvements in voice and speech. Pubertal changes deserve consideration for both sexes. Puberty onset occurs between ages eight and 15 in females and $9\frac{1}{2}$ and 14 in males. Completion of these changes are observed by age 12 to $16\frac{1}{2}$ in females and $13\frac{1}{2}$ to 18 in males. The most intense changes occur between ages $12\frac{1}{2}$ and 14 and last for about $1\frac{1}{2}$ years.[12] A comprehensive medical evaluation by otolaryngologists, speech and language pathologists, pediatricians, and audiologists should be initiated. Occasionally, additional specialists in neurology, gastroenterology, genetics, endocrinology, psychology and social work may be obtained.

A thorough history and physical examination should include a fiberoptic evaluation of the velopharynx, and larynx. This examination is tolerated by most pediatric patients if the environment is conducive to the exam.[13] Distal-chip flexible laryngoscopes have significantly improved the visualization of the larynx and are easier to tolerate than rigid laryngoscopy in the pediatric patient. For children under three, smaller endoscopes (2.3–3.2 mm) are utilized while in older patients, 4.0 mm endoscopes are utilized.[14] Evaluation should include connected speech, natural breathing, and sustained phonation. The ability to playback video of these evaluations is critical as assessment during evaluation is challenging. Rarely, direct laryngoscopy in the operating room is required when children do not tolerate fiberoptic evaluation or when detailed viewing is required for assessment of immobility or small lesions or when surgical intervention is required. Even with a cooperative patient, edema from laryngopharyngeal reflux may mask hyperfunction or a mass lesion to an extent that diagnosis is delayed.

### Outpatient Management

The various etiologies of voice abnormalities seen in pediatric population require a multi-disciplined approach. If possible, an audiogram should be performed prior to the visit if hearing loss is believed to be a contributing factor — a school audiogram is usually sufficient. Speech and language pathologists familiar with pediatric voice disorders should attempt to see the patient on the same day as the child's otolaryngology visit. Communication with these colleagues will significantly aid in both accurate diagnosis and determination of potential outpatient treatment methodologies. Assessment of developmental growth, speech and language delay or other medical conditions may significantly affect management and often prompt referral to additional specialists.

### Inpatient Management

Inpatient management of voice disorders is rare but is likely secondary to congenital disorders in the newborn or sequelae from other procedures in the child admitted for other purposes. Most commonly, these disorders are a result of vocal cord paralysis, edema, or hemorrhage due to intubation. Infectious croup may also present with voice changes and is addressed in another chapter. Primary concern for any inpatient voice evaluation is the assessment of the airway.

### Emergency Evaluation and Treatment

As discussed above, voice abnormalities may be secondary to edema of the vocal cords, partially obstructive masses or paralyzed vocal structures. Assessment of the child's respiratory status using pulse oximetry, careful physical exam noting chest movement, accessory muscle use, perfusion, and auscultation of chest and neck are a few of the most important exam findings to note on your initial assessment. A "Hot Potato" voice or inability to vocalize often indicates significant oropharyngeal and airway swelling. Inspiratory or expiratory stridor indicates obstruction.

Evaluation with imaging (chest X-ray, lateral soft tissue neck films, or CT), bedside fiberoptic exam, operative management with direct laryngoscopy or tracheostomy may be required.

### Complications and Their Management

Voice changes in children are frequently self limited or correctable with minor surgical procedures or voice therapy. Acute airway complications are possible during any operative intervention within the airway. Children and particularly, infants have low physiologic reserve so careful preoperative planning is required.

### Operative Interventions

Operative interventions are both diagnostic and corrective in a majority of cases. Of the greatest importance is management of the child's airway. Additionally, intubation caries its own risks to causation of voice abnormalities. Postoperative instructions such as voice rest are particularly difficult in pediatric populations. A careful assessment of the goals of the intended surgery is required prior to informed consent.

## ETIOLOGIES OF CONGENITAL PEDIATRIC VOICE DISORDERS

### Unilateral Vocal Fold Immobility

Unilateral vocal cord immobility may present with a weak breathy voice and aspiration or a nearly normal voice and swallowing function.

Together with bilateral immobility, this entity accounts for about 10% of the congenital abnormalities of the larynx. Immobility of the arytenoids complex can be caused by a variety of insults. In children this is usually neurogenic in origin. Although complete immobility is more frequently observed, subtle motion abnormalities causing mild voice changes may be observable on video stroboscopy due to partial paresis. With any immobility disorder, palpation of the arytenoid unit is often an important step to confirm diagnosis. Imaging of the course of the recurrent laryngeal nerve may uncover a causative mass lesion or cerebral abnormality. Laryngeal EMG may be considered and can be performed in the operating suite under light sedation using equipment found in most operating rooms.[15]

*Treatment*: Unilateral cord weakness treatment includes voice therapy, medialization thyroplasty, arytenoid adduction, and reinnervation. Reinnervation is ideal in this patient population however; timing of this treatment is an ongoing controversy. Following neurogenic paralysis, delay in treatment to await potential recovery results in vocal fold atrophy with reduction in the reinnervation potential. After five years, reinnervation rarely occurs. Complicating this is the finding that children with neurogenic vocal cord paralysis have a far greater potential for recovery of function but have a prolonged recovery timeline when compared to adults. Reports of over two years from date of onset to recovery is described in the literature. In fact, 50% of children who recover from iatrogenic paralysis do not improve until over one year after onset.[16] Voice therapy and temporary medialization with injection laryngoplasty is prudent while waiting for potential return of function. Close follow-up is recommended to ensure appropriate procedures are selected for long term management.

### Bilateral Vocal Fold Immobility

As in adults, bilateral immobility patients may present with a normal voice. However, airway issues may develop if abductory movement is significantly compromised. Newborns with bilateral cord paralysis frequently have near normal respirations and cry. Inspiratory stridor may not become symptomatic until six to 12 months after birth when increases in their activity cause greater respiratory demand. Like unilateral immobility, neurogenic causes are most common in the pediatric patient. Thoracic surgery, traumatic delivery, and CNS abnormalities such as Arnold-Chiari malformation are the leading causes.

*Treatment*: Tracheostomy may be required. Interventions such as arytenoidectomy or cordotomy should be delayed up to two years if recovery is possible.

## Laryngeal Web

This uncommon condition may go unnoticed if airway issues are not observed during the first year of life. Voice problems are frequently the presenting symptom when webs occlude less than 35% of glottic airway. These often require no intervention as surgical procedures may not significantly improve voice function. Airway compromise with webs of less than 50% of the glottic airway is rare. Webs larger than this, however, often require tracheostomy. These findings were classified by Cohen into the grading criteria in Table 2.[17]

*Treatment*: Options include tracheostomy, dilation, division (either open or laser technique) with or without a keel, or observation.[18] Mitomycin application is frequently utilized to prevent scar formation recurrence. As surgery does not always improve vocal function, patient selection is critical. Genetic consultation is recommended if findings are consistent with velocardiofacial syndrome. Figure 3 shows a laryngeal keel made from reinforced silastic prior to placement and in position. The right vocal cord may be seen to the right of the keel.

## Anterior and Posterior Laryngeal Cleft

Laryngeal clefts are rare congenital disorders resulting from failed fusion or chondrification of the cricoid lamina. Posterior clefts are

**Table 2. Laryngeal web classification system, symptoms and treatment.**

| | | | | |
|---|---|---|---|---|
| Type I | <35% | TVC visible, no subglottic web | Mild voice changes | Observe to age 3 or 4 |
| Type II | 35%–50% | TVC dysfunction, small subglottic extent | Airway changes rare, moderate voice changes | May require endoscopic keel or staged dilation |
| Type III | 50%–75% | Thick anterior web with subglottic extent, possible cricoid abnormalities | Severe airway dysfunction | Tracheostomy, laryngotomy, keel |
| Type IV | 75%–90% | Thick anteriorly and posteriorly, unable to visualize TVC, often coexisting cricoid abnormalities | Aphonia, emergency airway required | Tracheostomy, laryngotomy, keel or laryngotracheal reconstruction |

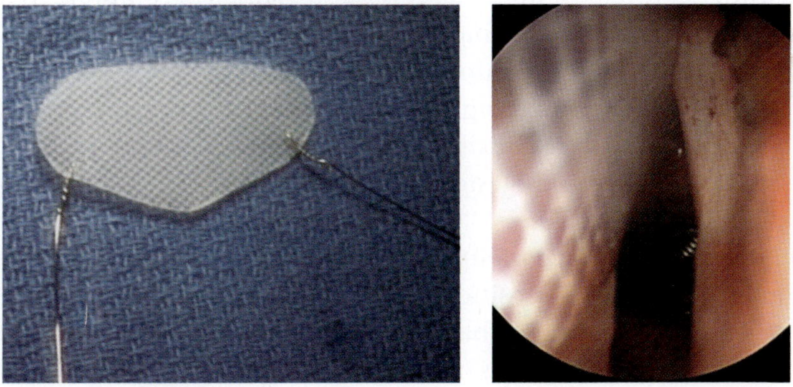

**Fig. 3.** Keel made from reinforced silastic with intraoperative view of placement following laser supraglottic web resection. Tracheostomy is required prior to placement. Removal is performed during direct laryngoscopy ten to 14 days following surgery. Photos courtesy of Dr. Howard.

**Table 3. Posterior laryngeal cleft classification and symptoms.**[20]

| | | |
|---|---|---|
| Type 1 | Supraglottic interarytenoid cleft is located above the vocal cord level | May be asymptomatic or mild aspiration, stridor, cough, or feeding abnormalities |
| Type 2 | Cleft extends below the vocal cords into the upper cricoid cartilage | More pronounced symptoms of aspiration and pneumonia |
| Type 3 | Cleft extends through the cricoid cartilage and possibly into the cervical trachea | Similar to Type 3 with greater airway compromise |
| Type 4 | Cleft extends into the thoracic trachea and extends variably toward the carina | Early respiratory distress; can lead to a child's death before a diagnosis is made |

far more common accounting for nearly 1.5% of laryngeal pathology in children. Table 3 represents a classification method introduced by Benjamin and Inglis. Anterior laryngeal clefts are exceedingly rare.[19] Both are associated with other aerodigestive tract abnormalities such as tracheoesophogeal fistula, tracheomalacia and subglottic stenosis. A high degree of suspicion is required in any infant with stridor, swallowing disorders, recurring pneumonia, or a weak cry. On flexible examination, the posterior glottis may appear normal or full. Direct laryngoscopy with palpation of the posterior glottis is diagnostic as flexible fiberoptic exam frequently misses these occasionally subtle lesions.

*Treatment*: Early management options include medical management of reflux, dietary and positional changes during feeding or use of nasogastric tubes and intubation to allow the child to mature and grow. Long segment clefts may require specialized endotracheal tubes. When surgical correction is indicated, Type 1 and some Type 2 posterior clefts are amenable to endoscopic treatment. $CO_2$ lasers or microscissors are used to denude the intra-arytenoid mucosa and sutures are placed to reapproximate the tissues. Most Type 3 and some Type 2 clefts require open techniques. Anterior approach via laryngofissure avoids RLN injury and allows excellent visability of the defect.[21] Alternative approaches include lateral pharyngotomy or posterior pharyngotomy. Mucosal flaps may be rotated into the defect or free buccal grafts may be sutured in place for smaller defects. Delayed reconstruction via a laryngotracheal reconstruction trough allows bolsters to stay in place for close monitoring of mucosal flaps or grafts. Intrathoracic clefts require combined team approach with pediatric cardiothoracic surgeons.

### Laryngocele and Saccular Cyst

Laryngocele is an uncommon cause of lateral congenital neck mass in children with potential voice and airway changes. These develop from the laryngeal saccule, an anterior pouch within the laryngeal ventricle. Both congenital and acquired laryngoceles may be internal or external based upon its position relative to the thyrohyoid membrane. Internal laryngoceles do not present as a neck mass and extend from the saccule posteriorly and superiorly within the false vocal fold and aryepiglottic fold. These lesions may cause voice abnormalities through interruption in vocal cord closure or from interruption in the resonance of the voice. External laryngoceles pass through the thyrohyoid membrane into the neck. Most commonly these are found at the entrance of the superior laryngeal nerve and vessel — a weak point within the thyrohyoid membrane. Congenital laryngoceles are exceedingly rare and are usually external. Acquired laryngocele is associated with prolonged intralaryngeal pressure from woodwind or brass instrument playing and is more common in adults. Saccular cysts are smaller expansions of the saccule and are unlikely to cause symptoms.

*Treatment*: Laryngocele may be asymptomatic, particularly in adults. Symptoms range from mild voice changes, dyspnea, cough, stridor, or foreign body sensation. In symptomatic cases of congenital laryngocele, tracheostomy reduces the intraglottic pressure resulting in a reduction of growth potential. Delayed surgical correction to allow for laryngeal growth is recommended to age 5. Endoscopic procedures using the $CO_2$ laser are recommended for internal laryngoceles while open techniques are used for external or combined laryngoceles.[22]

## ETIOLOGIES OF ACQUIRED PEDIATRIC VOICE DISORDERS

### Laryngopharyngeal Reflux — LPR

Reflux is the retrograde movement of gastric and esophogeal contents to the larynx. Although this is an oversimplified description of the disorder, it will suffice for most cases in the pediatric patient. Symptoms in children may mimic adult findings, but are frequently masked by compensatory measures until secondary changes occur affecting speech, respiration, or swallowing function. Symptoms of dysphonia, globus sensation, chronic cough and throat clearing, excessive mucus production, and halatosis are frequently seen. Postcricoid and intraarytenoid/periarytenoid edema, vocal fold erythema, thick mucus, and pseudosulcus may be observed on video stroboscopy.

*Treatment*: This involves dietary changes, lifestyle and behavioral modifications, and medical intervention (proton pump inhibitors, motility agents, and H2 blockers). Rarely, GI surgery is considered in the pediatric patient. Dual channel pH probes and newer minimally invasive pH probes may be useful in confirming a diagnosis. However, negative testing does not always rule out LPR.

### Laryngeal Hyperfunction

As described above, the pediatric vocal cord's size and powerful respiratory function enable the child to produce excessive trauma to the vocal fold with ease. Any parent knows that a child can emit a high frequency blast of sound that will nearly deafen anyone nearby. This capability does come with a cost. Following injury to the laryngeal mucosa from irritants such as postnasal drip, allergies, reflux or upper respiratory infections — the child is able to compensate for the edema through greater respiratory pressures and laryngeal tone. This increase in subglottic pressure and volume of air rushing past the injured cords creates further injury manifesting as vocal fold nodules, cysts, or polyps.

Symptoms of hyperfunction include vocal harshness or breathiness, throat pain, or aphonia. Prolonged voice misuse is also habit forming as children do not have an accurate perception of loudness. Fiberoptic evaluation may demonstrate this tension as anterior–posterior compression or false fold phonation known as dysphonia plicae ventricullaris (phonation from false vocal fold approximation) due to their excessive supraglottic tension.

*Treatment*: Johnson and Child concluded that 85%–90% of childhood voice problems are secondary to laryngeal hyperfunction.[23] Prior to treatment of any secondary lesions, voice and behavioral therapy should be initiated to limit recurrence. In fact, speech therapy may be curative.

## Vocal Fold Fibrovascular Lesions (Nodules, Ulcers, Granulomas and Scar)

Nodules are the most common lesions found in the pediatric patient. They account for roughly 45% to 80% of childhood dysphonia cases in the preschool age range (four to five years old) and elementary age children (six to 11 years old).[24] They are seen as swellings, usually bilateral within the mid membranous cord. The mass of these lesions impairs the vibratory pattern of vocal cord causing harshness. When large enough, these can prevent adduction of the cords causing breathy voice changes. These lesions often fluctuate in size due to use and local inflammation. Incidence of nodules ranges from 38% to 78% in children with hoarseness and is more common in boys with aggressive vocal tendencies.

*Treatment*: Fifty-nine percent of otolaryngologists sampled in a study stated that voice therapy was the sole treatment modality of a majority of their patients with vocal nodules.[25] Most resolve without intervention due to the natural changes in the vocal cords (as child grows — changes in vocal cord length results in decreased pitch and decreased subglottic pressure result in less trauma to the mucosa). Underlying inflammation caused by allergy, reflux, or chronic sinusitis should be treated. Speech pathology is often beneficial to address abnormal voice use. Complete voice rest, Botox, and surgery can be effective but are less frequently indicated in pediatric patients.

Ulcers and granulomas are seen in the posterior glottis — usually at or near the vocal process. These lesions may be unilateral or bilateral and are due to repeated contact between the vocal processes with coexisting inflammation caused by allergy, reflux, or both. Ulcers frequently cause pain but granulomas are often asymptomatic. Granulomas can become large enough to cause airway compromise. Opposing surfaces of the granuloma may fuse and cause posterior commissure stenosis.

*Treatment*: Options for granuloma include voice rest with observation, Botox (resulting in forced voice rest), or excision. Treatment of the underlying inflammatory cause is important to obtain resolution of ulcers and granulomas. Speech therapy is often required to ensure these lesions do not return.

## Vocal Fold Cysts

Unlike many of the fibrovascular lesions discussed above, cysts within the vocal cord do not resolve with voice rest or time. These lesions are likely secondary to intracordal bleeding occurring during intense voice use. This blood resorbs leaving an inflammatory capsule behind. Continued voice use incites local inflammation of the cyst resulting in expansion of the cyst. Voice rest will frequently cause a significant decrease in size of these lesions however recurrence is inevitable. Vocal cord cysts are sometimes challenging to differentiate from nodules as the cyst can cause contra-lateral thickening. However, these lesions often disrupt the mucosal wave to a greater degree on stroboscopy particularly during high pitched phonation.

*Treatment*: Surgical excision is curative. Microflap surgery is required and should be performed by surgeons experienced in this technique. Allowing a child to mature so that they may comply with up to two weeks of voice rest following surgery is recommended. Failure to remove the entire cyst will result in recurrence or an opening of the cyst to the surface — sulcus vocalis.

**Recurrent Laryngeal Papillomas**

Recurrent respiratory papillomas (RRP) are the most common benign neoplasm of the larynx in children. Hoarseness is the most frequent presentation. This disorder is caused by local infection with the human papilloma virus (HPV) and may cause significant voice and respiratory complications. Immune dysfunction is proposed to have an influence over disease progression. Diagnosis at a younger age corresponds to increased disease severity, more frequent surgical procedures, and greater risk of progressive disease.[26] Persistent voice abnormalities frequently last beyond remission of this disorder as scar formation caused by surgical modalities persists.

*Treatment*: For this disorder treatment is further specified in a previous (subsequent) chapter. Attempts to minimize vocal fold lamina propria injury may result in better long term vocal function.

**Hypernasality and Velopharyngeal Incompetence (VPI)**

Hypernasality is the finding of excessive nasal sounds during speech. VPI is defined as an excessive separation of the oral and nasal mucosa during phonation or deglutition. Nasal regurgitation of liquids and food may occur. These symptoms are frequently coexisting due to either an absence of appropriate contraction of the levator veli palatine muscle or pharyngeal constrictors. These muscles cause elevation of soft palate or medial movement of the lateral pharyngeal walls. Anatomic factors that influence this condition include short palate, cleft palate, submucus cleft, and motor abnormalities. Velocardiofacial syndrome describes inadequate motion (hypotonia) of the palate, cardiac and vascular abnormalities, small stature, and learning disability and is the most common syndrome with VPI symptoms. Care is required during tonsillectomy and adenoidectomy in these patients as the carotid artery may be very close to the operative field. VPI and hypernasality frequently coexist with other articulation or voice abnormalities. For comparison, hyponasality is a lack of nasal resonance during /m/, /n/, and /ng/ sounds. It is found in patients with excessive adenoid hypertrophy, nasal obstruction or in patients with overcorrection of VPI.

*Treatment*: Speech therapy is recommended for up to six months before surgical intervention is considered. Palatal appliances are not well tolerated in children, but may be helpful. Patients are followed closely for changes in voice and swallowing function. If speech therapy does not improve the VPI or a plateau is reached with continued dysfunction, surgical correction is considered. Superiorly based central flaps or lateral based pharyngeal flap surgery (sphincter pharyngoplasty) are selected based upon findings during fiberoptic evaluation. Fat injection or secondary procedures are occasionally required.[27]

## Laryngeal Trauma

Due to the high anatomic position of the larynx, flexibility of the cartilage, and protection from the mandible — external trauma to the larynx is rare in younger patients. As children age, the larynx becomes less resistant to external trauma. This is particularly true for adolescent males who are more likely to engage in contact sports or physical altercations. Fine cut CT imaging of the larynx is utilized to assess the laryngeal skeleton but is not as useful in children due to the limited calcification of the cartilage.

Intubation trauma is unfortunately common in young patients. Prolonged intubation, subglottic and vocal fold lacerations, excessive size of endotracheal tubes which can cause ulcers, or arytenoid injury from excessive force during intubation may result in dysfunction. Posterior glottis webs or stenosis due to bilateral granulomas has also been observed following long term intubation.

*Treatment*: Acute treatment for laryngeal injury is focused upon protection of the compromised airway. Secondary goals of voice and swallowing function are then considered. In a previously injured airway, tracheostomy under local anesthesia with light sedation may be indicated. Direct laryngoscopy is frequently required to assess the airway. Observation or surgical intervention is selected. Observation is usually best for asymptomatic patients with mild edema, small hematoma, or minor lacerations that do not involve the phonatory surface or the anterior commisure. Surgical management options include endoscopic and open approaches to stabilize laryngeal fractures or repair mucosal tears. Occasionally, laryngeal keels or T-Tubes are needed to prevent stenosis. Mitomycin may augment these treatments if abnormal healing may induce restrictions in vocal fold movement or stenosis.

## Paradoxical Vocal Fold Motion

Laryngospasm is the inappropriate adduction of the vocal folds during inspiration resulting in respiratory obstruction is an uncommon but distressing medical problem for children, parents, caregivers, and teachers. Frequently these children have had multiple visits to emergency rooms or have been placed on bronchodilators for presumed asthma prior to diagnosis. Although this disorder can coexist with asthma in up to 50% of patients, the two entities are distinctly

**Table 4. Comparison of laryngospasm (paradoxical vocal fold motion) and asthma.**

| | Laryngospasm (PVFM) | Asthma |
|---|---|---|
| Tightness | Neck/throat/larynx | Chest |
| Triggers | Exercise, temperature, irritants (smoke, PND, GERD), stress | Exercise, temperature, irritants (smoke, PND, GERD), allergy, stress |
| Recovery | Rapid | Longer |
| Night time symptoms | Rare except for reflux induced | Frequent |
| Bronchodilators | Not effective | Effective |
| Stridor | To and fro (inspiratory and expiratory) | No |
| Expiratory wheeze | No | Yes |
| Fiberoptic evaluation (when symptomatic) | Paradoxical motion; anterior compression seen during inspiration, possible diamond shaped posterior gap | Normal laryngeal exam; no paradoxical motion or adduction during respiration |

different. Table 4 details some of the similarities and differences of these disorders.

Laryngospasm usually has a rapid onset and offset of symptoms. The sensation of the throat "shutting off," with significant anxiety differs from the onset of asthma symptoms. Voice is usually unaffected but patients will not be able to complete full sentences due to inability to fully inspire. Laryngospasm is often triggered by a hyperresponsive laryngeal mucosa which can be observed on fiberoptic evaluation. Although rarely symptomatic, treatment for reflux aids in treatment.[28]

*Treatment*: Speech therapy with biofeedback is the principal treatment for these patients. Relaxation techniques, breathing exercises,[29] and anxiolytics are useful. Simple sniffing exercises or deep abdominal breathing can be used to break the adductor tone. Botulinum toxin may be used to restrict laryngospasm but therapy is still required to avoid recurrence of symptoms. Medications and dietary changes to limit reflux reduce laryngeal sensitivity.

## Dystonia

Laryngeal dystonias may affect voice (either speaking or singing) or respiration. Respiratory dystonia has similarities to both spasmodic dysphonia and laryngospasm with centrally based neurological causes of inspiratory adduction. These disorders are often accompanied by other focal dystonias such as writers cramp, blephrospasm, oromandibular dystonia, palatal myoclonus, or tremor. These spasms usually improve with sleep and worsen with stress. Central nervous system disorders must be ruled out in these patients.

*Treatment*: The approach to treatment for laryngeal dystonias in pediatric patients is similar to laryngospasm however they are more responsive to small doses of Botulinum toxin.[30] Voice therapy and psychological intervention to reduce stress is also a valuable intervention. Surgical treatment for adductor dystonia is not recommended until age 16.

## Articulation and Phonologic Disorders

The pattern of language development is influenced by many factors — genetics, culture, social environment, socioeconomic status, and parental involvement to name only a few. As coordination of the respiratory, laryngeal and articulatory movements are learned there will be a high amount of variability in the rate of progress. Speech production can be divided into voice, fluency, and speech intelligibility. Fluency disorders include apraxia, stuttering and cluttering. Stuttering is the repitition of words or parts of words, prolongation of sounds, or temporary blockage of speech with prevalence near 1%.[31] Cluttering is far less common

**Table 5. Screening recommendations by the American Academy of Pediatrics.**[34]

- Lack of babbling, pointing, or other gestural communication by age 12 months.
- Lack of use of single words by age 16 months.
- Lack of two-word novel phrases by age 24 months.
- Loss of language or social skills at any age.

and results in "rapid, dysrhythmic, sporadic, unorganized, and frequently unintelligible [speech]."[32]

Speech intelligibility involves the coordination of articulation and resonance. Developmental delay, cleft palate, autism, hearing loss and several syndromes affect intelligibility. It is common for children to slowly develop more refined speech. By age 36 months, most children will be attempting most speech sounds with conversational speech anticipated by age 4. Autism is one of the most common disorders of intelligibility with nearly one in every 150 children affected.[33] Table 5 details screening recommendations for autism.

*Treatment*: Fluency and articulation disorder treatment should include a team of providers — general pediatricians, audiologists, head and neck surgeons, and speech therapists. Although treatment of these diverse disorders is outside the scope of this article, parental involvement in the process is critical.

## CONCLUSION

Voice disorders in children may be divided into abnormalities in respiratory drive, vocal cord function, resonance, fluency and speech intelligibility. A team approach involving the family, teachers, speech therapist, audiologist, pediatrician, and surgical and medical specialists will aid in diagnosis and treatment. High quality fiberoptic evaluation with video playback capability is critical to success with this patient population. Surgical evaluation is required in many; however, early surgical management is rare for voice isolated disorders.

## REFERENCES


1. Merati AL, Keppel K, Braun NM, Blumin JH, Kerschner JE. Pediatric voice-related quality of life: findings in healthy children and in common laryngeal disorders. *Ann Otol Rhinol Laryngol* 2008;117(4): 259–262.
2. Carding PN, Roulstone S, Northstone K. The prevalence of childhood dysphonia: a cross-sectional study. *J Voice* 2006;20(4):623–630.
3. Kreiman J, Garrett BR, Kempster GB, Erman A, Berke GS. Perceptual evaluation of voice quality: review, tutorial, and a framework for future research. *J Speech Hear Res* 1993 Feb;36(1):21–40.
4. Powell M, Filter M, Williams B. A longitudinal study of the prevalence of voice disorders in children from a rural school division. *J Commun Disord* 1989;22:375–382.
5. Kahane JC. Growth of the human prepubertal and pubertal larynx. *J Speech Hear Res* 1982 Sep;25(3):446–455.
6. Boudoux C, Leuin SC, Oh WY, Suter MJ, Desjardins AE, Vakoc BJ, Bouma BE, Hartnick CJ, Tearney GJ. Optical microscopy of the pediatric vocal fold. *Arch Otolaryngol Head Neck Surg* 2009;135(1):53–64.
7. Kahane JC. Growth of the human prepubertal and pubertal larynx. *J Speech Hear Res* 1982 Sep;25(3):446–455.
8. Wiatrak BJ. Congenital anomalies of the larynx and trachea. *Otolaryngol Clin North Am* 2000 Feb;33(1):91–110.
9. Fried MP, Kelly JH, Strome M. Comparison of the adult and infant larynx. *J Fam Pract* 1982 Sep;15(3):557–558, 561.
10. Kahane JC. A morphological study of the human prepubertal and pubertal larynx. *Am J Anat* 1978;151:11–20.
11. Hoit JD, Hixon TJ, Watson PJ, *et al.* Speech breathing in children and adolescents. *J Speech Hear Res* 1990;33:51–69.
12. Spiegal JR, Sataloff RT, Emerich KA. The three ages of voice: the young adult voice. *J Voice* 1997;11(2):138–143.
13. Leeper HA, Leonard JE, Iverson RL. Otorhinolarngologic screening of children with vocal quality disturbances. *Int J Pediatr Otorhinolaryngol* 1980;2:123–131.
14. Hartnick CJ, Zeitels SM. Pediatric video laryngo-stroboscopy. *Int J Pediatr Otorhinolaryngol* 2005;69:215–219.

15. Scott AR, Chong PS, Randolph GW, Hartnick CJ. Intraoperative laryngeal electromyography in children with vocal fold immobility: a simplified technique. *Int J Pediatr Otorhinolaryngol* 2008;72:31–40.
16. Daya H, Hosni A, Bejar-Solar I, Evans JN, Bailey CM. Pediatric vocal fold paralysis: a long term retrospective. *Arch Otolaryngol Head Neck Surg* 2000;126(1):21–25.
17. Cohen SR. Congenital webs in children: a retrospective review of 51 patients. *Ann Otol Rhinol Laryngol* 1985;121(suppl):2–16.
18. Cohen SR, Thompson JW. Ventral cleft of the larynx: a rare congenital defect. *Ann Otol Rhinol Laryngol* 1990;99:281–285.
19. Hughes CA, Miller KA, Holinger LD, Miller RP. Anterior submucus laryngeal cleft. *Int J Ped Otorhinolaryngol* 2000;54:153–158.
20. Benjamin B, Inglis A. Minor congenital laryngeal clefts: diagnosis and classification. *Ann Otol Rhinol Laryngol* 1989 Jun;98(6):417–420.
21. Froehlich P, Truy E, Stamm D, *et al.* Cleft larynx: management and one-stage surgical repair by anterior translaryngotracheal approach in two children. *Int J Pediatr Otorhinolaryngol* 1993;27(1):73–78.
22. Dursun G, Ozgursoy OB, Beton S, Batikhan H. Current diagnosis and treatment of laryngocele in adults. *Otolaryngol Head Neck Surg* 2007;136:211–215.
23. Johnson TS, Child DR. Voice disorders in the child. In: Lass NJ, McReynolds LV, Northern JL, Yoder DE, eds. *Handbook of Speech-Language Pathology and Audiology*. Toronto: BC Decker Inc., 1988.
24. Hooper C. Treatment of voice disorders in children. *Lang Speech Hear Serv Schools* 2004;35:320–326.
25. Moran M, Pentz A. Otolaryngologists' opinions of voice therapy for vocal nodules in children. *Lang Speech Hear Serv Schools* 1987;18: 172–178.
26. Ruparelia S, Unger ER, Nisenbaum R, *et al.* Predictors of remission in jeuvenile-onset recurrent respiratory papillomatosis. *Arch Otolaryngol Head Neck Surg* 2003;129:1275–1278.
27. Boseley ME, Hartnick CJ. Assessing the outcome of surgery to correct velopharyngeal insufficiency with the pediatric voice outcome survey. *Int J Ped Otorhinolaryngol* 2004;68:1429–1433.
28. Sandage Mj, Zelany SK. Paradoxical vocal fold motion in children and adolescents. *Lang Speech Hear Serv Schools* 2004;35(4):353–362.

29. Martin RJ, Blager FB, Gay ML, Wood RP II. Paradoxical vocal cord motion in presumed asthmatics. *Sem Resp Med* 1987;8:332–337.
30. Altman K, Mirza N, Ruiz C, Sataloff R. Paradoxical vocal fold motion: presentation and treatment options. *J Voice* 2000;14:99–103.
31. Baker BM, Blackwell PB. Identification and remediation of pediatric fluency disorders. *J Ped Health Care* 2004 Mar-Apr;18(2):87–94.
32. Daly D. Helping the clutterer: therapy considerations. In: Myers FL, St. Louis KO, eds. *Cluttering: A Clinical Perspective.* Kibworth, Great Britain: Far Communications, 1992, p. 107.
33. American Academy of Pediatrics. Autism A.L.A.R.M. (2007). http://aap.org/healthtopics/Autism.cfm.
34. American Academy of Pediatrics. Autism A.L.A.R.M. (2007). http://aap.org/healthtopics/Autism.cfm.

# 10

# Dysphagia in Children

*N. Scott Howard and Dinesh K. Chhetri*

## INTRODUCTION

Dysphagia is defined as impaired swallowing and is a common symptom in infants and children with neuromuscular and developmental disorders. These abnormalities in swallowing and feeding mechanisms are frequently met with confusion by pediatricians and may require interventions from speech and language pathologists, occupational therapists, otolaryngologists, gastroenterologists, nutritionists, psychologists and other allied health providers. Interventions such as feeding tubes, intubation, or tracheostomy may be required. As a child grows, other swallowing disorders may surface that require intervention or therapy. The purpose of this chapter is to describe the anatomy and physiology of swallowing, describe evaluation tools, provide a list of common causes of dysphagia, and to provide a streamlined diagnostic and treatment algorithm.

## ANATOMY

The critical function of swallowing involves the mouth, oral cavity, palate, oropharynx, larynx, pharynx, and esophagus. More detailed anatomy of these structures may be found elsewhere in this book, but the interaction of these systems during swallowing is discussed here.

## The Mouth, Oral Cavity, Nasopharynx and Oropharynx

The mouth is the first sphincter in the digestive tract, and oral competence is critical to the first phase of swallowing. Buccal musculature tone and dental occlusion are important to enable bolus formation. In the newborn, fat pads (also known as sucking pads) supplement the buccal musculature until the buccinator muscles are developed. In the older child and adult, the primary or secondary dentition enables mastication and solid food consumption. Primary dentition usually erupts between the sixth and 28th months.

The oral cavity and oropharynx are defined by the soft mobile structures and hard boundaries contained within. The tongue occupies the majority of the space within the oral cavity and is critically important to bolus formation. The tongue receives motor innervation from the hypoglossal nerve, sensory innervation from the trigeminal, glossopharyngeal, and vagus nerves, and special sensory innervation (taste) from the glossopharyngeal and facial nerves (chorda tympani). The soft palate or velum enables closure of the nasopharynx during swallowing. The hard palate and mandible help define the boundaries of the oral cavity. Abnormalities in the size or growth of these bony structures can cause relative tongue glossoptosis causing swallowing abnormalities such as those seen in Pierre–Robin Sequence.

## The Larynx, Pharynx, Hypopharynx and Esophagus

The larynx is intimately involved with the pharyngeal phase of swallowing and is positioned anterior and superior to the esophogeal inlet. In infants, the larynx is positioned higher in the neck, allowing the infant to breathe while nursing. This elevated position provides some protection from aspiration, but as the child ages the larynx descends and provides less protection. Therefore, dysphagia caused by congenital vocal fold paralysis may not present until four to six months of age when the larynx descent makes it more vulnerable to incomplete glottic closure.

The pharynx is a muscular tube extending from the posterior portion of the nasal cavity down to the esophageal inlet. The superior constrictor, middle constrictor, and inferior constrictor are overlapping muscular layers that create this muscular funnel leading to the esophagus. The oropharynx extends from the level of the palate to the level of the tip of the epiglottis. The vallecula is a space between the base of tongue and epiglottis and is one of the key landmarks during fiberoptic evaluation. It is divided into a right and left side by the median glosso-epiglottic fold. The soft palate elevates and apposes the posterior pharyngeal wall to prevent reflux of food into the nasopharynx during swallowing.

The hypopharynx is the lowest portion of the pharynx. It extends from the tip of the epiglottis down to the cricopharyngeus muscle. The two piriform sinuses are located on either side of the larynx and are potential spaces formed by the inferior constrictor muscle attachments to the thyroid cartilage and thyrohyoid laterally and the arytenoid-aryepiglottic fold complex medially. Pooling of secretions in the piriform sinuses often suggests a swallowing disorder.

The cricopharyngeal muscle (CP) is the second sphincter enroute to the stomach and is commonly known as the upper esophageal sphincter (UES). Relaxation of the cricopharyngeal muscle allows the food bolus to pass from the hypopharynx into the esophagus. The esophagus is a muscular tube extending from just below the cricopharyngeal muscle to the stomach. The lower esophageal sphincter (LES) resides at the junction of the esophagus and stomach (gastro-esophageal junction). The esophagus is a multi-layered tubular organ with an inner lining of non-keratinized stratified squamous mucosa. Surrounding the mucosa are the lamina propria, smooth muscle muscularis mucosa, submucosa, muscularis externa, and adventitia. The composition of the muscularis externa varies, with striated muscle in the upper one-third and smooth muscle in the lower two-third of the esophagus. Anatomic, functional, and inflammatory disorders of the esophagus may result in feeding difficulties but will not be covered in this chapter.

## NEUROANATOMY AND PHYSIOLOGY

The phases of swallowing are listed in Table 1. The pharyngeal phase is a pattern-generated response enabling the fastest, most critical and coordinated swallowing phase. The action of the pharyngeal musculature during swallowing is termed a pattern-generated response because it receives input from cortical centers of the frontal lobe, basal ganglia, cerebellum, and the central pattern generator in the nucleus ambiguus of the medulla. Once initiated, a complete pharyngeal swallow pattern is involuntarily elicited.[1]

Intact sensory and motor control is required for the initiation and coordination of swallowing. These learned responses develop in the newborn into a suck-swallow-breathe pattern allowing the neonate to feed. A part of this pattern is elicited with help of a few reflexes associated with swallowing: gag, root, reflexive sucking, and phasic bite. These reflexes differ considerably from the patterned response of swallowing. For example, the gag reflex is a true reflex, controlled at the

**Table 1. Key phases of swallowing.**

| Phase | Key components of phase | Time/rate |
|---|---|---|
| Oral preparatory | Lip closure/labial seal<br>Buccal tone<br>Mastication and tongue movement<br>Development of bolus | Depends upon consistency of food type |
| Oral | Anterior to posterior tongue movement<br>Maintain intact labial seal<br>Bolus presentation to oropharynx | About 1 second |
| Pharyngeal | Elevation/retraction of velum to close nasopharynx<br>Initiation of superior constrictor squeeze<br>Elevation/closure of larynx (epiglottic inversion, contraction of aryepiglottic folds, closure of false and true vocal folds)<br>Relaxation of CP muscle (UES) | 1 second (measured from anterior tonsil pillar through CP junction) at rate of 10–40 cm/second |
| Esophageal | Peristaltic movement from UES to LES | 8–20 seconds at rate of 1–4 cm/second[2] |

level of the brainstem. All of these feeding reflexes are present before birth. Most of these reflexes are present 18 weeks following conception and either increase or diminish over time after birth.[2] Inhibition of these reflexes can occur early in life with sensory alterations caused by tape on the face, feeding tubes, laryngopharyngeal reflux, or intubation. Such sensory changes may result in the airway remaining open and unprotected during swallowing causing aspiration.

In neonates, sucking is performed by closure of the lips, occlusion of the back of the oral cavity through approximation of the base of tongue and soft palate, and followed by rhythmic downward movement of the mandible and depression/retraction of the tongue. The sub-atmospheric pressure developed by this process enables fluid to flow into the oral cavity.[3] Later in life, mastication develops, with the maturation of the phasic bite reflex beginning at about six months of age. The gag reflex is diminished during this time frame to allow for larger bolus transfer into the pharynx.

The muscles involved in the oral preparatory phase include the tongue (CN XII) and muscles of mastication innervated by the trigeminal nerve (CN V). The muscles of mastication include: the temporalis muscle which elevates, retracts, and assists in closing the mandible, the masseter muscle which elevates and closes the mandible, the medial pterygoid which elevates the mandible and aids in its closure, and the lateral pterygoid which depresses, opens, and protrudes the mandible, and moves it laterally for grinding. Other muscles involved in the oral preparatory phase are the lip and cheek muscles: orbicularis oris, zygomaticus and the buccinator which holds food in contact with the teeth. All three are innervated by the facial nerve (CN VII).

Following bolus formation, five muscles control the movements of the palate to ensure the bolus does not travel into the nasopharynx. Elevation of the palate is performed by the palatoglossal and the levator veli palatini muscles (CN X). The tensor veli palatini tenses the palate (CN V). The palatopharyngeus depresses the palate and constricts the pharynx and the muscularis uvula shortens the palate. Both are innervated by the cranial portion of the spinal accessory nerve traveling within the vagus.[4]

Laryngeal closure is mediated by CN X in response to bolus movement. The airway closure occurs at the level of the true vocal cords, the false vocal folds, and the supraglottis. Supraglottic closure occurs with vertical movement of the larynx causing flexion of the epiglottis, bringing this tissue into approximation with the arytenoids and aryepiglottic folds. In newborns, fluid collects in the vallecula following sucking efforts, and the swallow patterned response is triggered. In normal infants, spillover into the piriform prior to initiation of the swallow or supraglottic penetration is not observed.[5] Also, the high laryngeal position in newborns makes laryngeal penetration less likely.

The esophageal phase of swallowing occurs after relaxation of the CP muscle, which allows bolus transfer into the esophagus. The three pharyngeal constrictors, the longitudinally oriented stylopharyngeus and salpingopharyngeus muscles, and the base of tongue first help move food toward the cricopharyngeus. The CP muscle opening is assisted by the movement of the larynx in an upward and anterior direction. Following passage of the bolus into the esophagus, peristalsis moves the bolus to the stomach under autonomic control. In adults, the esophagus extends approximately 23–25 cm to the gastro-esophogeal junction. In neonates and children the length of the esophagus is variable, and shorter esophageal length has been associated with a higher rate of reflux.[6] Unlike other muscles along the digestive tract, the CP muscle has inherent contractile properties. Thus, denervation of the CP muscle through neurologic injury can cause abnormally high tone of this muscle during swallowing that may cause an inability of food to pass into the esophagus and may result in aspiration.

## EVALUATION

A systematic history and examination of the pediatric patient with concern for feeding abnormalities should be performed (Table 2). The developmental level of the child should be assessed along with their alertness, general nutrition and hydration status, posture and head control. Discussion with the caregiver of proper positioning

**Table 2. Assessment of swallowing disorders in children.**

| Assessment | Tool |
|---|---|
| Adequacy of oral motor skills | Physical exam |
| Abnormal gag reflex | Physical exam |
| Ability to achieve and sustain airway protection | FEES, videofluoroscopy |
| Integrity of upper aerodigestive tract | FEES, videofluoroscopy |
| Hypopharyngeal sensation | Endoscopy |
| Pharyngeal and esophageal motility | Manometry, videoflouroscopy, esophagram |
| Suck swallow breathe pattern | Physical exam, non-nutritive sucking |
| Physiologic abnormalities not seen on other evaluations | Direct laryngoscopy and esophagoscopy in OR setting |

during feeding should be performed. For example, observation has shown that extension of the neck may cause feeding abnormalities in normal children. Preterm infants nursed in a head elevated and tilted position leads to fewer abnormal feeding events compared with a more horizontal position.[7]

The size and tone of the tongue and size and position of the mandible should be evaluated. A retracted or large tongue may prevent adequate sucking as seen in Pierre–Robin Sequence or Beckwith–Wiedemann syndrome. The oral cavity examination of a newborn should evaluate the suck and root reflex as well as the gag reflex. The gag reflex in neonates is located in the middle third of the tongue and moves to the posterior third by age six to seven months.[1]

In neonates, evaluation of the suck-swallow-breathe bursts can be made with use of a stethoscope on the lateral neck during feeding. The normal ratio of these bursts is 1:1:1. Increased work of breathing, cyanosis, oxygen desaturations, fussiness, recurrent regurgitation or pauses in feeding is abnormal. These abnormal feeding patterns should be further evaluated by a speech pathologist during normal feeding or by investigational tools such as videofluoroscopic swallowing examination or fiberoptic endoscopic evaluation of swallowing (FEES).

Videoflouroscopic swallow evaluation is the gold standard in pediatric dysphagia evaluation and involves imaging the child during swallowing of radio-opaque barium of various consistencies. The study is performed in a 45-degree reclined position in newborns or an upright "feeding" position at three to seven months of age. This test can diagnose nasal regurgitation, laryngeal penetration, aspiration, CP muscle abnormalities and other oropharyngeal and upper esophageal motor and structural abnormalities. In addition to diagnostics, therapeutic measures such as introduction of low flow nipples, thickening the ingested liquid, and changes in positioning may be done during the test to evaluate changes in swallowing efficiency and safety. Unfortunately, there is significant subjectivity in the evaluation with these studies showing significant inter- and intra-rater variability.

To limit the radiation dose to the child, short pulses of radiation limited to 30–60 seconds total are used to observe the phases of swallowing.[8] Unfortunately, pediatric aspiration is frequently observed several minutes into a feeding cycle. Therefore, due to the limited time duration of this evaluation, a study may miss swallowing dysfunction.

Functional Endoscopic Evaluation of Swallowing or FEES has been performed in children since 1995. Many studies have demonstrated that it can be performed safely in children and it is well correlated with videofluoroscopic findings.[9] Advantages of FEES are that it does not involve radiation exposure and it allows direct visualization of anatomic defects such as laryngeal clefts, vocal fold paralysis, laryngomalacia, velopharyngeal incompetence or reflux findings. Although the validity of FEES is also limited by subjectivity, there have been attempts to reduce this by the creation of score sheets such as the Penetration-Aspiration Scale (PAS). Like videofluoroscopy, therapeutic measures may be taken during the exam to gauge potential improvement of swallowing.

Additional radiographic imaging may be appropriate in some patients. Arnold Chiari malformation, neural tube defects, or other neurologic deficits that may contribute to dysphagia can be evaluated with MRI imaging. Chest X-rays may be used to assess the potential complication of aspiration such as pneumonia.

Gastroesophogeal Reflux Scintigraphy or "milk scan" evaluates gastric emptying and reflux with technetium 99m sulfur colloid fed to the infant in a formula. Reflux and aspiration of the substance can be seen when viewing the chest or neck within a several hour period after feeding. The study is a good tool to assess aspiration but does not evaluate reflux or the phases of swallowing well. In one study, the incidence of penetration, aspiration, and nasal regurgitation in infants referred for evaluation by a speech pathologist were 40%, 21%, and 30% respectively.[10] These abnormalities were associated with prematurity, neurologic disorders, history of pneumonia, apnea events, and a history of tube feeding. Patients who had unexplained respiratory problems and concerns for dysphagia had significantly higher incidence of aspiration (nearly 60%). Premature infants were far more likely to have nasal regurgitation, and all patients with abnormalities demonstrated delayed pharyngeal response to bolus transit.[11] This was usually seen on fluoroscopy as material entering the piriform sinuses before initiation of the swallow. Interestingly, the first abnormal swallowing event was seen in most cases nearly one minute into the feeding, and would be missed with a short evaluation.

As discussed, complex and coordinated sensorimotor patterns are required for normal swallowing. Abnormal patterns such as tongue and jaw thrusting or retraction, lip retraction, tonic bite, and nasal regurgitationmay result in poor feeding efficiency. Infants may have difficulty initiating movements such as sucking or coordinating those movements with their breathing pattern, causing rapid fatigue. Neurologic abnormalities such as cerebral palsy or seizure disorder can explain some abnormal swallowing patterns seen in these children. Table 3 provides a list of common causes of disorders.

## OUTPATIENT MANAGEMENT

The prevalence of feeding disorders is estimated to be 25%–45% and is significantly higher in children with known developmental, physiologic or neurological delay such as craniofacial anomalies,

Table 3. Common causes of dysphagia in children.

| Congenital | Infectious | Neurologic |
|---|---|---|
| Choanal atresia | Acute pharyngitis/tonsillitis | CNS injury (TBI, Arnold Chiari, stroke) |
| Nasal masses | Peritonsillar abscess | Cranial nerve deficit |
| Cleft lip and palate | Retropharyngeal abscess | Neuromuscular junction disease |
| Laryngomalacia | Epiglottitis | Neuro-muscular disease |
| Laryngeal clefts | Esophagitis incl. eosinophilic esophagitis | |
| Tracheoesophogeal fistula | | |
| Esophogeal atresia | **Neoplastic** | **Trauma** |
| Vascular rings | Hemangioma | Caustic ingestion |
| | Lymphangioma | GERD |
| **Psychogenic** | Papilloma | Foreign bodies |
| Abnormal child-caregiver interaction | Leiomyoma | |
| | Neurofibroma | |

history of prematurity, genetic syndromes, or neurologic insults.[12] Furthermore, Rommel *et al.* evaluated over 700 children referred for feeding disorders with a mean age of 25 months and found that 50% of the children at risk of having feeding problems due to prematurity, developmental abnormalities or physiologic insults had multiple causes contributing to their feeding difficulty.[13]

Pediatric swallowing disorders include chronic generalized findings such as failure to thrive or parental concern over the child's feeding habits. These parental concerns may include long duration of feeding (over 30 minutes), oral defensiveness or refusal, abnormal changes in feeding, recurrent upper respiratory symptoms or airway concerns during feeding such as choking or cough. Cough, however, is not a common observation after aspiration in very young children due to immaturity of this reflex.[14]

Surveys of parents of children with feeding disorders recall frustration when pediatricians refused to initiate diagnostic procedures.

The parents report that the physicians did not evaluate the feeding difficulties, stating that the children were "normal" and would quickly "outgrow" the problems observed.[15] But once the patient does come to the appropriate clinician for evaluation, the symptoms reported by parents frequently help the clinician diagnose the phase of swallowing involved. In addition, exam findings or testing results may identify the phase of dysfunction. For example, drooling or weak suck may indicate poor oral phase control. Hyperactivity of the gag reflex can cause choking symptoms. Pauses in feeding may be caused by severe nasal congestion or adenoid hypertrophy. Failure in velopharyngeal closure can result in reflux into the nasal cavity. Inability to fully relax the CP muscle may cause pooling of liquids in the vallecula, resulting in a wet sounding cry and a serious risk of aspiration.

## INPATIENT MANAGEMENT

Improvements in infant survival following premature birth have resulted in an increase in the diagnosis of infant swallowing disorders.[16] While advances have been made in understanding adult swallowing disorders, pediatric swallowing continues to be poorly studied. This is likely due to the anatomic, physiologic, and neurologic developmental differences discussed above as well as difficulty in studying these patients. Patients who are admitted to the hospital for evaluation of feeding disorders frequently have severe airway protection concerns and may require immediate intervention such as feeding tube insertion, intubation, or tracheostomy. Patients who are admitted for other concerns can develop pulmonary disease caused by aspiration and may further exacerbate health disorders if the feeding issue is not addressed.[17]

## EMERGENCY EVALUATION AND TREATMENT

Children with severe dysphagia may require airway protection or resuscitation efforts due to poor oral intake and dehydration.

Resuscitation may begin with 20–60 ml/kg boluses of isotonic saline through an IV or intraosseous line. Serum glucose and electrolytes must be managed as well — 2.5 ml/kg of 10% dextrose as needed to maintain blood sugar levels, 2–3 mEq/kg/d sodium and 2–3 mEq/kg/d potassium to maintain normal levels. Severely depleted patients require hospital admission for monitoring and intervention.[18]

## MANAGEMENT OF DYSPHAGIA INCLUDING OPERATIVE INTERVENTIONS

Unfortunately, there are few studies looking at outcomes or research examining the effectiveness of diagnostic procedures and management of dysphagia in children. Therefore, many of the proposed treatments for pediatric dysphagia were developed for adult patients. Prior to any therapy, the goals of the therapy should be discussed with the caregiver to ensure realistic expectations. Unfortunately, sometimes the goal of therapy in severely disabled children is not to normalize swallowing. For example, a goal for a child with severe aspiration may be to provide taste stimulation without satisfying their nutrition and hydration needs. In another child with aspiration and drooling, bilateral submandibular and parotid duct ligation, possibly with tracheostomy for improved pulmonary toilet may be required. Nutrition support may be required in some children who are unable to quickly improve their swallowing. Rarely, surgical procedures such as a Nissen fundoplication, cricopharyngeus muscle myotomy, or G-tube insertion are required for refractory cases.

Treatments that do seem to work for pediatric patients with mild to moderate dysphagia include altering the positioning during feeding to a more vertical position, slowing the pace of feeding with a low flow nipple, feeding more frequently with a smaller volume per feed, and thickening of feeds. Infants with nasal congestion who have oxygen desaturations during feeding may improve with administration of nasal steroids. Occupational therapists or speech and language therapists may offer specialized oro-motor and feeding therapy that is beyond the scope of this chapter. However, non-nutritive sucking therapy is notable in assisting neonates to develop coordinated suck-swallow-breathe patterns. Specialized trainers such as the NTrainer have been created for this purpose.

The relationship between GERD, micro-aspiration, and respiratory disease is also well known, and children appear to have more frequent reflux events as suggested by their frequent regurgitation events. The exposure of the sensitive mucosa to acid reflux is theorized to cause functional anesthesia of the larynx.[19,20] Many children outgrow reflux within the first year of life without intervention.[21] However, studies evaluating neurologically intact children have found that gastroesophogeal reflux disease, sensory changes and swallowing disorders are correlated and may persist for three to four years or much longer.[22] Pharmacologic treatment of this disorder is usually with proton pump inhibitors, H2 blockers, or pro-motility agents. In patients who are refractory to treatment or have evidence of esophageal food impaction, eosinophilic esophagitis must be considered. Biopsy of the effected mucosa reveals elevated eosinophil counts (greater than 20 per high-powered field). Treatment with topical or systemic corticosteroids is usually successful.

## CONCLUSION

Swallowing is a basic function but has complex physiology with potential alterations caused by musculoskeletal, cardio-respiratory, oral-sensory, developmental, neurologic or behavioral disorders. Diagnosis and treatment of dysphagia in children is difficult, even with knowledgeable therapists and clinicians. Although there is an extensive list of potential causes of dysphagia, the anatomic and physiologic changes seen can frequently guide the clinician to the appropriate investigative tool and therapeutic measures. A clinical algorithm is enclosed to assist the clinician in determining when appropriate investigative tools may be appropriate to assist in diagnosis.

# CLINICAL ALGORITHM 1

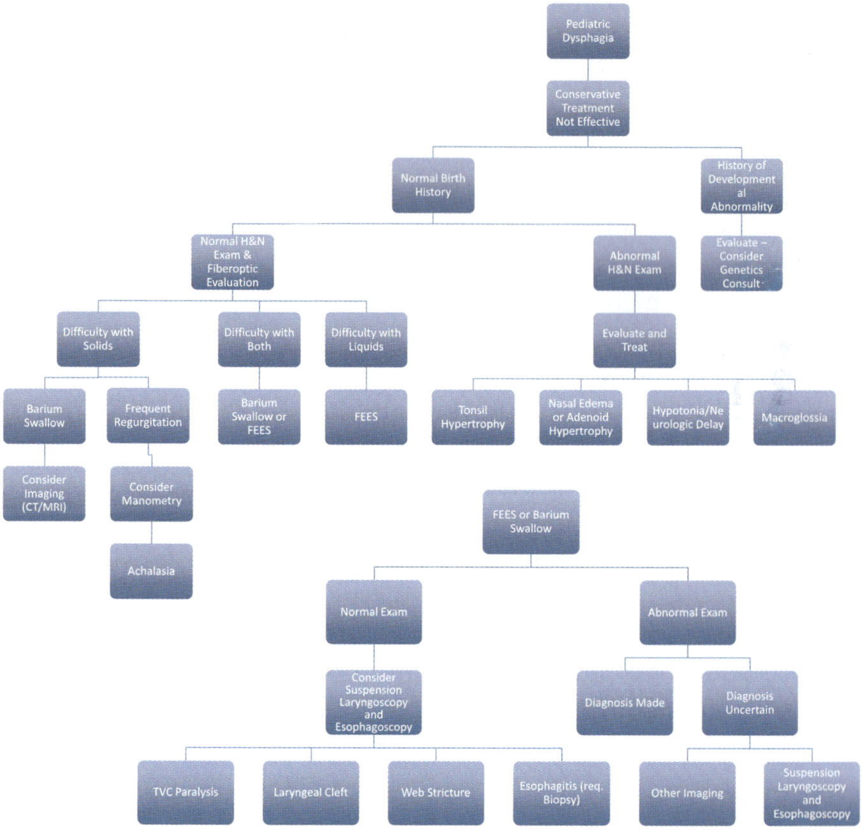

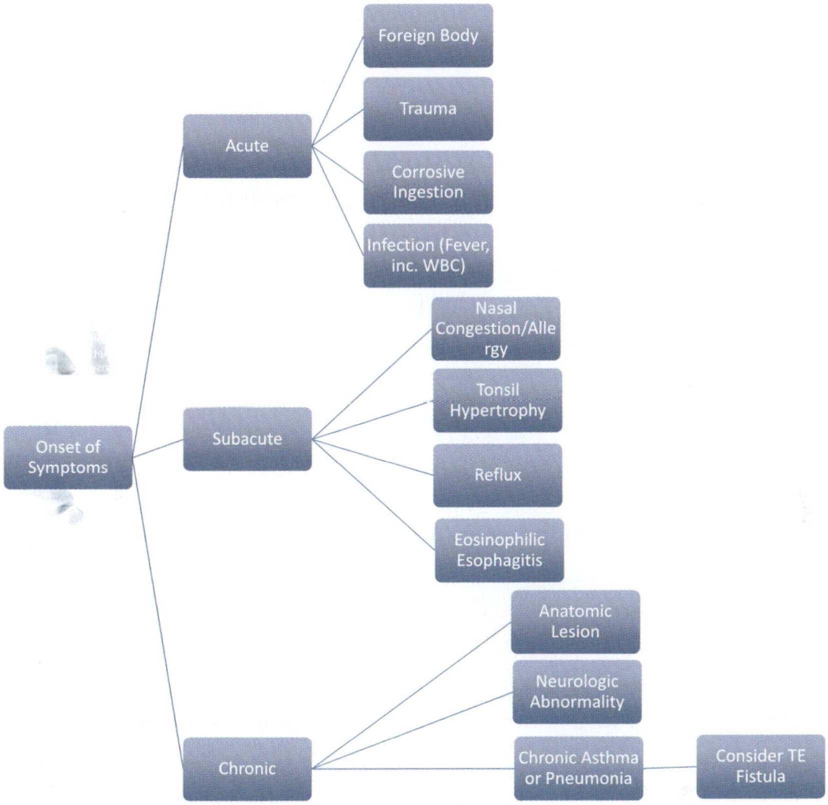


## REFERENCES


1. Dusick A. Investigation and management of dysphagia. *Semin Pediatr Neurol* 2003 December;10(4):225–264.
2. GI Motility Online. *Physiology of Oral Cavity, Pharynx and Upper Esophageal Sphincter.* www.nature.com/gimo.
3. Massey BT. *Physiology of the Oral Cavity, Pharynx, and Upper Esophogeal Sphincter.* GI Motility Online (2006) http://www.nature.com/gimo/contents/pt1/full/gimo2.html.
4. The Neuroanatomy of Swallowing (Zemlin, 1997; Logemann, 1998, 1989; Morrell, 1984; Dobie, 1978)
5. Newman LA, Cleveland RH, Blickman JG, Hillman RE, Jaramillo D. Videoflouroscopic analysis of infant swallow. *Invest Radiol* 1991;26: 870–873.

6. Koumanidou C, Vakaki M, Pitsoulakis G, Anagnostara A, Mirilas P. Sonographic measurement of the abdominal esophagus length in infancy: a diagnostic tool for gastroesophageal reflux. *Am J Roentgenol* 2004;183:801–807.
7. Jennie OG, von Siebenthal K, Wolf M, Matthias K, Duc G, Buchr HU. Effect of nursing in the head elevated tilt position (15 degrees) on the incidence of bradycardic and hypoxemic episodes in preterm infants. *Pediatrics* 1997;100:622–625.
8. Rogers BT, Arvedson J, Msall M, Demerath RR. Hypoxemia during oral feeding of children with severe cerebral palsy. *Dev Med Child Neurol* 1993 Jan;35(1):3–10.
9. Leder S, Karas DE. Fiberoptic endoscopic evaluation of swallowing in the pediatric population. *Laryngoscope* 2000;110:1132–1136.
10. Newman LA, Keckley C, Petersen MC, Hamner A. Swallowing function and medical diagnoses in infants suspected of dysphagia. *Pediatrics* 2001;108:1–4.
11. Lefton-Greif MA, Carroll JL, Loughlin GM. Long-term follow-up of oropharyngeal dysphagia in children without apparent risk factors. *Pediatr Pulmonol* 2006;41:1040–1048.
12. Miller CK. Updates on pediatric feeding and swallowing problems. *Curr Opin Otol Head Neck Surg* 2009;17:194–199.
13. Rommel N, DeMeyer A, Feenstra L, Veereman-Waters G. The complexity of feeding problems in 700 infants and young children presenting to a tertiary care institution. *J Pediatr Gastroenterol Nutr* 2003;37:75–84.
14. Arvedson J, Rogers B, Buck G, *et al.* Silent aspiration prominent in children with dysphagia. *Int J Pediatr Otorhinolaryngol* 1994;28:173–181.
15. Lefton-Greif MA, Carroll JL, Loughlin GM. Long-term follow-up of oropharyngeal dysphagia in children without apparent risk factors. *Pediatr Pulmonol* 2006;41:1040–1048.
16. Newman, LA, Keckley C, Petersen MC, Hamner A. Swallowing function and medical diagnoses in infants suspected of dysphagia. *Pediatrics* 2001;108:1–4.
17. Taniguchi M, Moyer R. Assessment of risk factors for pneumonia in dysphagia children: significance of videofluoroscopic swallowing evaluation. *Dev Med Child Neurol* 1994;36:495–502.

18. Boluyt N, Bollen CW, Bos AP, Kok JH, Offringa M. Fluid resuscitation in neonatal and pediatric hypovolemic shock: a Dutch Pediatric Society evidence-based clinical practice guideline. *Intensive Care Med* 2006;32:995–1003.
19. Aviv JE, Liu H, Parides M, Kaplan ST, Close LG. Laryngopharyngeal sensory deficits in patients with laryngopharyngeal reflux and dysphagia. *Ann Otol Rhinol Laryngol* 2000;109:1000–1006.
20. Thompson DM. Laryngopharyngeal sensory testing and assessment of airway protection in pediatric patients. *Am J Med* 2003;115(suppl 3A): 116S-168S.
21. Nelson SP, Chen EH, Syniar GM, Christoffel KK. Prevalence of symptoms of gastroesophageal reflux during infancy. A pediatric practice-based survey. Pediatric Practice Research Group. *Arch Pediatr Adolesc Med* 1997;151:569–572.
22. Suskinf DL, Thompson DM, Gulati M, Huddleston P, Liu DC, Baroody FM. Improved infant swallowing after gastroesophogeal reflux disease treatment: a function of improved laryngeal sensation? *Laryngoscope* 2006 Aug;116:1397–1403.

# 11

# Adenotonsillar Disease and Sleep-Disordered Breathing in Children

*Anita Jeyakumar, Jennifer Veraldi and Ron B. Mitchell*

## INTRODUCTION

Over the last 20 years there has been a shift in the way adenotonsillar disease in children presents to the otolaryngologist. Prior to the last two decades recurrent throat infections were the predominant reason for an adenotonsillectomy (T&A). Indications for T&A have evolved due to increasing recognition of the role of adenotonsillar hypertrophy in sleep-disordered breathing (SDB) in children. Restless sleep, frequent night-time awakenings, apneas, and hypopneas all characterize SDB. Several studies have shown that SDB has a dramatic effect on children's quality-of-life, behavior and school performance.[1–3] T&A is effective at improving sleep as well as these other important parameters. Consequently, more children present for T&A because of SDB than for recurrent throat infections. This chapter will summarize our current knowledge of the clinical presentation and management of adenotonsillar disease in children.

## EPIDEMIOLOGY OF ADENOTONSILLAR DISEASE

T&A is the most common major surgical procedures performed in children.[4] Between 1915 and the 1960s, T&A was the most frequently performed surgical procedure in the United States. Studies by Derkay and by Rosenfeld & Green reported that the overall incidence of adenotonsillar procedures decreased in the late 1970s and early 1980s, only to subsequently increase in incidence.[4,5] In fact, the overall incidence rates have nearly doubled in the past 35 years. The surge in the incidence of T&A in very young children accompanied by a slight increase in the incidence of T&A in older children and young adults is due to the change in indications for the procedures. There has been a dramatic trend toward T&A for SDB rather than for infectious reasons. The incidence of SDB is known to peak during early childhood and to affect 1%–4% of children.[6] In addition, older children and young adults are more frequently being treated for SDB with T&A.[7,8]

At least 400,000 children undergo an adenoidectomy each year in the United States. This number, however, likely underestimates the true incidence by at least 25% since it does not include those performed at free standing ambulatory surgery centers.[4] Roughly half of adenoidectomies are done for the indication of nasal obstruction and the other half for either recurrent or persistent otitis media or recurrent adenoiditis/rhinosinusitis. Tonsillectomy alone is performed infrequently in children younger than one year of age, whereas adenoidectomy alone is performed infrequently in individuals older than 14 years of age.

## ANATOMY AND PHYSIOLOGY

The palatine tonsils, adenoids (pharyngeal tonsils) and lingual tonsils, comprise a collection of lymphoid tissue named Waldeyer's ring. Waldeyer's ring is located at the cranial end of the pharynx. This collection of lymphatic tissue is thought to be involved in helping fight off pharyngeal and upper respiratory tract infections as part of the immune system. The immune function of these tissues is most active during childhood and declines with age.

The palatine tonsils lie at the entrance to the oropharynx between the palatoglossus (anterior tonsillar pillar) and palatopharyngeus (posterior tonsillar pillar). The palatine tonsils are lined by non-keratinized stratified squamous epithelium. The adenoid tissue lies at the superior aspect of the nasopharynx, extending laterally to the eustachian tubes and the walls of the pharyngeal recess. Pseudostratified ciliated columnar epithelium (respiratory epithelium) lines the surface of the adenoids.

## CLINICAL PRESENTATION

Adenotonsillar disease is broadly caused by either infectious disease or hypertrophic tissue leading to airway obstruction. The disease processes can affect the adenoid tissue, tonsils, or both.

### Adenoids

Infectious problems include acute and chronic adenoiditis, and otitis media. Adenoid hypertrophy has been associated with allergic rhinitis, otitis media, higher prevalence of SDB, and increased incidence of lower respiratory infections.

Acute adenoiditis often presents as a sudden onset of symptoms which are difficult to distinguish from those of generalized upper respiratory tract infections and rhinosinusitis. Symptoms can include nasal obstruction, rhinorrhea (purulent or clear), elevated temperatures, postnasal drainage, cough, mouth breathing, and possible concomitant otitis media. Chronic adenoiditis has a longer duration (greater than three months) of symptoms, and can result in the adenoid harboring bacteria, serving as a reservoir of infection for sinusitis.

Adenoid tissue plays an important role in the development of otitis media. The anatomical relationship of the middle ear, eustachian tube, and the adenoid tissue in the nasopharynx predisposes the child to otitis media via eustachian tube obstruction. The presentation of the classic complaints of otitis media, with or without effusion, in a child with acute or chronic nasal obstruction, rhinorrhea, mouth breathing, and postnasal drainage should prompt evaluation of the nasopharynx in addition to the middle ears.

Adenoid hypertrophy may occur in the presence or absence of infection. Hypertrophy of the adenoid tissue leads to upper airway obstruction that is more likely to be partial than complete. The characteristic complaints associated with SDB may present with adenoid hypertrophy and include daytime somnolence, hypopneic breathing, snoring, arousals, and enuresis.

## Tonsils

Infectious problems include acute tonsillitis, chronic tonsillitis, and peritonsillar abscess. Hypertrophic tonsils with or without hypertrophic adenoids can lead to SDB. Asymmetric tonsils or sudden growth of the tonsils should include a differential diagnosis of malignancy.

Acute tonsillitis is one of the most common infections in children. Symptoms can include sore throat, fever, dysphagia, tender cervical adenopathy, erythema of the tonsils and pharyngeal walls, and possibly tonsillar exudate or enlargment. The duration of symptoms depends on the etiology of the infection, which can be bacterial or viral. The commonly agreed definition of recurrent acute tonsillitis is four to seven episodes in one year, five episodes in each of two consecutive years, or three episodes per year for three consecutive years.[9]

Viral causes of tonsillitis include rhinovirus, influenzavirus, parainfluenza, adenovirus and Epstein-Barr virus (EBV). EBV causes infectious mononucleosis, a distinct constellation of symptoms including enlarged tonsils covered with a gray exudate, high fevers, and malaise. Other features of infectious mononucleosis are posterior cervical lymphadenopathy, enlarged spleen, petechiae along the line between the hard and soft palate and maculopapular rash on administration of amoxicillin.

Bacterial tonsillitis is most commonly caused by group A beta-hemolytic *Streptococcus pneumoniae*, the pathogen associated with "strep throat." *Haemophilus influenza* and *Moraxella catarrhalis* are the next most common bacterial causes of the classic tonsillitis-pharyngitis. Less common causes of tonsillitis include *Neisseria gonorrhoeae*, and *Corynebactierium diphtheria*. Diptheria can lead to edema of the airway with a sloughing exudate causing airway obstruction, requiring emergent airway management.

Tonsillar infection with *Candida* species, usually presents as adherent white plaques at the oral and pharyngeal mucosa, which can be scraped off to reveal a raw, bleeding mucosal base. Patients are often immunocompromised or recently treated with antibiotics.

Peritonsillar abscess (PTA) is the most common deep space infection of the neck. It usually occurs in children older than 12 years but can occur at any age.[10,11] The peak incidence is in early winter and spring which coincides with a high incidence of streptococcal tonsillitis and pharyngitis. The symptoms are a sore throat with fever, malaise and dysphagia. In addition the sore throat is usually worse on the side of the abscess and there may be ipsilateral otalgia. Physical findings include unilateral enlargement of the soft palate and tonsil, contralateral deviation of the uvula, trismus, drooling, muffled voice, and neck lymphadenopathy. The diagnosis is based on clinical findings. Rarely, computed tomography (CT) is helpful if the diagnosis is in doubt, if the child is young and cannot be fully evaluated or to look for recurrence or complications. Unilateral PTA is far more common than bilateral PTAs (<5%).

The treatment of a PTA includes drainage of the abscess, antibiotics (to cover aerobic and anaerobic bacteria), and hydration with pain control. If the swelling is severe enough to cause airway compromise, steroids are often added. Drainage of a PTA can be performed by needle aspiration, incision and drainage, or immediate tonsillectomy. Over the last 20 years there has been a move towards incision and drainage and away from immediate tonsillectomy. Most children with a PTA can be treated as outpatients with hospitalization reserved for those requiring hydration and pain control. Approximately 30% of children with a PTA satisfy criteria for a tonsillectomy and approximately 10% will have a second abscess. The tonsillectomy is usually performed as a routine procedure after the PTA has resolved.

Adenotonsillar hypertrophy can cause SDB, snoring, dysphagia, and altered craniofacial growth. Very severe cases of SDB may lead to pulmonary hypertension, cor pulmonale, and hypoventilation syndromes.

The presentation of new onset unilateral tonsillar hypertrophy is most likely due to infection, but the differential should include malignancy. Also, if a patient has sudden enlargement of Waldeyer's ring, lymphoma should be considered.

## CLINICAL EVALUATION

Adenoid hypertrophy is a common cause of nasal obstruction in children. Physical examination often elicits mouth breathing, hyponasal voice and the classic "adenoid facies" (open mouth, flat midface, dark discoloration under the eyes). However these findings can be seen with other causes of nasal obstruction. Evaluation of the adenoids in a child can be difficult and was often done using lateral skull radiographs. More recently, an increasing number of children have been evaluated using flexible fibreoptic nasopharyngoscopy. This allows for direct visualization without radiation exposure. Parikh *et al.* proposed a grading system for endoscopic examination of adenoid hypertrophy that is validated and user-friendly.[12] It ranges from adenoids not in contact with adjacent structures (Grade 1), to, the most severe, adenoid tissue in contact with the palate at rest (Grade 4).[12] Other methods such as video fluoroscopy have been shown to be effective at assessing adenoid size but are less commonly used.

Acute tonsillar enlargement results from acute infection or, less commonly, from a peritonsillar abscess that is usually unilateral. Throat cultures are considered the "gold standard" for the diagnosis of group A beta-hemolytic streptococcus (GABHS). Many clinicians advocate formal throat cultures for children with suspected streptococcal disease who have negative rapid streptococcus tests.

Chronic tonsillar hypertrophy has received increasing attention over the last 20 years because of its association with SDB in children. Tonsillar size is commonly measured on a scale of 1 to 4: 1 represents

0%–25% airway obstruction, 2 represents 25%–50% airway obstruction, 3 represents 50%–75% airway obstruction, and 4 represents 75%–100% airway obstruction.[13]

The "gold standard" for the diagnosis and quantification of SDB is polysomnography. Often otolaryngologists will perform a T&A based on clinical symptoms in a child with adenotonsillar hypertrophy. However, clinical evaluation will yield 25%–75% success rates in predicting who has significant SDB. It is worth noting that this poor predictive value of clinical assessment does not improve with the use of questionnaires or nocturnal home video recordings.[14]

## MANAGEMENT

Management of a patient with adenotonsillar disease depends on the underlying etiology and can include medical and surgical approaches. Acute infections in the form of acute adenotonsillitis, and some cases of SDB need appropriate antibiotics and possibly continuous positive airway pressure (CPAP). However the majority of persistent adenotonsillar disease is considered a surgical problem.

T&A in children has generated controversy among health professionals for many years. The indiscriminate reliance on these operations during the early and middle decades of the 20th century led many pediatricians to oppose their performance under any and all circumstances. Nonetheless, T&A has retained support throughout the professional and lay communities for a number of reasons. Many clinicians remained convinced — based on their training, experience, or evidence from clinical trials — that the operations were efficacious in relieving certain recurrent or persistent upper-respiratory and middle-ear disorders. It also has become clear that hypertrophy of the adenoids, tonsils, or both, can obstruct the upper airway and result in SDB, alveolar hypoventilation and cor pulmonale. There is evidence that these conditions respond well to T&A.[1,15–18] Many dentists and orthodontists also argue that chronic upper airway obstruction results in abnormal craniofacial and dental growth — the "adenoid facies" — and that this too can be modified favorably by adenoidectomy or T&A. Many parents of children who underwent T&A continue to report satisfactory resolution of their children's presenting problems.[19]

## SURGICAL TECHNIQUES

### Tonsillectomy

Since its description in the first century, surgery to remove tonsils has evolved considerably. However, tonsillectomy continues to have a significant morbidity and mortality for a predominately young patient population. Children still suffer from prolonged painful recoveries with odynophagia, otalgia, dehydration, and poor oral intake. The recovery from tonsillar surgery is not only difficult for the child but also for their caregivers who lose sleep and time from work. Over the last two decades, in order to reduce some of the morbidity and speed up recovery time, there has been renewed interest and research in different surgical techniques and instruments for tonsillectomy. The first description of a tonsil surgery is attributed to Cornelius Celsus, a Roman encyclopedist, in the first century around 30AD. He described the use of a finger or knife to remove the tonsil. Subsequent surgeons and authors advocated various other instruments including knives, fingers, guillotines, wires, and strings. These techniques removed only a portion of the tonsil, leaving residual tissue behind.

The complete removal of the tonsil and its capsule had its origin in the early 20th century in the United States.[20] With improvements in anatomical understanding and identification of the tonsil capsule, surgeons began to advocate for its complete removal. Complete removal of the tonsil, however, leaves the musculature of the pharynx exposed to heal from secondary intention. Patients experience significant pain and risk of bleeding as the exposed muscle is slowly re-mucosalized. Multiple modalities have evolved in an attempt to minimize patient discomfort during the healing process. Since 1980 electrocautery has become the instrument of choice for tonsillectomy as surgeons can perform a faster procedure with minimal bleeding. According to the latest survey of members of the

American Academy of Otolaryngology and the American Society of Pediatric Otolaryngology, electrocautery is the preferred method for tonsillectomy by roughly 55% of Otolaryngologists.[21] Coblation tonsillectomy is estimated to be the preferred method by 20%–25%, cold steel techniques by 10% and other techniques including microdebrider partial tonsillectomy by the remaining 10%. Although popular, the electrocautery technique has its drawbacks as it has been shown to be a more painful surgery than cold techniques, due to the additional thermal injury inflicted upon the exposed musculature.

Recently, there has been increasing interest in performing a partial tonsillectomy, or tonsillotomy, to maintain the tonsillar capsule and reduce postoperative pain and bleeding. As with every surgical technique, intracapsular tonsillectomy also has its drawbacks. Large case series have shown that tonsillar regrowth occurs in about 0.5%–6% of patients with a smaller percentage requiring completion tonsillectomy. The operation takes several minutes longer than electrocautery tonsillectomy, which adds to the surgical costs. Intraoperative blood loss is greater but appears to not be clinically significant. The role of intracapsular techniques for managing children with recurrent tonsillitis is still unproven though initial studies are encouraging for this indication.[22]

**Adenoidectomy**

Traditional adenoidectomy techniques involved use of adenoid curettes or adenotomes with hemostasis achieved with packing, topical hemostatic agents like bismuth or tannics, neosynephrine or oxymetazoline or use of suction electrocautery. Although the equipment for this method are relatively inexpensive and reusable, there are concerns with excessive bleeding, difficulty in teaching the technique to inexperienced surgeons, transmission of Creutzfeld-Jakob disease (also known as CJD and mad cow disease), and leaving residual tissue around the Eustachian tube orifice and/or posterior choana. In response to these concerns, new methods such as suction bovie cautery, use of a microdebrider or coblation are widely used for removal of adenoids and have been shown to be effective, less time consuming, and associated with a low morbidity.

## OUTCOMES

### The Efficacy of T&A for Recurrent Tonsillitis

The efficacy of T&A for recurrent tonsillitis has been studied in a number of ways including randomized controlled trials comparing T&A with non-surgical treatment, studies comparing quality-of-life parameters before and after surgical intervention and surveys of parental satisfaction with surgical therapy. There is anecdotal evidence that some children's well-being is transformed by the surgery, which may be caused by a combination of factors that include the tendency of the recurrent tonsillitis to resolve over time and the elimination of a source of infection and of obstructive symptoms. The evidence for tonsillectomy for recurrent infections remains, perhaps surprisingly, less than satisfactory.

Randomized clinical trials comparing the benefits of T&A to observation and medical treatment have resulted in controversy about the efficacy of surgical therapy.[9,23] Paradise *et al.* compared a randomized and non-randomized group of children undergoing T&A for recurrent tonsillitis to control groups.[9] The study included severely affected children with good clinical documentation of tonsillitis. There was a significant decrease in throat infections in the surgical group compared to the control group for the first and second years following T&A but no difference by the third year (Fig. 1).[9] In a follow-up study of less severely affected children, both the surgical and control group had a significant decrease in infections over time without any statistical differences between the two groups.[24] Paradise *et al.* concluded that surgical intervention was not indicated for less severe recurrent tonsillitis.[24] There are a number of limitations to these studies. Firstly, children with recurrent sore throats are heterogeneous in both causation and severity. Furthermore, distinguishing tonsillitis from pharyngitis is difficult if not impossible and long-term data are unavailable. Nonetheless, these studies have raised concerns that a

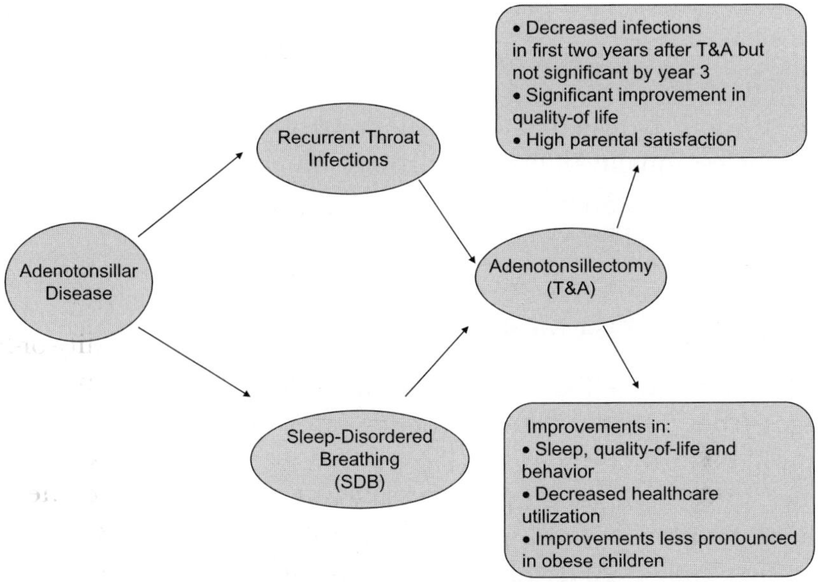


**Fig. 1.** Adenotosillectomy (T&A) for children.

large number of children undergo unnecessary surgery when only a relatively small number benefit.

Surgical outcomes of T&A for recurrent tonsillitis have also been studied by using quality-of-life and parental satisfaction measures. Several studies have shown that parental satisfaction with T&A for recurrent tonsillitis is very high (90%–100%).[19,25] Stewart *et al.* measured the health status of children with either recurrent tonsillitis or SDB using a validated global quality-of-life instrument.[25] Their results showed that these children had significantly worse scores than the controls and similar scores to children with chronic asthma or juvenile rheumatoid arthritis. Goldstein *et al.*, in a multicenter, prospective observational outcomes-based study, reported that children had significant improvements in disease specific and global quality-of-life parameters following a T&A for recurrent tonsillitis.[19] Improvements in airway and breathing, infection, healthcare utilization, cost of care, eating and swallowing were noted.

T&A for recurrent tonsillitis is effective at significantly reducing the number and severity of sore throats in children who are severely affected. In less severe cases of recurrent tonsillitis the difference in sore throats between T&A and controls is less pronounced. Nonetheless, quality-of-life is improved dramatically after T&A even in less severe cases and parental satisfaction with the procedure is extremely high (Fig. 1).

### The Efficacy of T&A for SDB

The success rate of T&A for SDB, as measured by polysomnography, ranges from 20%–90% and depends on a number of parameters that will be further discussed (Fig. 1). Two factors contribute to outcomes: the criteria used to define SDB and the comorbidities of the patient population. For example, SDB can be defined as an apnea-hypopnea index (AHI) of 1, 2, or 5. The higher the AHI used in defining SDB the higher the success rate. Resolution of SDB is higher than 80% in normal-weight children but lower than 20% in obese children.[26] Children with allergies, craniofacial, neuromuscular and genetic problems are at high risk for persistent postoperative SDB. It is therefore important to interpret the results of studies in the light of the definition used for SDB and the characteristics of the study population.

## BEHAVIOR, QUALITY OF LIFE AND HEALTHCARE UTILIZATION

Pediatric SDB is known to be associated with behavioral problems that include hyperactivity, aggression, anxiety, depression and somatization. Approximately 30%–40% of children with SDB have behavioral problems that are considered abnormal. Mitchell and Kelly have reported a significant improvement after T&A for SDB in a high proportion of children with behavioral problems.[18] The improvement was dramatic, was maintained for up to 18 months after surgery and was seen regardless of gender, age, ethnicity, parental education or parental income.[27] The degree and severity of behavioral problems in children with SDB as well as improvements after T&A were similar regardless of the severity of the sleep disorder.

Consequently, it is not surprising that healthcare costs are higher in children with SDB.[28] Tarasiuk *et al.* compared healthcare costs in children from three groups: children with SDB who had a T&A, children with untreated SDB, and healthy controls.[28] They reported that total healthcare costs were reduced by one-third in children with SDB following T&A.[28] This change was not seen in the control or untreated group. The reduction in healthcare costs was a result of a reduction in outpatient and emergency room visits, hospitalizations and pharmacy costs.

## CHILDHOOD OBESITY AND SDB

The prevalence of obesity in children in the US has doubled in the last two decades, and there is evidence that this trend is likely to continue. Approximately 30% of children in the US are overweight and 50% of overweight children are considered obese. The prevalence of SDB in obese children, at 30%, is ten times higher than in normal-weight children. The increasing prevalence of childhood obesity implies that more children will present for treatment of SDB in the future. In obese children, a number of factors in addition to adenotonsillar hypertrophy may compromise surgical therapy and associated improvements in quality-of-life and behavior. Adipose tissue immediately adjacent to the pharynx may decrease the cross-sectional area and cause compression of the upper airway that is further decreased by enlarged tonsils and adenoids. Also, therapeutic options directed at weight reduction are rarely successful. Furthermore, T&A for SDB improves but does not resolve the sleep disorder in the majority of obese children.[29]

## OTHER "HIGH-RISK" CHILDREN FOR SDB

Surgical management of SDB is more complicated in children with neuromuscular or craniofacial disorders, Down's syndrome, mucopolysaccharidoses, cerebral palsy, Prader-Willi syndrome, achondroplasia, Arnold-Chiari malformations and sickle-cell disease. These children are considered high-risk because SDB is multifactorial in etiology and have the additional risk of increased perioperative complications and persistent postoperative SDB. Surgical management in complicated cases requires a multidisciplinary approach.

## SURGICAL COMPLICATIONS

Any physician who recommends T&A must weigh the possibility that harm will result. The possible adverse consequences range from death to non-fatal direct and indirect anesthetic and surgical complications to hypothetical interference with immunologic defense mechanisms. It is unfortunate that accurate statistics regarding mortality and morbidity in large patient populations are not readily available.

Complications after T&A are divided into perioperative and postoperative complications. Perioperative complications include mechanical difficulties during intubation causing laryngeal trauma, laryngospasm, laryngeal edema, respiratory compromise, cardiac arrest, aspiration, malignant hyperthermia, trauma to the teeth, pharyngeal wall or soft palate injuries and hemorrhage; postoperative complications include hemorrhage, infections, postoperative pain, edema and hematoma of the uvula, pulmonary complications, postoperative scarring of the soft palate and tonsillar remnants.

Hemorrhage, either primary (within 24 hours of surgery) or secondary (more than 24 hours after surgery), rarely requires transfusion. In published reports, the rate of primary hemorrhage has ranged from 0.2% to 2.2% and the rate of secondary hemorrhage from 0.1% to 3%.[30] Postoperative infections following tonsillectomy can range from local cellulites, bronchitis, pneumonia, pulmonary edema, septicemia, and deep neck abscesses. Local anesthetic injections into the major vessel of the neck may cause hemiplegia, loss of vision, anaphylaxis and even death due to cardiac arrest. These complications are exceedingly rare.

Velopharyngeal insufficiency can sometimes develop after adenoidectomy even in children who preoperatively showed no evidence of palatal insufficiency. Airway complications include both obstructive and central apnea, the latter particularly likely to occur in children younger than three years of age who had had obstructive symptoms preoperatively. Postobstructive pulmonary edema is a particularly serious entity that may follow T&A in severely affected children and tends to occur more frequently in the morbidly obese children with severe preoperative SDB. Otitis media has been reported as a not infrequent postoperative complication, but it is not clear that the risk is higher than in comparable patients not undergoing T&A. Rare complications of tonsil or adenoid surgery include nasopharyngeal stenosis, and refractory torticollis (Grisel's syndrome).

The death of a child as a consequence of T&A is especially tragic as the surgery is usually elective. Mortality from tonsillectomy is rare.[31] Studies of mortality in the US have indicated a rate of approximately one per 16,381 tonsillectomies with about one-third attributable to bleeding. When death occurred, these unfortunate outcomes have been related to bleeding, aspiration, electrolyte imbalance or anesthetic agents.[30]

## CONTRAINDICATIONS

Contraindications to T&A include coagulation abnormalities that should be addressed prior to surgery. Patients with hereditary coagulopathies as well as conditions such as leukemia, sickle cell disease or agranulocytosis need hematology involvement prior to surgery.[32] A patient with a cleft palate is predisposed to velopharyngeal insufficiency, and should rarely undergo adenoidectomy. Patients with acute illnesses or acutely decreased reserve that might impair the ability to maintain adequate postoperative hydration should defer elective surgery.

## CONCLUSIONS

T&A is the most common major surgery performed in children and is highly effective in carefully selected patients. Generally, there are two reasons why a child may need a T&A — obstruction or infection.

The most frequent current indication for T&A is SDB related to obstruction. T&A in the US is commonly performed on an outpatient basis. There are many different surgical techniques for performing T&A and the evidence to-date indicates none to be superior. Appropriate patient selection, good surgical skills, and cautious postoperative management are the keys to successful treatment of children with adenotonsillar disease.

## REFERENCES

1. Mitchell RB, Kelly J. Behavior, neurocognition and quality-of-life in children with sleep-disordered breathing. *Int J Pediatr Otorhinolaryngol* 2006;70(3):395–406.
2. Leiberman A, Stiller-Timor L, Tarasiuk A *et al.* The effect of adenotonsillectomyon children suffering from obstructive sleep apnea syndrome (OSAS): the Negev perspective. *Int J Pediatr Otorhinolaryngol* 2006;70:1675–1682.
3. Gozal D. Sleep-disordered breathing and school performance in children. *Pediatrics* 1998;102:616–620.
4. Derkay CS. Pediatric otolaryngology procedures in the United States: 1977–1987. *Int J Pediatr Otorhinolaryngol* 1993;25(1–3):1–12.
5. Rosenfeld RM, Green RP. Tonsillectomy and adenoidectomy: changing trends. *Ann Otol Rhinol Laryngol* 1990;99(3 Pt 1):187–191.
6. Ali N, Pitson D, Stradling J. Snoring, sleep disturbance, and behaviour in 4–5 year olds. *Arch Dis Child* 1993;68:360–366.
7. Mattila PS, Tahkokallio O, Tarkkanen J *et al.* Causes of tonsillar disease and frequency of tonsillectomy operations. *Arch Otolaryngol Head Neck Surg* 2001;127:37–44.
8. Guilleminault C, Lee JH, Chan A. Pediatric obstructive sleep apnea syndrome. *Arch Pediatr Adolesc Med* 2005;159:775–785.
9. Paradise JL, Bluestone CD, Bachman RZ, Colborn DK, Bernard BS, Taylor FH, Rogers KD, Schwarzbach RH, Stool SE, Friday GA *et al.* Efficacy of tonsillectomy for recurrent throat infection in severely affected children. Results of parallel randomized and nonrandomized clinical trials. *N Engl J Med* 1984;310(11):674–683.

10. Galioto NJ. Peritonsillar abscess. *Am Fam Physician* 2008 15 Jan; 77(2):199–202.
11. Herzon FS, Harris P. Mosher Award thesis. Peritonsillar abscess: incidence, current management practices, and a proposal for treatment guidelines. *Laryngoscope* 1995 Aug;105(8 Pt 3 Suppl 74):1–17.
12. Parikh SR, Coronel M, Lee JJ, Brown SM. Validation of a new grading system for endoscopic examination of adenoid hypertrophy. *Otolaryngol Head Neck Surg* 2006 Nov;135(5):684–687.
13. Brodsky L, Moore L, Stanievich J. A comparison of tonsillar size and oropharyngeal dimensions in children with obstructive adenotonsillar hypertrophy. *Int J Pediatr Otorhinolaryngol* 1987;13:149–156.
14. Brietzke SE. Can history and physical examination reliably diagnose pediatric obstructive sleep apnea/hypopnea syndrome? A systematic review of the literature. *Otolaryngol Head Neck Surg* 2004 Dec;131(6):827–832.
15. Baldassari CM, Mitchell RB, Schubert C, Rudnick EF. Pediatric obstructive sleep apnea and quality of life: a meta-analysis. *Otolaryngol Head Neck Surg* 2008 Mar;138(3):265–273.
16. Mitchell RB, Call E, Yao N, Kelly J. Quality of life after adenotonsillectomy for obstructive sleep apnea in children. *Arch Otolaryngol Head Neck Surg* 2004 Feb;130(2):190–194.
17. Mitchell RB, Call E, Yao N, Kelly J. Long-term changes in quality of life after surgery for pediatric obstructive sleep apnea. *Arch Otolaryngol Head Neck Surg* 2004 Apr;130(4):409–412.
18. Mitchell RB, Kelly J. Quality of life after adenotonsillectomy for SDB in children. *Otolaryngol Head Neck Surg* 2005 Oct;133(4):569–572.
19. Goldstein NA, Stewart MG, Witsell DL, Hannley MT, Weaver EM, Yueh B, Smith TL, Orvidas LJ. Quality of life after tonsillectomy in children with recurrent tonsillitis. TO TREAT Study Investigators. *Otolaryngol Head Neck Surg* 2008 Jan;138(1 Suppl):S9–S16.
20. Koempel JA. On the origin of tonsillectomy and the dissection method. *Laryngoscope* 2002 Sep;112(9):1583–1586.
21. Maddern BR. Electrosurgery for tonsillectomy. *Laryngoscope* 2002; 112:11–13.
22. Chang KW. Intracapsular vs subcapsular coblation tonsillectomy. *Otolaryngol Head Neck Surg* 2008;138:153–157.

23. van Staaij BK, van den Akker EH, Rovers MM, Hordijk GJ, Hoes AW, Schilder AG. Effectiveness of adenotonsillectomy in children with mild symptoms of throat infections or adenotonsillar hypertrophy: open, randomised controlled trial. *BMJ* 2004 18 Sep;329(7467):651–653.
24. Paradise JL, Bluestone CD, Colborn DK, Bernard BS, Rockette HE, Kurs-Lasky M. Tonsillectomy and adenotonsillectomy for recurrent throat infection in moderately affected children. *Pediatrics* 2002 Jul;110(1 Pt 1):7–15.
25. Stewart MG, Friedman EM, Sulek M *et al.* Quality of life and health status in pediatric tonsil and adenoid disease. *Arch Otolaryngol Head Neck Surg* 2000;126:45–48.
26. Mitchell RB. Adenotonsillectomy for obstructive sleep apnea in children: outcome evaluated by pre- and postoperative polysomnography. *Laryngoscope* 2007 Oct;117(10):1844–1854.
27. Mitchell RB, Kelly J. Long-term changes in the behavior of children after adenotonsillectomy for obstructive sleep apnea. *Otolaryngol Head Neck Surg* 2006 Mar;134(3):374–378.
28. Tarasiuk A, Simon T, Tal A, Reuveni H. Adenotonsillectomy in children with obstructive sleep apnea syndrome reduces health care utilization. *Pediatrics* 2004;113:351–356.
29. Costa DJ, Mitchell R. Adenotonsillectomy for obstructive sleep apnea in obese children: a meta-analysis. *Otolaryngol Head Neck Surg* 2009 Apr;140(4):455–460.
30. Windfuhr JP, Chen YS, Remmert S. Hemorrhage following tonsillectomy and adenoidectomy in 15,218 patients. *Otolaryngol Head Neck Surg* 2006;132(2):281–286.
31. Windfuhr JP, Schloendorff G, Seserhenn AM, Prescher A, Kremer B. A devastating outcome following adenoidectomy and tonsillectomy: ideas for an improved prevention and management. *Otolaryngol Head Neck Surg* 2009;140:191–196.
32. Kay DJ, Mehta V, Goldsmith AJ. Perioperative adenotonsillectomy management in children: current practices. *Laryngoscope* 2003 Apr;113(4): 592–597.

# HEAD AND NECK

# 12

# Congenital Neck Masses

*Andrew R. Scott and Michael J. Cunningham*

## INTRODUCTION

Most neck masses in children are benign lesions of inflammatory origin that either respond to medical therapy or resolve spontaneously. Excisional biopsy is usually indicated for diagnostic or cosmetic purposes in the case of recurrent or persistent neck masses. Therapeutic surgical intervention is warranted for lesions that cause airway symptoms, dysphagia or present with other worrisome features. This chapter will focus on pediatric neck masses of congenital etiology.

The term congenital literally means present at birth, however, many of the lesions described in this chapter do not become apparent until later in childhood and occasionally in adulthood. A working knowledge of the embryonic events leading to the formation of these lesions improves understanding of their pathophysiology and enhances their effective surgical removal.

The following is a review of the presentation, work-up and management of the more common congenital neck masses organized according to the characteristic age of presentation during childhood. Congenital vascular anomalies also arise in the head and neck region in children; details regarding such infantile hemangiomas and vascular malformations of lymphatic and venous origin can be found elsewhere in this book.

# NECK MASSES PRESENTING IN THE FETAL OR NEONATAL PERIOD

## Teratomas and Congenital High Upper Airway Obstruction (CHAOS)

Teratomas refer to tumors that are composed of cells from all three germ cell layers — ectoderm, mesoderm, and endoderm — in various stages of maturity and are comprised of tissue that is foreign to the site of origin. Teratomas most commonly occur in the sacrococcygeal and cervicofacial regions. Cervical teratomas are characteristically benign lesions. They are frequently diagnosed *in utero* with a 20% to 50% incidence of maternal polyhydramnios thought to be related to extrinsic esophageal obstruction; additionally alpha fetal protein levels may be elevated.[1]

The fetal presentation of a teratoma may be associated with congenital high upper airway obstruction syndrome (CHAOS), a rare *in utero* condition characterized by complete or near complete obstruction of the upper airway. Potential etiologies of CHAOS include laryngeal atresia or stenosis, tracheal atresia or stenosis, or extrinsic upper airway compression due to a large mass in the neck or upper aerodigestive tract. While there are case reports of foregut duplication cysts and lymphatic vascular malformations causing such upper airway obstruction, teratomas represent the vast majority of congenital tumors associated with CHAOS.[2]

The diagnosis of CHAOS is usually made during prenatal ultrasound. Characteristic findings include polyhydramnios, lung expansion, inversion of the diaphragm and cardiac compression. When due to extrinsic compression, the large cervical or upper aerodigestive tract mass is typically identifiable.

Further work-up necessitates the assistance of a maternal-fetal medicine specialist or perinatologist in addition to the potential consultative services of a medical geneticist, a pediatric surgeon, and a pediatric otolaryngologist. Fetal echocardiogram and amniocentesis for karyotype may be obtained. Magnetic resonance imaging allows for excellent soft tissue definition without the potential morbidity associated with radiation to the developing fetus. Such high resolution fetal MRI of the head and neck can prove particularly useful in cases of extrinsic airway compression from large neck masses that may need to be addressed at birth.

Ultimately an airway must be established at the time of delivery. This is typically accomplished via a so-called *ex utero* intrapartum treatment (EXIT) procedure. Such an EXIT procedure is often performed after 30 weeks gestation if possible, balancing early intervention with the survival benefit afforded by maximizing fetal size and lung maturity. Other factors such as fetal hydrops or congestive heart failure may necessitate earlier delivery. During the EXIT procedure, the mother is maintained under general anesthesia while the head and neck of the fetus is partially delivered through an incision in the uterus. The placenta remains intact, and fetal perfusion is maintained through the umbilical circulation, a scenario analogous to extracorporeal membrane oxygenation (ECMO). This technique allows for up to 90 minutes of time in which the fetal airway can be secured either through endoscopic-assisted intubation or by surgical means. Additionally there are reports of subtotal resection of cervical teratomas during the EXIT procedure in order to facilitate establishment of an airway.[3]

Those cervical teratomas not identified prenatally are typically evident at the initial neonatal assessment. Examination usually reveals a firm, anterolateral neck mass which may display nodularity and focal areas of discoloration (Fig. 1). These masses are often quite large with secondary tracheal compression or deviation.

Radiographic evaluation of a cervical teratoma with computed tomography (CT) or magnetic resonance imaging (MRI) allows for high resolution evaluation of the mass itself and definition of the tumor's relationship to adjacent structures. These imaging modalities typically reveal a well-encapsulated, heterogeneous lesion with both solid and cystic components; there may be speckled calcifications on CT imaging.

Surgical resection is the treatment of choice for cervical teratomas. Complete excision, if feasible, is ideal. These masses are usually poorly vascularized. Operative morbidity includes potential paresis or paralysis of the vagus and recurrent laryngeal nerves on the affected side. The

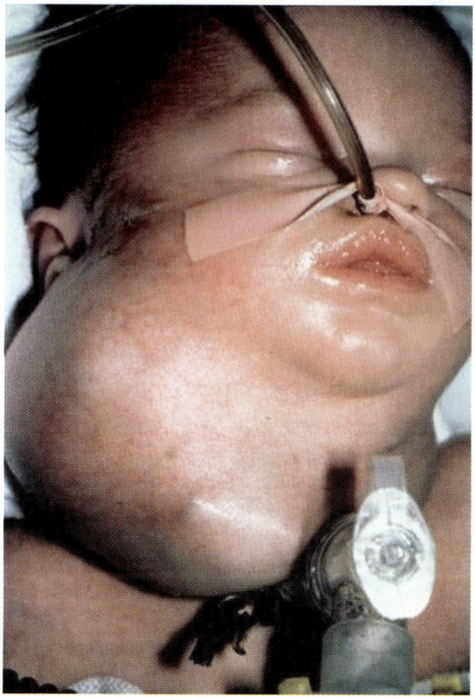

**Fig. 1.** Infant with a cervical teratoma requiring tracheotomy for airway securement at birth.

recurrent laryngeal nerve is at particular risk due to the fact that these tumors are often intimately related to the thyroid gland. Near total thyroidectomy may be required to achieve adequate tumor margins. Postoperatively these patients should be followed with regular examinations to assess for recurrence and to monitor for hypothyroidism.[1]

## Fibromatosis Colli

Pseudotumor of infancy (POI) is a unilateral contracture of the sternocleidomastoid (SCM) muscle that may be evident at birth or become manifest within the first six weeks of life. The SCM contracture causes a characteristic posture in which the chin is rotated away from the lesion and the occiput is rotated towards the affected side, hence the term congenital muscular torticollis.

On physical examination a firm, non-tender mass is palpable within the body of the contracted SCM muscle. This mass, known as fibromatosis colli, occurs when muscle tissue is replaced by fibrosis. The exact cause is unknown but several theories exist. The intrauterine theory postulates that compressive forces lead to abnormal fetal positioning of the neck causing fibrosis and contracture of the SCM. The traumatic theory poses that there is damage to the SCM during a difficult delivery that leads to intramuscular hematoma and scarring. Other etiologies such as compartment syndrome, vascular occlusion leading to ischemia and infarction, and even a genetic influence have been postulated. Although the clinical presentation is typically straightforward, ultrasound is the diagnostic study of choice to confirm the mass in question is truly intramuscular.[4] A solid mass within the sternocleidomastoid muscle is consistent with fibromatosis colli. Surgical biopsy is necessary only when the ultrasonographic evaluation alternatively documents an extramuscular lesion raising concern of a more worrisome diagnosis such as a peripheral nerve sheath tumor or a cervical neuroblastoma.

The natural history of fibromatosis colli is usually one of spontaneous regression. Pseudotumor of infancy and congenital muscular torticollis are therefore best managed expectantly. Physical therapy for passive range of motion exercises may enhance recovery. Surgery is indicated only in those infrequent cases in which the torticollis fails to resolve after 12 to 18 months.[5] Facial asymmetry and plagiocephaly may become apparent in these children over time. Surgical intervention is in the form of a sternocleidomastoid tenotomy to release the contracture.

## NECK MASSES PRESENTING IN INFANCY AND CHILDHOOD

### Midline Neck Masses

#### *Thyroid gland anomalies*

During the third week of gestation, the thyroid gland develops from a diverticulum arising from the floor of the pharynx and becomes bilobed as it descends into the anterior neck. Throughout its migration, the primitive gland remains attached to its origin within the pharynx by a hollow canal, the thyroglossal duct, which ultimately involutes by weeks 5 to 8 of gestation. The pharyngeal site of attachment persists as the foramen cecum of the tongue and the glandular site of attachment may remain as the pyramidal lobe of the thyroid. Arrest in the normal descent of the gland results in ectopic thyroid tissue, whereas failure of a portion of the epithelial-lined embryonic duct to involute is the cause of a thyroglossal duct cyst. These remnants may present in the anterior neck anywhere along the path of descent. This path extends from the foramen cecum through the base of tongue, anterior to or through the hyoid bone, and inferiorly over the thyrohyoid membrane and laryngeal cartilages.

## Ectopic thyroid tissue

The incidence of ectopic thyroid tissue in a sublingual or thyrohyoid location is rare, accounting for only 1% to 2% of thyroid ectopia.[6] Such ectopic cervical thyroids usually become manifest because the ectopic gland enlarges in response to the increasing metabolic demands of the growing child. Thyroid function studies reveal these children to be typically euthyroid with elevated thyroid stimulating hormone (TSH) levels. Radiographic evaluation by either thyroid ultrasound or thyroid scintiscanning is necessary to evaluate for the presence or absence of additional functional orthotopic glandular tissue (Fig. 2).

The surgical removal of asymptomatic ectopic thyroid tissue is typically not warranted. Symptomatic lesions may be managed by hormonal suppression therapy. A standard open approach is used for those rare cases of symptomatic ectopic cervical thyroid unresponsive to such medical management. Lifelong thyroid hormone replacement therapy is necessary in such cases.

## Thyroglossal duct cysts

Thyroglossal duct cysts (TDCs) are comparatively very common. Cadaveric studies suggest that TDCs are present in approximately

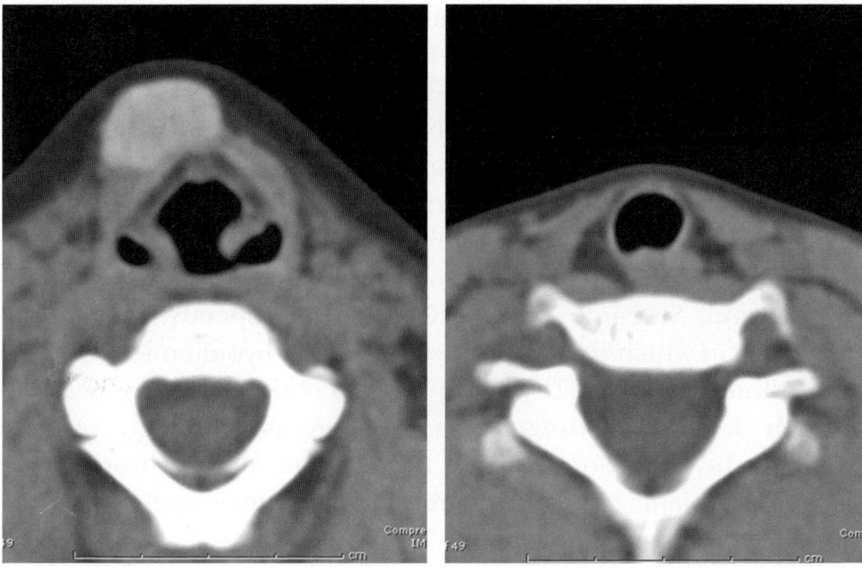

(a) (b)

**Fig. 2.** Axial CT scans without contrast demonstrating (a) ectopic cervical thyroid overlying the thyroid lamina, and (b) an absence of orthotopic thyroid tissue at the level of the cervical trachea.

7% of the population. Most of these TDCs never become symptomatic, but when they do present, two thirds manifest before age 30 and half present before the age of ten years.[7] The classic presentation is that of a painless, midline neck mass near the hyoid bone that moves with swallowing and tongue protrusion. Inflammatory presentations are, however, common with up to 25% of patients presenting with an indurated mass from which a draining sinus can develop due to spontaneous rupture or following attempted surgical drainage.[8] A variety of aerobic and anaerobic bacteria have been isolated from such lesions, reflective of a persistent pharyngeal communication via the foramen cecum.

Apart from a thorough history and physical examination, the work-up of a suspected TDC should involve some form of imaging to establish the presence of a normal orthotopic thyroid gland. Cervical ultrasound is ideal for this purpose; CT or MRI also certainly suffice.

Although all these studies distinguish between cystic and solid masses, absolute differentiation of a TDC from a dermoid cyst may not be preoperatively possible. A TSH level is not typically obtained unless the cervical ultrasound is abnormal or the clinical history suggests the need to do so. An abnormal TSH level would suggest the need for thyroid scintiscanning prior to surgical intervention.

The surgical management of TDCs has evolved over time. Due to a high rate of recurrence approximating 50% following simple cyst excision, Sistrunk in 1920 described an operative technique used today in which the central portion of the hyoid bone is excised in continuity with the TDC.[9] Removal of a contiguous core of tissue through the base of tongue was also suggested, though Sistrunk modified the procedure so as to transect the superior tract in the submucosal plane beneath the foramen cecum, thereby avoiding oropharyngeal communication.[10] Numerous studies have supported the use of this technique in terms of a markedly decreased rate of recurrence ranging from 4% to 6%.[7,11] Failure to follow the surgical principles of the Sistrunk procedure increases the risk of recurrence, as does intraoperative cyst rupture. Factors that contribute to intraoperative cyst violation include previous inflammation, prior incision and drainage, and skin involvement. Revision surgery mandates a modification of the Sistrunk procedure incorporating an *en bloc* anterior dissection with removal of approximately 3 to 4 cm of strap muscles down to the pretracheal and prelaryngeal fascia, and wider resection of the hyoid bone in continuity with a 5 to 10 mm core of tongue tissue. Recurrence rates are significantly lower utilizing this technique for revision surgery.[12]

### *Cervical dermoid cysts*

Dermoid cysts arise from nests of trapped epithelial elements along embryonic lines of fusion. In the neck they commonly occur at the junction of the first and second branchial arches, particularly in the submental, submandibular, and thyrohyoid regions. Dermoid cysts are lined by epithelium and contain epithelial appendages such as hair, hair follicles, and sebaceous glands. Although histopathologically cystic lesions, dermoids are typically firm subcutaneous masses to palpation. Midline cervical dermoids are difficult to clinically differentiate from thyroglossal duct cysts, and may not be easily distinguishable radiographically.[13]

Dermoid cysts are amenable to simple cyst excision. The removal of a thyrohyoid dermoid may, however, require resection of a portion of the hyoid for thorough diagnostic and therapeutic purposes. In fact, a formal Sistrunk procedure is recommended for all midline masses deep to the cervical strap musculature due to the difficulties of preoperative TDC versus thyrohyoid dermoid cyst differentiation.

*Foregut duplication cysts and bronchogenic cysts*

Foregut duplication cysts and bronchogenic cysts are two comparatively rare clinical entities that also deserve mention. Both of these anomalies develop from rests of epithelium of endodermal origin, and both may give rise to cystic structures within the upper aerodigestive tract or within the soft tissues of the neck. The clinical presentation and radiographic characteristics of these masses may mimic more common entities such as thyroglossal duct cysts and branchial cleft cysts. Hence their diagnoses is typically not made clinically but rather established by histopathologic evaluation following excision.

Foregut duplication cysts are often lined by gastric mucosa. They most commonly manifest as a cystic mass in the floor of mouth or adjacent to the anterolateral tongue (Fig. 3). Depending on the size of the lesion, airway compromise or swallowing dysfunction may be evident. Complete excision is curative. Such can be accomplished at any age, but may be necessary in the neonatal period to relieve airway obstruction and dysphagia.[14,15]

Bronchogenic cysts contain both respiratory epithelium and cartilage elements. They can present anywhere along the tracheobronchial tree, more commonly in the chest, although they may manifest in the cervical region, most frequently in a suprasternal location. Unlike foregut duplication cysts, these masses tend to present later in childhood or young adulthood.[16,17]

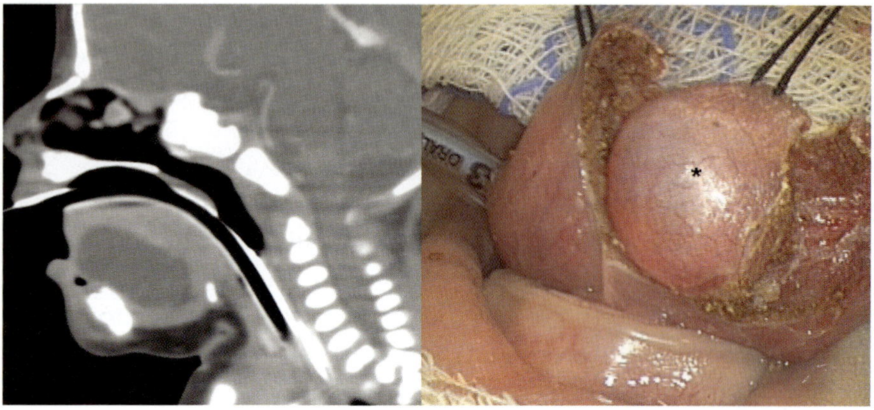

(a) (b)

**Fig. 3.** (a) Sagittal MRI scan demonstrating a cystic sublingual mass in a neonate. (b) Intraoperative photograph demonstrating mass (*) excision via a midline glossotomy approach; histopathologic evaluation confirmed a foregut duplication cyst.

*Cervical (plunging) ranula*

A ranula is a mucus retention cyst or mucocele that arises secondary to ductal obstruction of one of the sublingual glands. The term originates from the Latin word *rana,* meaning frog, alluding to how the blue translucency of an intraoral ranula has a similar appearance to the underbelly of a frog. A plunging ranula refers to the anterior neck mass which develops when a sublingual mucocele traverses the myelohyoid muscle and extends from the sublingual space into the submandibular area. The resultant cervical mass is usually soft, compressible, and painless. Histopathologically the lining of a plunging ranula is composed of fibrous connective tissue, indicative of a pseudocyst filled with mucoid saliva.

The clinical presentation of a plunging ranula can be confused with that of a lymphatic vascular malformation. Both of these lesions may appear as fluid-filled macrocysts on cervical imaging. A plunging ranula, however, will demonstrate a communication between the sublingual space and the submandibular space via a communication through or around the myelohyoid muscle. Therefore a cystic mass with components on either side of the myelohyoid muscle should raise suspicion that the lesion in question is a plunging ranula.

A plunging ranula is best managed by surgical excision. Removal of the ipsilateral sublingual gland, the source of the ranula, is recommended to prevent recurrence. Some authors have suggested that transoral removal of the offending sublingual gland alone is adequate for treating both simple and plunging ranulas.[18] The more traditional surgical approach for a plunging ranula involves transcervical excision of both cyst and sublingual gland, typically including removal of the ipsilateral submandibular gland to enhance floor of mouth access. The transcervical approach provides greater exposure for identification and protection of both the hypoglossal and lingual nerves than is possible transorally.[19]

## Anterocervical Neck Masses

### *Branchial remnants*

The branchial system appears during the fourth week of development, giving rise to many of the symmetrically paired structures of the head and neck. The branchial system is composed of five paired arches, referred to as such due to their resemblance to the gill arches of fish. Each arch is composed of mesodermal tissue which will go on to form mesenchymal derivatives including cartilage, bone and muscle. The arches are separated by each other by internal and external invaginations. The external cleft is of ectodermal origin and the internal pouch is of endodermal origin. The clefts and pouches are separated from each other by a thin epithelial plate.

A branchial system anomaly exists as a sinus tract, a fistula tract, or a cyst. Sinus tracts arise from incompletely closed clefts or pouches, depending on the presence of an internal or external opening. A complete fistula tract forms when both openings remain and there is dissolution of the intervening epithelial plate. A cyst may occur anywhere along these potential sinus or fistula tracts.

Branchial sinuses or fistulae with external openings are typically detected at birth or soon thereafter on routine physical examination.

In contrast, internal sinus tracts and branchial cleft cysts may not become apparent until later in childhood or adulthood, presenting often in the context of acute infection. Imaging with CT and MRI may provide valuable information in regards to location and size of the branchial remnant as well as its relation to vital anatomic structures.

## First branchial cleft anomalies

First branchial cleft anomalies may be divided into two distinct anatomic types according to a classification schema described by Work.[20] A type I first branchial cleft cyst or sinus opening is located inferior, medial, or posterior to the auricle above the level of the mandible (Fig. 4). The sinus tract, if present, is superficial to the parotid gland and parallels the external auditory canal. In type II first branchial cleft anomalies, the cyst or sinus opening is located in the anterior neck below the level of the mandible and superior (cephalad) to the hyoid bone (Fig. 5). The sinus tract, if present, courses over the angle of the mandible and through the parotid gland, terminating in the inferior external auditory canal in the region of the bony-cartilaginous junction. The course of a type II first branchial cleft tract relative to the facial nerve is highly variable.

A standard preauricular face-lift like approach is advocated for the removal of type I branchial cysts or sinus tracts as the branchial remnant in such cases is always superficial to the parotid gland and hence to the facial nerve (Fig. 4). Type II anomalies, on the other hand, are typically intraparotid. Superficial or subtotal parotidectomy with facial nerve dissection is required in order to accomplish complete, safe excision of these lesions (Fig. 5).

## Second branchial cleft anomalies

In second branchial cleft anomalies, the cyst or sinus opening is located inferior (caudal) to the level of the hyoid bone along the anterior border of the sternocleidomastoid muscle, often near the junction of its middle and inferior two thirds. The sinus tract or

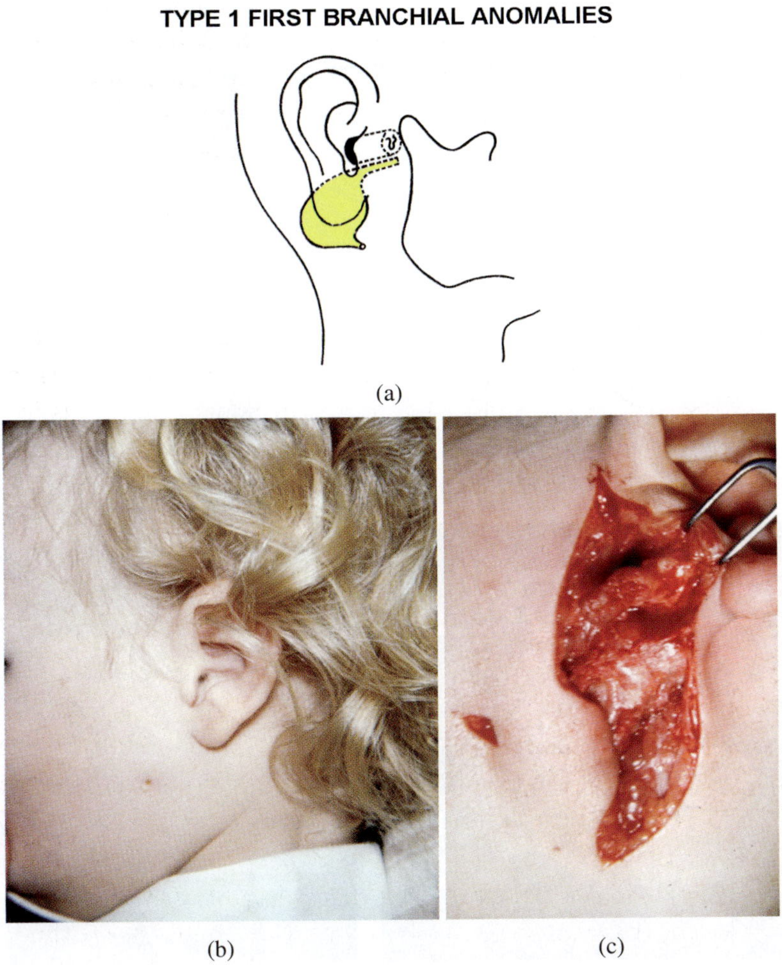


**Fig. 4.** (a) Diagrammatic representation of a type 1 first branchial anomaly. (b) Classic clinical presentation. (c) Surgical approach for excision.

complete fistula tract, if present, courses from the external skin to an internal opening in the tonsillar fossa, passing over the hypoglossal and glossopharyngeal nerves before passing through the carotid bifurcation. Cysts may occur anywhere along this potential path, however, they are most common in the anterior neck deep to the SCM muscle (Fig. 6).

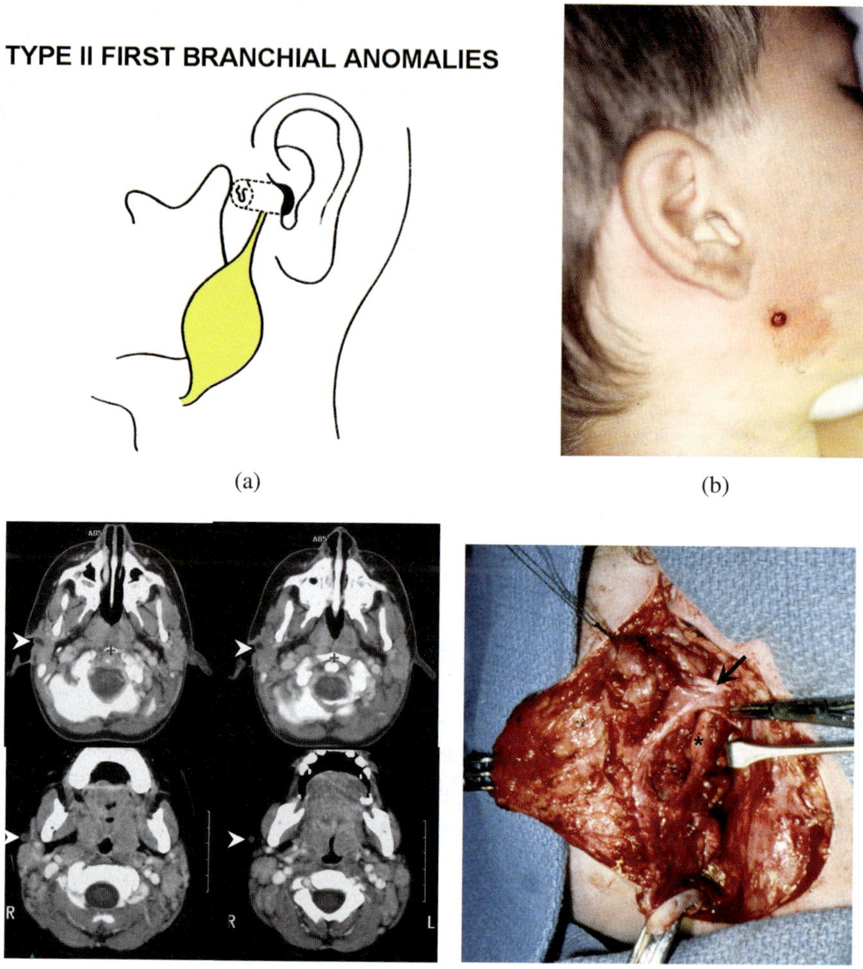


(a) (b) (c) (d)

**Fig. 5.** (a) Diagrammatic representation of a type 2 first branchial anomaly. (b) Classic clinical presentation with sinus punctum located at angle of the mandible. (c) Axial CT scan of the same child with a type 2 first branchial cleft tract extending from the cartilaginous canal through the parotid gland to the infra-auricular skin (arrow head). (d) Intraoperative findings of a similar case on the left side demonstrating the sinus tract (duplication of the external auditory canal)* passing deep to the facial nerve (black arrow).

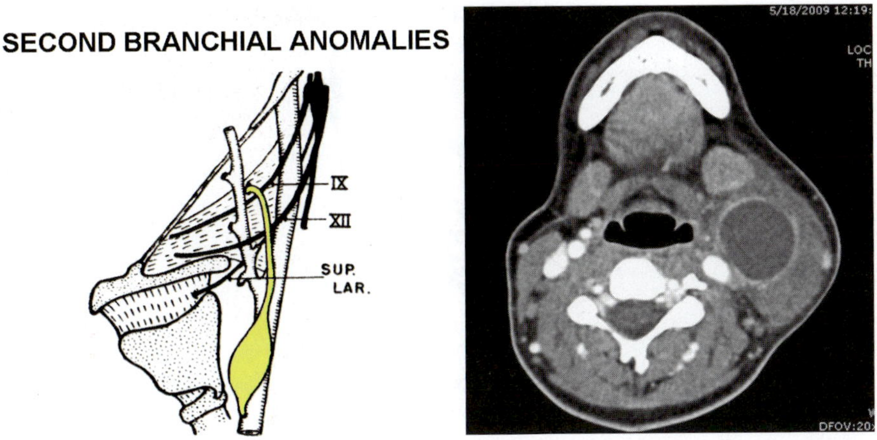


(a) (b)

**Fig. 6.** (a) Diagrammatic representation of a second branchial anomaly. (b) Axial contrast-enhanced CT scan of a second branchial cleft cyst.

## Third and fourth branchial cleft anomalies

The external cervical openings of third and fourth branchial cleft anomalies are found in a similar location to that of second branchial cleft derivatives along the anterior border of the SCM muscle, although often more inferior (caudal). Internal openings arise from the ipsilateral pyriform sinus. In third branchial anomalies, a complete fistula tract would course superiorly through the thyrohyoid membrane just above the superior laryngeal neurovascular bundle, over the hypoglossal nerve and under the glossopharyngeal nerve, descend behind the internal carotid and along the common carotid, and terminate in the anterior neck (Fig. 7). The theoretical course of a complete fistula tract of fourth arch derivation would originate near the apex of the ipsilateral pyriform sinus, course under the thyroid ala and inferior constrictor muscle, then travel superficial to the course of the recurrent laryngeal nerve adjacent to the thyroid gland, eventually terminating in the anteroinferior region of the neck.[7]

The clinical presentation of third and fourth branchial anomalies is typically along two principal lines. Cleft remnants present as

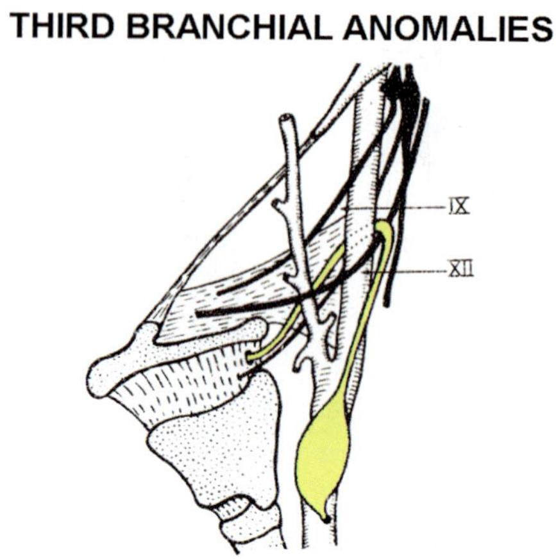


**Fig. 7.** Diagrammatic representation of a third branchial anomaly.

external sinuses opening in the lower third of the lateral neck, whereas common presenting manifestations of pouch remnants include suppurative thyroiditis and cervical abscesses.

The external sinus openings of third and fourth branchial cleft anomalies are frequently asymptomatic. Drainage, when present, typically occurs in older children and is often seromucoid in character. Recurrent or persistently draining external tracts require excision. Such tracts are of variable length. Short tracts may terminate at the level of the superficial layer of the deep cervical fascia at the border of the sternocleidomastoid muscle. A potentially deep sinus tract must, however, be anticipated based upon the complex embryologic origin of these lesions. Preoperative sinus tract contrast studies or MRI assessment can occasionally be helpful from a tract delineation standpoint.

Operative hypopharyngoscopy and laryngoscopy for identification of a possible communication within the pyriform sinus is advocated when a third or fourth branchial pouch anomaly is suspected (Fig. 8). Chemical and thermal cauterization of such pyriform sinus entry point has been advocated as treatment by some authors.[21] The complete excision of a third or fourth branchial pouch fistula tract may require partial pharyngectomy with or without

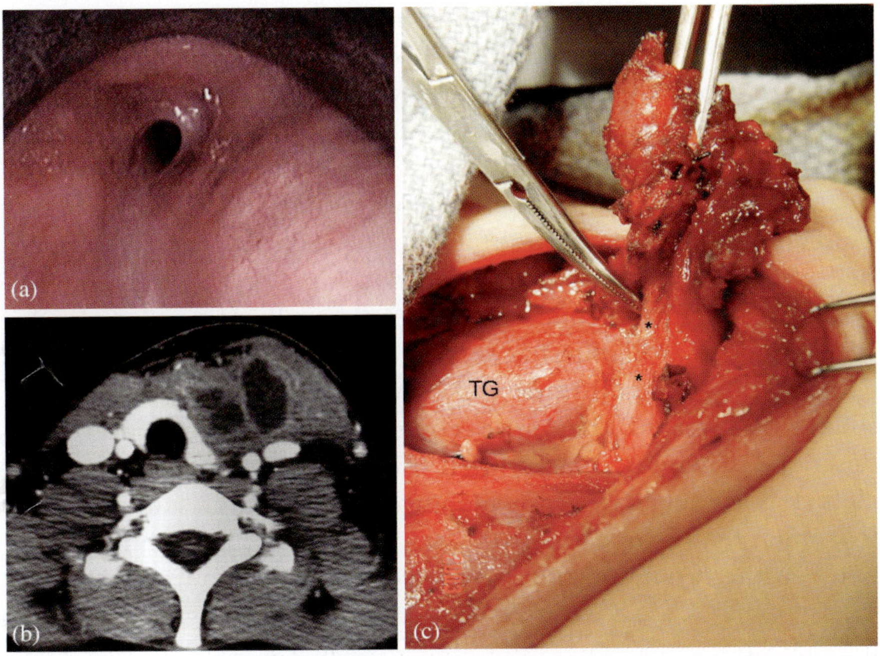


**Fig. 8.** (a) Fourth branchial pouch sinus tract opening evident at the apex of the left pyriform sinus on operative pharyngoscopy. (b) Axial contrast-enhanced CT scan demonstrating a left-sided neck abscess effacing the left thyroid lobe. (c) Intraoperative photograph demonstrating thyroid gland (TG) and fistula tract (*) arising from lateral aspect of the cricothyroid region.

thyroid alatomy for exposure, as well as hemithyroidectomy to prevent recurrence. Interestingly the vast majority of third and fourth branchial pouch anomalies reported in the literature have occurred on the left side.[22]

### *Thymic gland anomalies*

The thymus gland arises bilaterally from the fourth and primarily the third branchial pouches and contains elements from all three germ layers. These thymic primordia elongate from the pharynx in a medial and caudal direction, originating from the pyriform sinuses, passing through the thyrohyoid membrane and descending along both carotid sheaths, eventually joining at the midline in the mediastinum. Congenital thymic anomalies, therefore, may present anywhere from the level of the pyriform sinuses to the chest, although the inferior aspect of the neck is the more common location.[23] During thymic gland descent, potential connections to the pharynx remain as hollow, epithelially-lined structures known as thymopharyngeal ducts. These thymopharyngeal ducts eventually degenerate as part of normal thymic development. A persistent duct results in a cervical thymic cyst, whereas partially-descended glandular elements may manifest as cervical ectopic thymus.

Cervical ectopic thymus and cervical thymic cysts present in a similar fashion to the more common neck masses previously described. Thymic cysts are often initially confused with branchial cleft cysts as they have nearly identical clinical manifestations owing to similar embryonic origins (Fig. 9). The distinguishing factor between the two lies in the presence of thymic tissue within the cyst

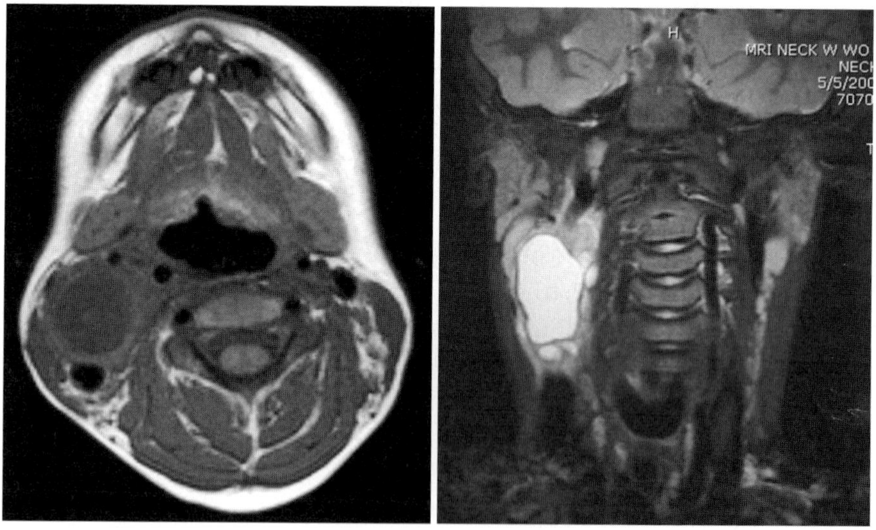


(a) (b)

**Fig. 9.** (a) Axial (T1) and (b) coronal (T2) MRI scans of a young child with a thymic cyst; notice the similar appearance to a branchial cleft cyst and the close relationship of the cystic mass to the great vessels.

wall of thymic cysts, a characteristic appreciated only upon pathological evaluation. Solid cervical ectopic thymus may clinically resemble a lymph node or benign-appearing neoplastic lesion; histopathologic examination demonstrating Hassall's corpuscles and tissue architecture of normal thymus gland provides the definitive diagnosis.

## REFERENCES

1. Martino F, Avila LF, Encinas JL, Luis AL, Olivares P, Lassaletta L, Nistal M, Tovar JA. Teratomas of the neck and mediastinum in children. *Pediatr Surg Int* 2006;22:627–634.
2. Hartnick CJ, Barth WH, Cote CJ, Albrecht MA, Grant PE, Geyer JT. A pregnant woman with a large mass in the fetal oral cavity. *N Engl J Med* 2009;360:913–921.
3. Hirose S, Sydorak RM, Tsao K, Cauldwell CB, Newman KD, Mychaliska GB, Albanese CT, Lee H, Farmer DL. Spectrum of intrapartum management strategies for giant fetal cervical teratoma. *J Pediatr Surg* 2003 Dec;38(12):1846, comment in: *J Pediatr Surg* 2003 Mar;38(3):446–450 (discussion on 446–450).
4. Maddalozzo J, Goldenberg JD. Pseudotumor of infancy — the role of ultrasonography. *Ear Nose Throat J* 1996;75:248–254.
5. Wei JL, Schwartz KM, Weaver AL, Orvidas LJ. Pseudotumor of infancy and congenital muscular torticollis: 170 cases. *Laryngoscope* 2001;111:688–695.
6. Wong RJ, Cunningham MJ, Curtin HD. Cervical ectopic thyroid. *Am J Otolaryngol* 1998;19:397–399.
7. Acierno SP, Waldhausen JH. Congenital cervical cysts, sinuses and fistulae. *Otolaryngol Clin North Am* 2007;40:161–176.
8. Foley DS, Fallat ME. Thyroglossal duct and other congenital midline cervical anomalies. *Semin Pediatr Surg* 2006; 15:70–75.
9. Sistrunk WE. The surgical treatment of cysts of the thyroglossal tract. *Ann Surg* 1920;71(2):121–124.
10. Sistrunk WE. Technique of removal of cysts and sinuses of the thyroglossal duct. *Surg Gynecol Obstet* 1928;46:109–112.
11. Cunningham MJ. The management of congenital neck masses. *Am J Otolaryngol* 1992;13:78–92.

12. Kim MK, Pawel BR, Issacson G. Central neck dissection for the treatment of recurrent thyroglossal duct cysts in childhood. *Otolaryngol Head Neck Surg* 1999;121:543–547.
13. DeMello DE, Lima JA, Liapis H. Midline cervical cysts in children: thyroglossal anomalies. *Arch Otolaryngol Head Neck Surg* 1987;113:418–420.
14. Eaton D, Billings K, Timmons C, Booth T, Biavati JM. Congenital foregut duplication cysts of the anterior tongue. *Arch Otolaryngol Head Neck Surg* 2001;127:1484–1487.
15. Kim JK, Park KK. Foregut duplication cyst of the hypopharynx: a rare cause of upper airway obstruction. *J Pediatr Surg* 2007;42:E5–E7.
16. Teissier N, Elmaleh-Bergès M, Ferkdadji L, François M, Van den Abbeele T. Cervical bronchogenic cysts: usual and unusual clinical presentations. *Arch Otolaryngol Head Neck Surg* 2008;134:1165–1169.
17. Mehta RP, Faquin WC, Cunningham MJ. Cervical bronchogenic cysts: a consideration in the differential diagnosis of pediatric cervical cystic masses. *Int J Pediatr Otorhinolaryngol* 2004;68:563–568.
18. Yoshimura Y, Obara S, Kondoh T. A comparison of three methods used for treatment of ranula. *J Oral Maxillofac Surg* 1995;53:280–282 (discussion on 283).
19. Cunningham MJ. Salivary gland surgery. In: Bluestone CD, Rosenfeld RM, eds. *Surgical Atlas of Pediatric Otolaryngology*. Hamilton, Ontario: BC Decker, 2002, pp. 532–535.
20. Work WP. Newer concepts of first branchial cleft defects. *Laryngoscope* 1972; 82:1581–1593.
21. Verret DJ, McClay J, Murray A, Biavatt M, Brown O. Endoscopic cauterization of fourth branchial cleft sinus tracts. *Arch Otolaryngol Head Neck Surg* 2004;130:465–468.
22. Nicoucar K, Giger R, Pope HG Jr, Jaecklin T, Dulguerov P. Management of congenital fourth branchial arch anomalies: a review and analysis of published cases. *J Pediatr Surg* 2009;44:1432–1439.
23. Clark JJ, Johnson SM. Solid cervical ectopic thymus in an infant. *J Pediatr Surg* 2009;44:E19–E21.

# 13

# Infections of the Pharynx and Neck in Children

*Sofia Lyford-Pike and Emily F. Boss*

## ADENOTONSILLAR AND PHARYNGEAL INFECTIONS

In the United States, adenotonsillar infections and pharyngitis account for a high proportion of evaluations of children in ambulatory settings each year.

The pharynx is composed in part by a ring of lymphoid tissue. *Waldeyer's ring*, named after a 19th century German anatomist, is composed of the nasopharyngeal tonsil, palatine tonsils, tubal tonsils, lingual tonsils and lateral pharyngeal bands. The most prominent components are the nasopharyngeal tonsil and palatine tonsils, commonly referred to as adenoid and tonsils respectively.[1] The tonsils and adenoid are present at birth and grow to a maximum development at approximately five to six years of age at which point they begin to involute.[2,3] Tonsils and adenoids are secondary lymphatic organs primarily composed of B-lymphocytes that mediate immunoglobulin response to airborne and alimentary antigens.[1,3] With its universal exposure to aerodigestive pathogens, the pharynx thus becomes a primary location for infections. Acute pharyngitis, also referred to as acute tonsillitis in the presence of tonsils, is most commonly seen in the winter months when respiratory viruses are prevalent, and children are the major reservoirs for these pathogens.[4] Infectious causes of pharyngitis in children and their associated clinical features are listed in Table 1.

**Table 1. Infectious causes of pharyngitis in children.**

| | Clinical features |
|---|---|
| **Viruses** | |
| Rhinovirus | Common cold, winter months, cough and coryza |
| Coronavirus | Common cold, winter months, cough and coryza |
| Respiratory syncitial virus | Common cold, bronchiolitis |
| Adenovirus | Pharyngoconjunctival fever, upper respiratory illness |
| Parainfluenza | Common cold, ***croup***, cough, coryza, noisy breathing |
| Influenza A + B | Fever, myalgias, pharyngitis, cough |
| Epstein-Barr virus (EBV) | Infectious mononucleosis ("***mono***"), fever, malaise, tonsillar enlargement, exudative tonsillitis, cervical lymphadenophathy, hepatosplenomegaly |
| Cytomegalovirus (CMV) | Infectious mononucleosis, less common organism |
| Coxsackie virus | Herpangina, hand-foot-mouth disease, vesicular lesions posterior pharynx |
| Human immunodeficiency virus (HIV) | Primary HIV infection: fever, adenopathy, malaise, exposure history |
| **Bacteria** | |
| Group A beta-hemolytic streptococcus (GABHS) | Exudative pharyngitis, ***most common bacterial cause*** |
| Group C and G beta-hemolytic streptococcus | Pharyngitis with possible rash, respiratory and food borne transmission |
| Oral anaerobic bacteria | |
| *Fusobacterium necrophorum* | Pharyngitis, deep space abscess, Lemierre's syndrome |
| *Neisseria gonorrhea* | Sexually transmitted disease, oral-genital contact, adolescents |
| *Corynebacterium diphtheriae* | Diphthera, pseudomembranous pharyngitis, non-vaccinated/foreign exposure<br>Reportable disease |
| *Treponema species* | Necrotizing gingivopharyngitis, Vincent's angina, Trench mouth, poor oral hygiene |
| *Treponema pallidum* | Syphillis (primary/secondary), oropharyngeal chancres |
| *Chlamydia trachomatis* | Sexually transmitted disease, oral-genital contact, adolescents |

(*Continued*)

Table 1. (*Continued*)

| | Clinical features |
|---|---|
| *Mycoplasma pneumoniae* | Pharyngitis, pneumonia, bronchitis, atypical bacterium |
| *Fransicella tularensis* | Tuleremia, fever, lymphadenopathy, ulcerative/ exudative pharyngitis<br>Contaminated food/$H_2O$ ingestion |
| Arcanobacterium hemolyticum | Pharyngitis and rash, adolescents |
| **Others** | |
| Candida albicans | Thrush, white plaques over pharynx, immunocompromised host |

## Viral Pharyngitis

Viral infections are the most common cause of acute pharyngitis in the pediatric population. Respiratory viruses such as rhinovirus, coronavirus, parainfluenza virus and influenza virus are common culprits.[4–6] Viral infections are usually self-limited, and supportive therapy is warranted. It is important to differentiate viral etiologies from bacterial etiologies, as bacterial pharyngitis may have associated complications thus requiring further intervention. Pharyngitis, associated with the symptoms of coryza, cough, diarrhea, hoarseness, conjunctivitis and viral exanthems is commonly of viral etiology. The absence of fever is also suggestive of viral origin, however, some viral causes of pharyngitis, for example adenoviral infections and infectious mononucleosis, may manifest with fever.[5,6]

### *Epstein-Barr virus*

Infectious mononucleosis is caused by the Epstein-Barr Virus (EBV) and in adolescents and young adults often is manifested by acute pharyngitis. The symptoms associated with EBV infection may be difficult to differentiate from streptococcal pharyngitis. Patients present with fever and severe pharyngitis with constitutional symptoms of generalized malaise, anorexia, and weight loss. Physical findings include exudative tonsillitis, bilateral cervical lymphadenopathy, and possible palatal petechiae and hepatosplenomegaly. Fever and malaise generally precede the development of pharyngitis and lymphadenopathy.[7,8]

Absence of fatigue and cervical lymphadenopathy make the diagnosis of EBV less likely.[9] Work-up for EBV includes a differential blood count and the evaluation serum heterophile antibodies. Lymphocytosis, greater than 50% lymphocytes or an absolute lymphocyte count greater than 4500/μL, is found in mononucleosis. In addition, greater than 10% atypical lymphocytes may be seen.[10] Reactive heterophile antibodies are present in EBV infections. These antibodies can be tested for in the serum of patients by testing agglutination with horse red blood cells (the Monospot test), or sheep read blood cells (the Paul-Bunnell test). Testing may also be performed rapidly with enzyme-linked immunosorbent assay techniques (ELISA). False-negative heterophile antibody testing can be found in early stages of clinical infection, therefore cases highly suggestive of EBV infection should be further evaluated by serum EBV-specific antibody titers or PCR for EBV DNA.[9] Liver function testing may demonstrate elevated aminotransferases in patients with hepatomegaly, nausea and vomiting.

Acute symptoms of EBV generally resolve within one to two weeks, however, generalized fatigue may persist.[11] Management of infectious mononucleosis is supportive. There is no support for the routine use of corticosteroids or acyclovir.[12,13] Corticosteroids however have been used in severe cases of mononucleosis presenting or progressing to life threatening upper airway obstruction. A nasopharyngeal airway may be placed to stabilize the airway in this setting.

In severe cases of obstruction without response to high dose corticosteroids, surgical intervention through tonsillectomy has been advocated.[14–16] If surgery is warranted, a specific airway management algorithm must be agreed upon by the otolaryngologist and anesthesiologist prior to the induction of anesthesia. Cricothyroidotomy and tracheostomy sets should be available.

**Bacterial Pharyngitis**

*Group A streptococcal pharyngitis*

Group A beta-hemolytic streptococcus (GABHS), or *streptococcus pyogenes* accounts for 15%–30% of pharyngitis cases in children.[17] Children between the ages of five to 15 are primarily affected; however atypical presentation of GABHS infections, with the absence of characteristic pharyngitis, can be seen in younger children.[18,19]

Streptococcal pharyngitis presents with abrupt onset of fever and sore throat, typically in the winter or spring months. Patients may have constitutional symptoms of anorexia, nausea, and vomiting, and will have associated physical findings of erythematous tonsillitis, patchy exudates and tender cervical lymphadenopathy.[18] Supportive therapy is not appropriate for GABHS as the condition is associated with serious complications if left untreated, specifically, rheumatic fever and post-streptococcal glomerulonephritis. In addition, confirmation of streptococcal infection is important for the prevention of misuse and overuse of antibiotics.

The risk of GABHS may be assessed in patients by clinical and epidemiologic factors, and scoring algorithms support that patients determined to be low risk do not require throat culture.[4,20,21] These factors however do not reliably diagnose positive disease. Therefore, the Infectious Diseases Society of America (IDSA) and the American Academy of Pediatrics recommends that high risk cases, for example those with acute pharyngitis with lack of viral symptoms or acute pharyngitis with history of exposure, be confirmed with microbiologic testing.[4,22]

Throat culture is the gold standard for diagnosis of GABHS. Both tonsils (or tonsillar fossae) and the posterior pharynx must be swabbed without contact with areas of the mouth or pharynx.[4] Evaluation of the sample for other bacterial pathogens if suspected may have to be specifically requested, as they are not often tested. The limitation of throat culture is the time it takes to obtain result. For this reason, rapid antigen detection tests (RADTs) performed from throat swab specimens were developed. Several RADTs, commonly referred to as “rapid strep” tests have been developed with good specificities of greater than or equal to 95%.[23] However, sensitivities vary and with reports of significant false negative rates have been reported and thus negative results warrant confirmation with throat culture.[24–26] This need for confirmation adds additional cost and thus demonstrates the importance of targeting the use of RADTs to high risk patients. Confirmatory cultures are not necessary with negative RADT results in the adult population as there are low risks of serious complications of untreated GABHS in this population.[18]

Antibiotic treatment is required for throat cultures and RADT demonstrating the presence of GABHS. Penicillin is the antibiotic of choice for GABHS; however, amoxicillin suspension is used in the pediatric population due to its improved palatability.[18,21]

Once daily dosing of amoxicillin (≤40 kg 750 mg/day, >40 kg 1000 mg/day) has been studied due to its improved compliance and has been found to be both adequate in efficacy and comparable in side effects to penicillin and multi-dose amoxicillin therapy.[27–29] Oral erythromycin or cephalosporins, in the absence of history of immediate hypersensitivity to beta-lactams, may be used for penicillin-allergic patients.[4]

## Additional Etiologies of Acute Pharyngitis

Group C and G beta-hemolytic streptococci also cause acute pharyngitis with clinical presentation similar to that of GABHS. Both of these bacteria may be transmitted through droplets of food, and their role in acute pharyngitis may be undervalued due to current methods of throat culture evaluation. Both respond to penicillin.[4]

Other etiologies of acute bacterial pharyngitis, although less common, include gonococcal pharyngitis, Vincent's angina, syphilis and diphtheria. *Neisseria gonorrhoeae* may cause asymptomatic infection or may present with exudates, and is commonly transmitted through oral sex.[35] Vincent's angina is caused by spirochetes of the *Treponema* family. It arises from poor dental hygiene and presents with pharyngeal ulcerations. Primary and secondary syphilis may present with oropharyngeal chancres and is caused by the bacteria *Treponema pallidum*.

Pharyngeal *Corynebacterium diphtheriae* infection results in fever, pharyngitis and malaise. Its incidence has decreased due to effective vaccination. It is characterized by a progression from oropharyngeal erythema to a gray pseudomembrane that elicits bleeding if removed.[36] Diagnosis is obtained through throat culture, and in the United States positive cases should be reported to the Center for Disease Control. Diphtheria anti-toxin must be delivered early in the condition, and the patient should be monitored both for airway obstruction and possible cardiac or neurogenic complications.[37]

Acute human immunodeficiency virus (HIV) infection may present with sore throat, cervical lymphadenopathy and fever. Hyperemia and oropharyngeal edema are seen on physical examination, however tonsillar exudates or enlargement are not common.[38,39] Primary HIV is not commonly diagnosed in the acute setting as symptoms are non-specific and resolve.[39] In adolescents who prove to neither be EBV or GABHS positive, an HIV risk assessment is recommended. If there is a history of high risk behavior, serum HIV viral load and antibody titers should be considered.

## Role of Tonsillectomy

Tonsillectomy demonstrated a benefit in decreased rates of infection for the first two years after surgery in cases of severe recurrent acute GABHS pharyngitis characterized by fever, cervical adenopathy and tonsillar exudates. Recurrent infections are defined as at least seven documented severe infections in one year, five in two consecutive years and three in each of three consecutive years.[40,41] Chronic tonsillitis associated with foul taste and halitosis or recurrent tonsillitis in the setting of GABHS carrier state, which are unresponsive to medical therapy, are indications for tonsillectomy according to The American Academy of Otolaryngology-Head and Neck Surgery.[42]

## Complications of Pharyngitis

Complications of GABHS are both suppurative and non-suppurative. Suppurative complications including peritonsillar abscess (PTA) and other abscesses are discussed later in the chapter as deep space neck infections. Rheumatic fever (RF) and post-streptococcal glomerulonephritis (PSGN) are two complications that result from untreated GABHS pharyngitis, presenting one to three weeks after the resolution of pharyngitis.[30,31] RF is characterized by arthritis, carditis, chorea, subcutaneous nodules, and erythema marginatum. This can be prevented by starting appropriate antibiotic therapy within nine days of onset of GABHS pharyngitis symptoms.[31] PSGN has not been found to be prevented by antibiotic therapy of the initial infection. This complication however is commonly self-limited with large rates of spontaneous recovery.[32,33]

Scarlet fever, characterized by scarlatiniform rash in the setting of GABHS pharyngitis, may develop as a result of erythrogenic exotoxin released by the bacteria. Pediatric autoimmune neuropsychiatric disorder (PANDAS) has also been described as a complication of GABHS and is characterized by obsessive-compulsive or involuntary movement disorders in children after infection.[34]

### *Lemierre's syndrome*

A life threatening complication of oropharyngeal and deep neck space infections is internal jugular vein thrombophlebitis, also termed Lemierre's syndrome or post-anginal sepsis. This condition is characterized by a recent history of oropharyngeal infection, internal jugular vein thrombus and identification of *Fusobacterium necrophorum*. It is most commonly seen in adolescents and young adults but has affected younger children.[43] Ramirez *et al.* reported an increased number of serious infections caused by *F. necrophorum* in a pediatric children's hospital from 1995–2002.[44] A recent review reports the pooled mortality from the condition as 5%.[45] The most common findings at presentation are a recent history of sore throat and neck swelling and/or tenderness.[45]

Physical examination of the oropharynx may demonstrate a range of findings, from a benign exam to exudative or ulcerative pharyngitis.[46,47] Patients may frequently present with pulmonary

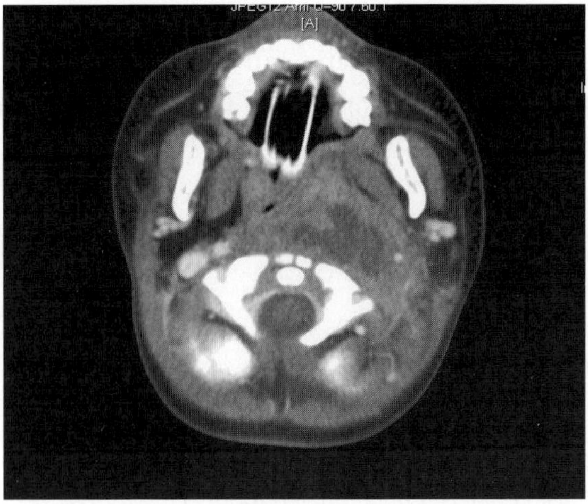


**Fig. 1.** Axial CT scan image showing loculated left parapharyngeal space abscess with thrombosis of the left internal jugular vein.

septic emboli.[46,47] Blood cultures and high resolution computed tomography (CT) with intravenous (IV) contrast are the two primary diagnostic tools for this condition (Fig. 1). Any isolation of *Fusobacterium* species in either throat or blood culture regardless of clinical picture warrants antibiotic therapy.[45] Metronidazole and clindamycin are the antibiotics of choice due to increasing rates of beta-lactamase resistance in *F. necrophorum.*[48] There is no clear consensus on the role of anticoagulation for Lemierre's syndrome. Surgical intervention is often warranted in addition to prolonged IV antibiotic therapy.[45,49]

## CERVICAL LYMPHADENITIS

Cervical lymphadenitis is commonly evaluated by the pediatric otolaryngologist. Although both infectious and inflammatory etiologies exist, infections are more commonly the cause of this finding in the pediatric population. In this chapter, infectious causes will be discussed. The submandibular and deep cervical lymph nodes are more commonly affected. The jugulodisgastric node, of the superior deep cervical nodes, is frequently involved.[50] Infectious causes of cervical lymphadenitis can be characterized as acute or subacute lymphadenitis.[51] Evaluation of a child who presents with cervical lymphadenitis is outlined in Table 2.

**Table 2. Evaluation of pediatric infectious lymphadenitis in the acute care setting.**

| |
|---|
| **History** |
| Onset, duration, progression |
| Associated symptoms |
|     *Cough, coryza, fever, malaise, weight loss, rash, pharyngitis, dental infection* |
| Exposures |
|     *Animals, sick contacts, contaminated foods, TB, HIV risk behavior* |
| Previous antibiotic therapy |
|     *Response, Progression, Recurrence* |
| Immunization history |
| **Physical examination** |
| Vital signs |
|     *Evaluate for fever, tachycardia* |
| Evaluate for respiratory distress |
| Examination of head, eyes, ears, nose, oral cavity and oropharynx |
| Examination of neck |
|     *Unilateral vs. bilateral* |
|     *Single node vs. multiple* |
|     *Greatest size* |
|     *Fluctuance* |
|     *Tenderness* |
|     *Associated skin changes* |
| **Diagnostic tests** |
| Complete blood count with differential |
| C-reactive protein and erythrocyte sedimentation rate |
| **Acute** |
| Bilateral |
|     *URI symptoms: supportive care* |
|     *Pharyngitis: throat culture, monospot* |

(*Continued*)

**Table 2. (*Continued*)**

| |
|---|
| Unilateral large solitary node |
| *Computed tomography scan with intravenous contrast (if not optimal, diagnostic ultrasound)* |
| *Consider needle aspiration for gram stain and culture* |
| *Tuberculin skin test* |
| **If febrile, ill appearing child, perform blood cultures |
| |
| **Subsacute/chronic** |
| Serologic testing based on pertinent history findings |
| *i.e. Bartonella, EBV, HIV, CMV* |

## Acute Lymphadenitis

Acute lymphadenitis most commonly represents reactive lymphadenitis. Reactive lymphadenitis is characterized by multiple bilateral minimally tender lymph nodes that lack associated skin inflammation and demonstrate reactive hyperplasia.[51] It is self-limited and subsides with the resolution of the acute illness. Most common causes are viruses resulting in upper respiratory infections (URIs).[52] Acute pharyngitis, as previously discussed, can also present with reactive lymphadenitis as seen with EBV and GABHS.

Acute, unilateral, tender lymphadenitis with associated inflammation may also be of bacterial etiology. Patients may have associated symptoms of fever, irritability and decreased appetite and may have developed suppuration. *Staphylococcus aureus* and GABHS account for 40% to 80%of infections in pre-school age children with this presentation.[50] The incidence of methicillin resistant *Staphylococcus Aureus* (MRSA) cervical infections in the pediatric population is rising and now comprises as many as 27%–29% of *S. aureus* isolates demonstrating antibiotic resistance.[53,54]

Group B streptococcus presents with acute facial or submandibular swelling and erythema in infants. Anaerobic bacteria, primarily *Bacteroides* species, *Peptococcus* species, and *Peptostreptococcus* species are causative organisms in children with associated periodontal disease.[55]

Bacterial organisms which cause cervical lymphadenitis less frequently include *Francisella tularensis, Pasteurella multocida, Yersinia pestis,* and *Haemophilus influenza* type b.[56]

Treatment is based on the severity of the illness at presentation and the antibiotic sensitivities of the most common organisms. Initial oral antibiotic therapy is recommended for suspected acute bacterial infections with fever and tender non-fluctuant lymphadenitis. Antibiotic choice is based on coverage for both *Staphylococcus* and *Streptococcus* species and beta-lactamase resistance. Amoxicillin-clavulanic acid, cephalosporins or clindamycin may be used. Clindamycin provides appropriate therapy in areas with high prevalence of community-acquired MRSA and for periodontal disease. Hospitalization and the administration of parenteral antibiotics must be considered for very young patients, patients with progression of symptoms and/or patients with presentation of severe illness, (characterized by high fever, cellulitis and fluctuance).[51,57] Initial empiric therapy should be initiated, and antibiotic therapy should be continued for five days after clinical improvement is obtained for a total of ten to 14 days. Persistent or severe clinical findings such as high fever, leukocytosis, or cellulitis suggest suppuration of the involved lymph nodes. Needle aspiration may be adequate for culture in suppurative lymphadenitis, however, surgical incision and drainage is typically warranted.[51] At this point, direct cultures may be obtained and antibiotic therapy may subsequently be tailored. A penrose drain may be placed into the abscess cavity once it is evacuated to prevent early closure.

## Subacute or Chronic Lymphadenitis

Subacute or chronic lymphadenitis is caused by different pathogens than acute lymphadenitis and is characterized by persistent lymphadenopathy or recurrent lymphadenopathy.[51] These infections are often not associated with cellulitis or acute inflammatory signs.

Non-tuberculous mycobacterial infections (also known as *atypical mycobacteria*) and cat scratch disease are the most common etiologies of subacute or chronic lymphadenitis. A unilateral firm node or cluster of nodes that slowly enlarge over weeks is characteristic of non-tuberculous mycobacterial lymphadenitis. Overlying skin may develop a pink or violacious discoloration, and suppuration may ultimately be seen with spontaneous drainage.[58] *Mycobacterium avium-intracellulare* and *Mycobacterium scrofulaceum* are the most commonly isolated strains.[51] A peripherally placed ppd, while not completely diagnostic, may be partially reactive. A CT scan may show intranodal calcifications. Treatment is based on high index of suspicion as definitive diagnosis is only available after positive culture obtained from fine needle aspiration or after surgical biopsy. Surgical excision results in resolution of disease and prevents cutaneous complications. Full excision of affected nodes should be performed. Curettage is also an option but may result in a higher rate of recurrence. Incision and drainage is not recommended.[59] Deep infections where cutaneous involvement is unlikely may be managed conservatively. Superficial infections will also typically self-resolve, however resolution may take six to 12 months and may result in significant cutaneous sequelae (Fig. 2).

Cat scratch disease presents with regional lymphadenitis after skin inoculation with *Bartonella henselae.* Lymphadenitis may develop up to two months after inoculation of the bacterium in the

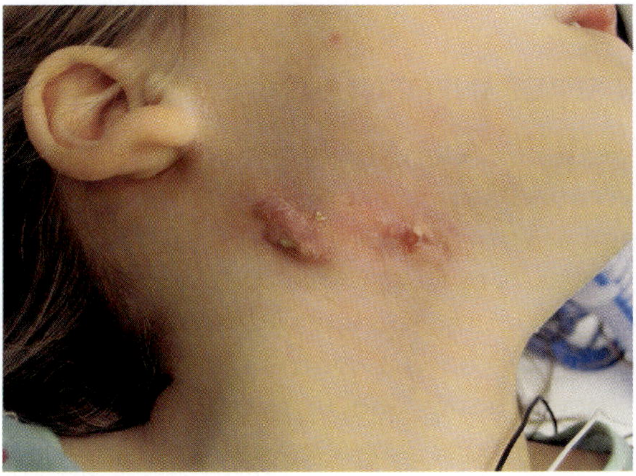

**Fig. 2.** Cutaneous erythema and fistula secondary to untreated atypical mycobacterial lymphadenitis.

region. History is often positive for exposure to cats.[60] A large tender lymph node is present on examination, and constitutional symptoms are generally mild. Fluctuance may be present. Diagnosis is confirmed through serologic testing for *Bartonella henselae.* The use of antibiotics for treatment is controversial, as non-systemic mild to moderate infections are self-limited. However, antibiotics, such as a five-day course of azythromycin, may prevent disseminated disease in a percentage of patients and may expedite the resolution of lymphadenopathy.[61]

*Mycobacterium tuberculosis* results in lymphadenitis with similar presentation to that of atypical mycobacterial infections and often cannot be differentiated clinically.[51] A positive PPD test, history of exposure to individuals infected with tuberculosis and/or an abnormal chest radiograph are consistent with tuberculous infection.[62] Extended multi-drug antibiotic therapy is indicated. Surgical excision is not generally necessary due to high rates of response to anti-tuberculous medications, but it may be indicated in the event of suppuration and associated cellulitis, or in the event that biopsy is necessitated to rule out malignancy.

HIV, cytomegalovirus (CMV), toxoplasmosis, nocardia and fungal infections are additional etiologies to consider in subacute or chronic lymphadenitis.

## DEEP NECK SPACE INFECTIONS

Deep neck space infections are suppurative infections that require urgent intervention. Unlike superficial suppurative infections of cervical lymphadenitis, these infections must be considered life-threatening as they can result in airway compromise. These infections result from the seeding of interfascial spaces with bacteria from infections in other regions of the head and neck, such as pharyngitis, periodontal infections and parotitis. Peritonsillar abscess, parapharyngeal abscess and retropharyngeal abscess require drainage by the otolaryngologist, and delay of intervention increases the risk of spontaneous rupture and aspiration.

**Peritonsillar Abscess**

The peritonsillar space is defined as the space between the tonsillar capsule, the superior constrictor, and the palatopharyngeus muscles. Peritonsillar abscess (PTA) is the most common deep neck space infection in children. PTA is seen in all ages but occurs most frequently in adolescents.[63,64] PTA has an association to GABHS pharyngitis and exudative tonsillitis and presents in the winter and spring months when the incidence of these infections is high. Inflammation of mucous salivary glands of the soft palate in this region may lead to the development of PTA.[65] Peritonsillar infections are polymicrobial with a predominance of group A streptococcus, *Staphylococcus aureus* (including MRSA), and oral anaerobes (*Prevotella, Porphyromonas, Fusobacterium* and *Peptostreptococcus* species).[66]

Common presentation includes severe unilateral sore throat, fever, voice change, drooling and decreased oral intake. Characteristic findings on examination are trismus, erythema of the oropharynx with palatal fullness and tonsillar swelling causing contralateral deviation of the uvula. Uvular deviation and trismus are two physical features that help distinguish this condition from acute pharyngitis, peritonsillar cellulitis, or parapharyngeal space abscess.[67] History and physical examination are typically adequate for the diagnosis of PTA. Computed tomography (CT) with intravenous contrast is indicated when the physical exam is limited and/or when other deep neck infections or complications are suspected. CT scanning should not be performed in children with respiratory symptoms, and the use of sedation for imaging should be carefully evaluated in mild cases as respiratory distress may be exacerbated. In such situations evaluation in the operating room may be warranted.

Patients will require supportive therapy with analgesics and intravenous hydration upon presentation. Unless symptoms are mild and the abscess is small and quickly responsive to antibiotics, decompression of the abscess is required. Controversy exists on the appropriate method, as it may be performed through needle aspiration or incision and drainage under local anesthetic.[68] Conscious sedation has been found to be safe for the drainage of peritonsillar abscesses in an appropriate monitored setting with the proper skilled personnel.[69–71] For pediatric patients who cannot tolerate drainage with the use of local anesthesia or when conscious sedation is not appropriate, drainage must be performed under general anesthesia. In this setting drainage may also be performed by either method, with or without tonsillectomy. Tonsillectomy at the time of drainage, also termed "quincy" tonsillectomy, is sometimes performed in patients with previous history of PTA or recurrent pharyngitis. Quincy tonsillectomies are safe and may decrease future interventions or hospitalizations in this subset of pediatric patients.[72] No consensus exists on the benefit of steroid therapy in the setting of PTA. Clindamycin or ampicillin-sulbactam are appropriate antibiotic therapies, and culture information can aid in medication selection.

Complications of PTA include airway obstruction, aspiration pneumonia, extension into the parapharyngeal space and Lemierre's syndrome.

## Parapharyngeal Abscess

The parapharyngeal space is lateral to the pharynx and extends from the base of the skull to the hyoid bone in the shape of an inverted pyramid. It is defined laterally by the medial parotid fascia, medially by the buccopharyngeal fascia and pharyngeal constrictors, anteriorly by the pterygomandibular raphe and posteriorly by the carotid sheath. Parapharyngeal infections develop from periodontal infections, PTAs, or rarely otitis, parotitis and mastoiditis.[73]

Patients will generally be ill-appearing and present with fever, sore throat, dysphagia, and possibly respiratory distress. Physical exam demonstrates trismus, and medial fullness of the lateral pharyngeal wall. As opposed to PTA, the uvula is typically not deviated, and the tonsils are largely symmetrical. Swelling and induration may be present in the neck, and flexible fiberoptic laryngoscopy will demonstrate asymmetry of the pharynx with bulging medially on the affected side. CT scan with intravenous contrast is the modality of choice to evaluate the extent of the abscess or other possible complications. Infections are also polymicrobial with organisms isolated as in PTA.[66]

Parenteral antibiotic therapy is required with empiric coverage for the common aerobic and anaerobic pathogens. If the abscess is large and the patient's symptoms are severe, surgical drainage is indicated. The CT scan will show the extent and location of the abscess as well as its orientation to the great vessels. Most commonly the abscess is medial to the vessels and judicious intraoral drainage may be performed. If the abscess extends far into the neck or lateral to the great vessels, external approach through a cervical incision is warranted.[74] Medical therapy with intravenous antibiotics and CT follow-up has been advocated for non-complicated parapharyngeal infections.[75]

Complications of parapharyngeal space abscess include airway obstruction, aspiration pneumonia, Lemierre's syndrome or carotid erosion from carotid sheath involvement.

**Retropharyngeal Abscess**

The retropharyngeal space is found posterior to the pharynx and anterior to the cervical vertebrae extending from the base of skull to the posterior mediastinum. It is defined anteriorly by the buccopharyngeal fascia, laterally by the carotid sheaths and parapharyngeal spaces, and posteriorly by the alar deep cervical fascia. Retropharyngeal lymph node chains are prominent in childhood and involute at puberty.[76] These drain several regions of the head and thus are susceptible to infection leading to higher rates of retropharyngeal abscesses in children. Preceding factors include upper airway infection, periodontal disease, penetrating pharyngeal trauma or cervical spine osteomyelitis.

Children present with fever, sore throat, neck pain, neck swelling, decreased oral intake, and decreased range of motion in the neck. Increased stertor and snoring is frequently appreciated, and frank respiratory distress may occur. Infants may present with stridor.[77] Physical exam findings can include cervical lymphadenopathy, torticollis and a retropharyngeal bulge. Diagnosis is confirmed and differentiated from retropharyngeal cellulitis or phlegmon by CT with IV contrast (Figs. 3a and 3b). As with the other deep neck space

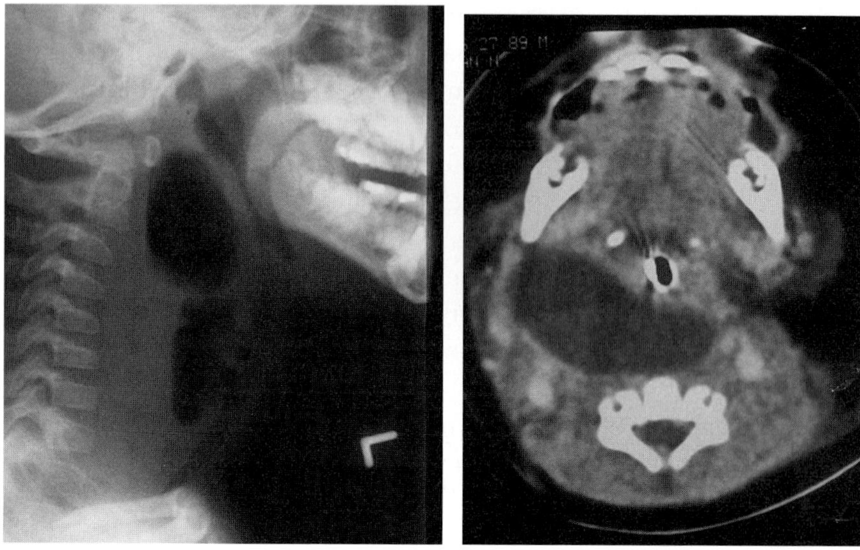

(a) (b)

**Fig. 3.** Large retropharyngeal abscess seen on lateral soft tissue plain film (a) and CT (b).

infections discussed, retropharyngeal abscesses are polymicrobial demonstrating *Streptococcus*, *Staphylococcus*, *Hemophilus* species and common oral anaerobes.[78]

Intravenous antibiotics are required and must account for the polymicrobial nature of infection and high incidence of beta-lactamase resistance in these strains. Some retropharyngeal space infections may be managed with parenteral antibiotics alone. Surgical drainage may be performed for a discrete abscess in a symptomatic patient. Traditionally a trans-oral approach is preferred, although an external anterior cervical approach may be required for extensive or recurrent abscesses.

Children may suffer from complications of retropharyngeal abscesses which include airway obstruction, aspiration pneumonia, mediastinitis, or less commonly Lemierre's syndrome, carotid artery erosion or atlanto-axial instability.

## REFERENCES


1. Brandtzaeg P. Immunology of tonsils and adenoids: everything the ENT surgeon needs to know. *Int J Pediatric Otorhinolaryngol* 2003; 67(Suppl 1):S69–S76.
2. Crelin ES. *Functional Anatomy of the Newborn.* London: Yale University Press, 1973.
3. Richtsmeier WJ, Shikhari AM. The physiology and immunology of the pharyngeal lymphoid tissue. *Otolaryngol Clin North Am* 1987;20:219–228.
4. Gerber MA. Diagnosis and treatment of pharyngitis in children. *Pediatr Clin N Am* 2005;52:729–747.
5. Bisno AL. Acute pharyngitis. *N Engl J Med* 2001;344:205–211.
6. Putto A. Febrile exudative tonsillitis: viral or streptococcal? *Pediatrics* 1987 Jul;80(1):6–12.
7. Evans AS, Niederman JC. Epstein-Barr virus. In: Evans AS, Kaslow RA, eds. *Viral Infections of Human Epidemilogy and Control.* New York: Plenum Publishing, 1989.
8. Ray PJ. Infectious mononucleosis. *Pediatr Rev* 1998 Aug;19(8):276–279.
9. Ebell MH. Epstein-Barr virus infectious mononucleosis. *Am Fam Physician* 2004;70:1279–1287.
10. Brigden ML, Au S, Thompson S, Brigden S, Doyle P, Tsaparas Y. Infectious mononucleosis in an outpatient population: diagnostic utility of 2 automated hematology analyzers and the sensitivity and specificity of Hoagland's criteria in heterophile-positive patients. *Arch Pathol Lab Med* 1999 Oct;123(10):875–881.
11. Buchwald DS, Rea TD, Katon WJ, Russo JE, Ashley RL. Acute infectious mononucleosis: characteristics of patients who report failure to recover. *SO Am J Med* 2000 Nov;109(7):531–537.
12. Candy B, Hotopf M. Steroids for symptom control in infectious mononucleosis. *Cochrane Database Syst Rev* 2006 19 Jul;3:CD004402.
13. Torre D, Tambini R. Acyclovir for treatment of infectious mononucleosis: a meta-analysis. *Scand J Infect Dis* 1999;31(6):543–547.
14. Stevenson DS, Webster G, Stewart IA. Acute tonsillectomy in the management of infectious mononucleosis. *J Laryngol Otol* 1992 Nov;106(11):989–991.

15. Chan SC, Dawes PJ. The management of severe infectious mononucleosis tonsillitis and upper airway obstruction. *J Laryngol Otol* 2001 Dec;115(12):973–977.
16. Irving JA, Cameron BR, Ludemann JP, Taylor G. Florid infectious mononucleosis: clinicopathological correlation in acute tonsillectomy. *Int J Pediatr Otorhinolaryngol* 2002 21 Oct;66(1):87–92.
17. Bisno AL, Gerber MA, Gwaltney JM Jr, Kaplan EL, Schwartz RH. Practice guidelines for the diagnosis and management of group A streptococcal pharyngitis. Infectious Diseases Society of America. *Clin Infect Dis* 2002 15 Jul;35(2):113–125.
18. Bisno AL, Gerber MA, Gwaltney JM, Kaplan EL, Schwartz RH. Practice guideline for the diagnosis and management of group A streptococcal pharyngitis. *Clin Infect Dis* 2002;35:113–125.
19. Powers GF, Boisvert PL. Age as a factor in Streptococcosis. *J Pediatr* 1944;25:481–504.
20. Wald ER, Green MD, Schwartz B, Barbadora K. A streptococcal score card revisited. *Pediatric Emerg Care* 1998;14:109–111.
21. Attia MW, Zaoutis T, Klein JD, Meier FA. Performance of a predictive model for streptococcal pharyngitis in children. *Arch Pediatr Adolesc Med* 2001;155:687–691.
22. Snow V, Mottur-Pilson C, Cooper RJ, Hoffman JR. Principles of appropriate antibiotic use of acute pharyngitis in adults. *Ann Intern Med* 2001;134:506–508.
23. Gerber MA, Shulman ST. Rapid diagnosis of pharyngitis caused by group A streptococci. *Clin Microbiol Rev* 2004;17:571–580.
24. Bisno AL, Gerber MA, Gwaltney JM Jr, Kaplan EL, Schwartz RH. Practice guidelines for the diagnosis and management of group A streptococcal pharyngitis. Infectious Diseases Society of America. *Clin Infect Dis* 2002 15 Jul;35(2):113–125.
25. McIsaac WJ, Kellner JD, Aufricht P, Vanjaka A, Low DE. Empirical validation of guidelines for the management of pharyngitis in children and adults. *JAMA* 2004 7 Apr;291(13):1587–1595.
26. Leung AK, Newman R, Kumar A, Davies HD. Rapid antigen detection testing in diagnosing group A beta-hemolytic streptococcal pharyngitis. *Expert Rev Mol Diagn* 2006 Sep;6(5):761–766.

27. Feder HM Jr, Gerber MA, Randolph MF. Once-daily therapy for streptococcal pharyngitis with amoxicillin. *Pediatrics* 1999 Jan;103(1): 47–51.
28. Shvartzman P, Tabenkin H, Rosentzwaig A, Dolginov F. Treatment of streptococcal pharyngitis with amoxycillin once a day. *BMJ* 1993;306:1170–1172.
29. Clegg HW, Ryan AG, Dallas SD, Kaplan EL, Johnson DR, Norton HJ, Roddey OF, Martin ES, Swetenburg RL, Koonce EW, Felkner MM, Giftos PM. Treatment of streptococcal pharyngitis with once-daily compared with twice-daily amoxicillin: a noninferiority trial. *Pediatr Infect Dis J* 2006 Sep;25(9):761–767.
30. Rammelkamp CH Jr, Stolzer BL. The latent period before the onset of acute rheumatic fever. *Yale J Biol Med* 1961 Dec–1962 Feb;34: 386–398.
31. Catanzaro FJ, Stetson CA, Morris AJ, *et al.* The role of streptococcus in the pathogenesis of rheumatic fever. *Am J Med* 1954;17:749–756.
32. Lewy JE, Salinas-Madrigal L, Herdson PB, Pirani CL, Metcoff J. Clinicopathologic correlations in acute poststreptococcal glomerulonephritis. A correlation between renal functions, morphologic damage and clinical course of 46 children with acute poststreptococcal glomerulonephritis. *Medicine (Baltimore)* 1971 Nov;50(6):453–501 (Review).
33. Tejani A, Ingulli E. Poststreptococcal glomerulonephritis. Current clinical and pathologic concepts. *Nephron* 1990;55(1):1–5.
34. Swedo SE, Leonard HL, Garvey M, Mittleman B, Allen AJ, Perlmutter S. *et al.* Pediatric autoimmune neuropsychiatric disorders associated with streptococcal infections: clinical description of the first 50 cases. *Am J Psychiatry* 1998;155:264–271.
35. Morris SR, Klausner JD, Buchbinder SP, Wheeler SL, Koblin B, Coates T, Chesney M, Colfax GN. Prevalence and incidence of pharyngeal gonorrhea in a longitudinal sample of men who have sex with men: the EXPLORE study. *Clin Infect Dis* 2006 15 Nov;43(10):1284–1289.
36. Farizo KM, Strebel PM, Chen RT, Kimbler A, Cleary TJ, Cochi SL. Fatal respiratory disease due to *Corynebacterium diphtheriae*: case report and review of guidelines for management, investigation, and control. *SO Clin Infect Dis* 1993 Jan;16(1):59–68.

37. MacGregor RR. Corynebacterium diphtheriae. In: Mandell GL, Bennett JE, Dolin R, eds. *Principles and Practice of Infectious Diseases*, 6th Ed. Philadelphia: Churchill Livingstone, 2005, p. 2457.
38. Valle SL. Febrile pharyngitis as the primary sign of HIV infection in a cluster of cases linked by sexual contact. *Scand J Infect Dis* 1987;19(1):13–17.
39. Schacker T, Collier AC, Hughes J, Shea T, Corey L. Clinical and epidemiologic features of primary HIV infection. *Ann Intern Med* 1996; 125:257–264.
40. Paradise JL, Bluestone CD, Bachman RZ, Colborn DK, Bernard BS, Taylor FH, Rogers KD, Schwarzbach RH, Stool SE, Friday GA, *et al.* Efficacy of tonsillectomy for recurrent throat infections in severely affected children. *N Engl J Med* 1984;310:674–683.
41. Baugh RF, Archer SM, Mitchell RB, Rosenfeld RM, Amin R, Burns JJ, *et al.* Clinical Practice Guideline: tonsillectomy in children. American Academy of Otolaryngology — Head and Neck Surgery Foundation. *Otolaryngol Head Neck Surg* 2011 Jan;144(1 Suppl):S1–30.
42. Anonymous. *1995 Clinical Indicators Compendium.* Alexandria (VA): American Academy of Otolaryngology–Head and Neck Surgery, 1995.
43. Sinave CP, Hardy GJ, Fardy PW. The Lemierre syndrome: suppurative thrombophlebitis of the internal jugular vein secondary to oropharyngeal infection. *Medicine (Baltimore)* 1989;68:85–94.
44. Ramirez S, Hild TG, Rudolph CN, Sty JR, Kehl SC, Havens P, Henrickson K, Chusid MJ. Increased diagnosis of Lemierre syndrome and other *Fusobacterium necrophorum* infections at a children's hospital. *Pediatrics* 2003 Nov; 112(5):e380.
45. Karkos PD, Asrani S, Karkos CD, Leong SC, Theochari EG, Alexopoulou TD, Assimakopoulos AD. Lemierre's syndrome: a systematic review. *Laryngoscope.* 2009 Aug;119(8):1552–1559.
46. Golpe R, Marin B, Alonso M. Lemierre's syndrome (necrobacillosis). *Postgrad Med J* 1999 Mar;75(881):141–144.
47. Sinave CP, Hardy GJ, Fardy PW. The Lemierre syndrome: suppurative thrombophlebitis of the internal jugular vein secondary to oropharyngeal infection. *Medicine (Baltimore)* 1989 Mar;68(2):85–94.
48. Appelbaum PC, Philippon A, Jacobs MR, Spangler SK, Gutmann L. Characterization of beta-lactamases from non-Bacteroides fragilis

group Bacteroides spp. belonging to seven species and their role in beta-lactam resistance. *Antimicrob Agents Chemother* 1990 Nov;34(11): 2169–2176.

49. Chirinos JA, Lichtstein DM, Garcia J, Tamariz LJ. The evolution of Lemierre syndrome: report of 2 cases and review of the literature. *Medicine (Baltimore)* 2002;81:458–465.
50. Kelly C, Kelly R. Lymphadenopathy in children. *Pediatr Clin North Am* 1998;45:875–888.
51. Gosche JR, Vick L. Acute, subacute, and chronic cervical lymphadenitis in children. *Semin Pediatr Surg.* 2006 May;15(2):99–106.
52. Peters T, Edwards K. Cervical lymphadenopathy and adenitis. *Pediatr Rev* 2000;21:399–404.
53. Guss J, Kazahaya K. Antibiotic-resistant *Staphylococcus aureus* in community-acquired pediatric neck abscesses. *Int J Pediatr Otorhinolaryngol.* 2007 Jun;71(6):943–948.
54. Inman JC, Rowe M, Ghostine M, Fleck T. Pediatric neck abscesses: changing organisms and empiric therapies. *Laryngoscope.* 2008 Dec;118(12):2111–2114.
55. Bodenstein L, Altman R. Cervical lymphadenitis in infants and children. *Semin Pediatr Surg* 1994;3:134–141.
56. Chesney P. Cervical lymphadenitis and neck infections. In: Long S, Pickering L, Prober C, eds. *Principles and Practice of Pediatric Infectious Diseases,* 2nd Ed. Philadelphia: *Churchill Livingstone,* 2003, pp. 165–176.
57. Khayr W, Taepke J. Management of peritonsillar abscess: needle aspiration versus incision and drainage versus tonsillectomy. PTA management. *Am J Ther* 2005 Jul–Aug;12(4):344–350.
58. Fraser L, Moore P, Kubba H. Atypical mycobacterial infection of the head and neck in children: a 5-year retrospective review. *Otolaryngol Head Neck Surg* 2008 Mar;138(3):311–314.
59. Lindeboom JA, Kuijper EJ, Bruijnesteijn van Coppenraet ES, Lindeboom R, Prins JM. Surgical excision versus antibiotic treatment for nontuberculous mycobacterial cervicofacial lymphadenitis in children: a multicenter, randomized, controlled trial. *Clin Infect Dis* 2007 15 Apr;44(8):1057–1064.
60. Carithers HA. Cat-scratch disease. An overview based on a study of 1,200 patients. *Am J Dis Child* 1985 Nov;139(11):1124–1233.

61. Rolain JM, Brouqui P, Koehler JE; Maguina C, Dolan MJ, Raoult D Recommendations for treatment of human infections caused by Bartonella species. *Antimicrob Agents Chemother* 2004 Jun;48(6):1921–1933.
62. Spyridis P, Maltezou H, Hantzakos A. *et al.* Mycobacterial cervical lymphadenitis in children: clinical and laboratory factors of importance for differential diagnosis. *Scand J Infect Dis* 2001;33:362–366.
63. Schraff S, McGinn JD, Derkay CS. Peritonsillar abscess in children: a 10-year review of diagnosis and management. *Int J Pediatr Otorhinolaryngol* 2001 Mar;57(3):213–218.
64. Ungkanont K, Yellon RF, Weissman JL, Casselbrant ML, Gonzalez-Valdepena H, Bluestone CD. Head and neck space infections in infants and children. *Otolaryngol Head Neck Surg* 1995 Mar;112(3):375–382.
65. Passy V. Pathogenesis of peritonsillar abscess. *Laryngoscope* 1994; 104(2):185–190.
66. Brook I. Microbiology and management of peritonsillar, retropharyngeal, and parapharyngeal abscesses. *J Oral Maxillofac Surg* 2004 Dec;62(12):1545–1550.
67. Szuhay G, Tewfik TL. Peritonsillar abscess or cellulitis? A clinical comparative paediatric study. *J Otolaryngol* 1998 Aug;27(4):206–212.
68. Khayr W, Taepke J. Management of peritonsillar abscess: needle aspiration versus incision and drainage versus tonsillectomy. *Am J Ther* 2005 Jul–Aug;12(4):344–350.
69. Suskind DL, Park J, Piccirillo JF, Lusk RP, Muntz HR. Conscious sedation: a new approach for peritonsillar abscess drainage in the pediatric population. *Arch Otolaryngol Head Neck Surg* 1999 Nov;125(11):1197–1200.
70. Bauer PW, Lieu JE, Suskind DL, Lusk RP. The safety of conscious sedation in peritonsillar abscess drainage. *Arch Otolaryngol Head Neck Surg* 2001 Dec;127(12):1477–1480.
71. Luhmann JD, Kennedy RM, McAllister JD, Jaffe DM. Sedation for peritonsillar abscess drainage in the pediatric emergency department. *Pediatr Emerg Care* 2002 Feb;18(1):1–3.
72. Yellon RF. Head and neck space infections. In: Bluestone CD, Casselbrant ML, Stool SE, *et al.*, eds. *Pediatric Otolaryngology*, 4th Ed. Philadelphia: Saunders, 2003, p. 1681.
73. Page C, Biet A, Zaatar R, Strunski V. Parapharyngeal abscess: diagnosis and treatment. *Eur Arch Otorhinolaryngol* 2008;265:681–686.

74. Sichel J-Y, Dano I, Hocwald E, Biron A, Eliashar R. Nonsurgical management of parapharyngeal space infections: a prospective study. *Laryngoscope* 2002;112:906–910.
75. Hammerschlag PE, Hammerschlag MR. Peritonsillar, retropharyngeal, parapharyngeal abscesses. In: Feigin RD, Cherry JD, eds. *Textbook of Pediatric Infectious Diseases,* 3rd Ed. Philadelphia: Saunders, 1992, pp. 166–171.
76. Thompson JW, Cohen SR, Reddix P. Retropharyngeal abscess in children. *Laryngoscope* 1988;98:589–592.
77. Asmar BI. Bacteriology of retropharyngeal abscess in children. *Pediatr Infect Dis J* 1990;9:595–597.
78. Gaglani MJ, Edwards MS. Clinical indicators of childhood retropharyngeal abscess. *Am J Emerg Med* 1995 May;13(3):333–336.

# 14

# Benign Salivary Gland Disorders in Children

*Diego A. Preciado and Sukgi S. Choi*

## INTRODUCTION

Salivary gland disorders, with the exception of inflammatory conditions, are infrequent in children when compared to adults.[1] Non-obstructive inflammatory and congenital conditions are generally more prevalent than neoplastic lesions in children.[2] The goal of this chapter is to review the evaluation and management of benign salivary gland conditions encountered in the pediatric population.

## ANATOMY AND PHYSIOLOGY

The salivary glands are derived from ectoderm and are grouped into major and minor glands. The major glands drain into the oral cavity through end-excretory ducts and include the paired parotid, submandibular, and sublingual glands. The histological characteristics of the salivary glands are identical in adults and children older than two years of age.[3] Their basic functional secretory units are comprised by an acinus, a secretory duct, and a collecting duct. The parotid and submandibular glands have a single large-caliber end-excretory extraglandular collecting duct with only a few major interlobular intraglandular collecting ducts. The interlobular ducts are connected to multiple small intralobular secretory ducts, which transport saliva from acini. In contrast to the parotid and submandibular glands, the sublingual glands empty through ten to 12 smaller and distinct end-excretory ducts. Acini are composed of a central lumen encircled pyramidal cells which can be either serous or mucinous. These cells are in turn surrounded by flat myoepithelial cells. The parotid gland acini are primarily comprised by serous cells, while the sublingual gland acini are chiefly comprised by mucinous cells. The submandibular glands have mixed cell acini.

The minor salivary glands are basically groups of individual secretory units distributed throughout the submucosa of the oral cavity with small, short convoluted end-excretory ducts. Like sublingual glands, their acini are primarily mucinous.[4]

The parotid glands are smaller and rounder in infants compared to adults. The facial nerve exits the skull base through the stylomastoid foramen and courses through the substance of the parotids branching into its main peripheral branches within the glandular tissue. In infants less than two, the nerve exits the skull base positioned in a superficial location just underneath the subcutaneous tissues posterior to the gland. With tympanic pneumatization and formation of the mastoid tip by two years of age, the facial nerve exits in a deeper location, but takes a more abrupt lateral turn than in adults. Injury to the facial nerve during parotidectomy is one of the most common causes of facial paralysis in children. The marginal mandibular branch of the facial nerve courses superficially just medial to the platysma and can be easily injured while surgically approaching the submandibular gland.

The secretion of saliva is under autonomic nervous system control. The bulk of salivary flow comes from the parotid and submandibular glands. At rest, salivary flow is maintained primarily by the submandibular glands. Saliva is important in preventing oral mucosal dryness and trauma, aiding normal deglutition, and maintaining orodental hygiene.

## EVALUATION AND MANAGEMENT

The evaluation of children with disorders of the salivary glands should begin with a thorough history and physical examination. Much like in other head and neck pathologies, of particular importance in the history is the onset, duration, magnitude and location of swelling. The presence of systemic symptoms should be determined. The physical examination should include careful bimanual palpation of the glands. In children, because salivary gland enlargement can often be misdiagnosed as cervical lymphandenopathy, care must be taken to distinguish these entities. Facial nerve function should be assessed for subtle or discrete weaknesses or asymmetries. Careful inspection of the salivary gland orifices should be performed focusing on the quantity and consistency of the salivary content. Repeat examination may be helpful and necessary to follow the natural history of the disease, especially in chronic recurrent conditions of the salivary glands seen in childhood.

Adjunctive evaluation techniques done on an outpatient basis include fine needle aspiration, ultrasonography, computed tomography (CT), magnetic resonance imaging (MRI), and sialography. CT may be especially useful in delineating lesions within the deeper portions of the parotid glands, and in distinguishing intraglandular lesions from cervical ones. MRI is more sensitive than CT in defining the nature and character of lesions within the salivary glands, but in children often requires the use of sedation and in some cases general anesthesia. Ultrasonography can be used alone to detect intrinsic vs. extrinsic masses, and distinguish solid from cystic lesions. Lesions can be measured and easily followed with repeat examinations. Advantages, especially in children, include low cost, avoidance of radiation, and avoidance of anesthesia. Sialography allows for recognition of sialectasis and can provide insights into the anatomic structure of the duct and gland, disclosing the presence of obstructions, duct narrowing, dilatations, or traumatic transactions. Siaolography should not be performed in the setting of acute infection. Sialendoscopy is a relatively new tool that allows for direct endoscopic evaluation of the end-excretory ducts.[5,6] It provides interventional access either for retrieval of sialoliths, or for dilatation of obstructed ducts.[7] Sialendoscopy has not replaced sialography and appears to be a complementary technique in managing obstructive salivary gland disorders.[8] In children, general anesthesia is required for sialendoscopy. The diagnostic yield of fine needle aspiration is dependent on institutional expertise with the technique, but in many cases can be useful in distinguishing benign from malignant pathologies and for guiding operative planning.[9]

Laboratory tests are helpful in some cases. Leukocyte count and differential can help distinguish bacterial from viral infections, assess severity of systemic involvement, and aid in following disease progression. Chest radiographs and purified protein derivative (PPD) skin tests are of importance when tuberculosis or atypical tuberculosis is a consideration. HIV testing is useful in instances of bilateral parotid cystic disease or in the presence of risk factors.

Biopsy of discrete salivary gland lesions in children most typically is excisional rather than incisional and should be considered when firm, solid lesions have persisted for more than six weeks or when FNA cannot rule out malignancy. The role of incisional biopsy is limited to defining cell type of known malignancy to direct medical management. In the parotid gland, excisional biopsy most often entails a superficial parotidectomy with careful dissection of the facial nerve. Excisional biopsy of submandibular gland lesions is accomplished by removal of the involved submandibular gland.

The outpatient, inpatient, emergency, and operative management of benign salivary conditions depends on the nature of the problem. Given that these conditions encompass a wide array of pathology, the ultimate management of these disorders is not uniform. However, many of the disorders can present with similar signs and symptoms. Adequate treatment is based first and foremost on accurate diagnosis. In general, benign pathologic conditions can be classified into non-neoplastic and neoplastic. Non-neoplastic lesions can be grouped into inflammatory, autoimmune, granulomatous, and congenital lesions. Neoplastic benign lesions in children in most cases are comprised of lymphatic or vascular malformations but can also include benign solid salivary gland tumors.

## INFLAMMATORY CONDITIONS

### Acute Viral Sialadenitis

Viral agents associated with acute salivary gland infection include mumps, Coxsackie A, parainfluenza 1 and 3, and Epstein-Barr and HIV. Previously, mumps was considered the most frequent cause of inflammatory parotitis, however with the routine usage of the MMR (mumps, measles, rubella) vaccine, the number of mumps cases has continued to decline. From 2001 to 2003, fewer than 300 cases of mumps were reported in the United States, a 99% decline from the 185,691 cases reported in 1968.[10] However, in 2005 there were large Midwest US and UK outbreaks of mumps in adolescents, suggesting possible waning of vaccine immunity and that mumps once again may become more prevalent.[11] The diagnosis of mumps is made on clinical grounds. The infection is characterized by painful swelling of the salivary glands, most often the parotids (Fig. 1), accompanied by malaise, loss of appetite, fever, chills, and sore throat. Orchitis, pancreatitis, and meninoencephalitis can also occur. Sensorineural hearing loss, frequently unilateral, can result in rare instances. The disease is rarely fatal. Laboratory screening reveals mild lymphocyotosis. Amylase levels, complement fixation, and hemagglutination tests can be used for diagnostic confirmation. Management is symptomatic in the form of hydration, fever, and pain control, and the infection usually resolves over a few weeks.

### Acute Suppurative Bacterial Sialadenitis

Acute bacterial sialadenitis in childhood may present in a similar manner to viral sialadenitis, however, the clinical picture is more prone to acute episodes of exacerbation and remission. In contrast to adults, children may have recurrent episodes of acute sialadenitis, especially of the parotid glands, that span many years which often subsides by puberty.[12] The pathogenesis results from salivary stasis secondary to obstruction or decreased salivary production. Predisposing factors include dehydration, calculi, duct strictures, and sialectasis. In children, trauma from repeated biting, dental appliances, or molar tooth

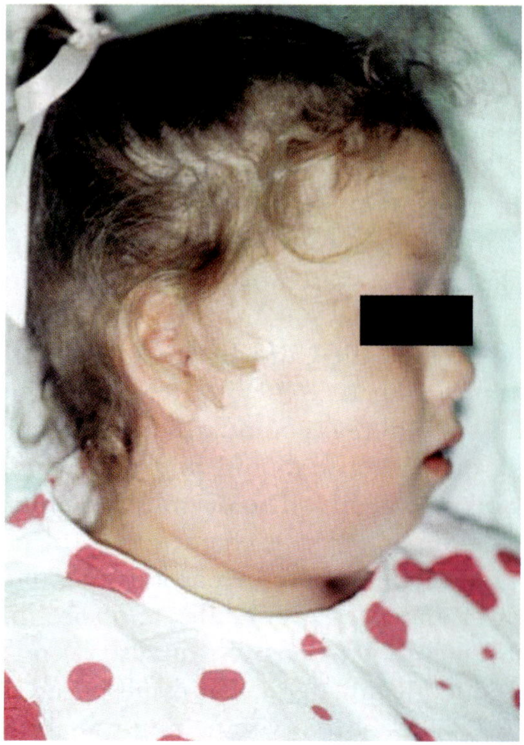

**Fig. 1.** Child with acute swelling of right parotid gland.

eruption can also result in the condition. Signs and symptoms include pain and swelling in the glands and overlying soft tissues. Purulent secretions can sometimes be expressed through the natural glands' orifice by manual "milking" of the involved gland. *Staphylococcus aureus* and *Streptococcus viridians* are the most commonly cultured organisms.[13] Treatment involves adequate hydration, massage, local heat, sialogogues, and appropriate administration of antibiotics with gram positive coverage, especially to *S. aureus* such as clindamycin, cefalexin, or vancomycin for severe infections administration. Recurrent attacks can lead to ductal metaplasia with increased mucous glands, resulting in formation of more viscous saliva. In turn, this leads to higher propensity of salivary stasis, and recurrent infection. The need for surgery in these children is rare. In some cases,

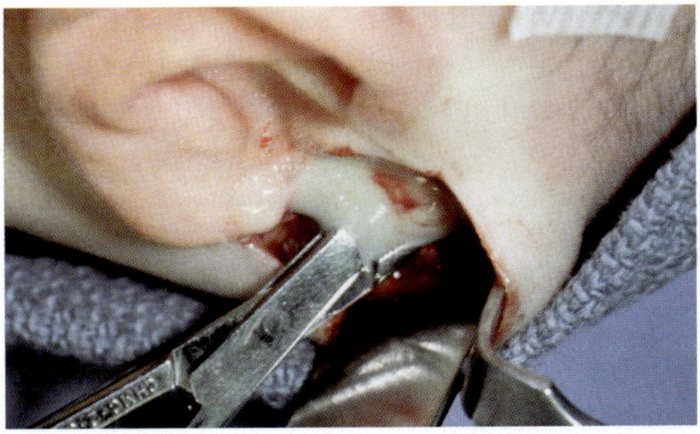

**Fig. 2.** Parotidectomy approach for drainage of a parotid abscess.

parotid abscess may form late in the disease. The abscess should be drained through a standard parotidectomy incision, raising of a preauricular subdermal facial rhytidectomy-type flap, and radial incisions along the parotid fascia in the direction of the facial nerve branches (Fig. 2).

Neonatal sialadenitis is a variation of acute bacterial sialadenitis. It occurs in otherwise healthy infants less than one year of age, and in premature neonates. Resolution occurs promptly, and recurrence is rare. The disease is usually limited to a single gland, and signs and symptoms of systemic disease may not be seen.

## Chronic Recurrent Sialadenitis

Children are at particular risk for developing recurrent sialadenitis. In the parotid gland, this condition is often termed "recurrent parotitis of childhood". The etiology of the condition is unclear, as stated previously, repeated infections may lead to ductal metaplasia ultimately leading to bacterial stasis. Colonization with opportunistic oral pathogens can then lead to chronic recurrent sialadenitis. Congenital ectasia of portions of the ductal system may also be a predisposing factor in this condition.[14] A familial form of recurrent parotitis of childhood has been described with autosomal dominant inheritance.[15] In addition, immunologic abnormalities with isolated

IgG or IgA deficiencies have been associated with recurrent parotitis. Autoimmune exocrinopathy can also present as recurrent parotitis.[16] Finally, viral infections may also play a role as many patients have preceding a history of mumps or EBV parotitis. Recurrent parotitis has a reported incidence of 20% in HIV infected children. End stage disease can be characterized by sialectasis, ductal ectasia, and progressive acinar destruction with massive lymphocytic infiltration. The treatment of the condition involves ruling out immunologic deficiencies or autoimmune causes and administration of prolonged courses of gram-positive antibiotic coverage often up to six weeks. In cases of recurrent, unmitigated parotid infections, with sialographic findings of altered ductal architecture, total parotidectomy during a period of quiescence may be necessary (Fig. 3). Superficial parotidectomy alone appears to increase the risk of recurrent sialadenitis.[17] Given the risk to the facial nerve of total parotidectomy and the fact that the recurrent nature of the condition seems to remit by puberty, a conservative approach is more frequently employed. Recurrent infections of the submandi-bular gland are treated with surgical extirpation of the involved gland.

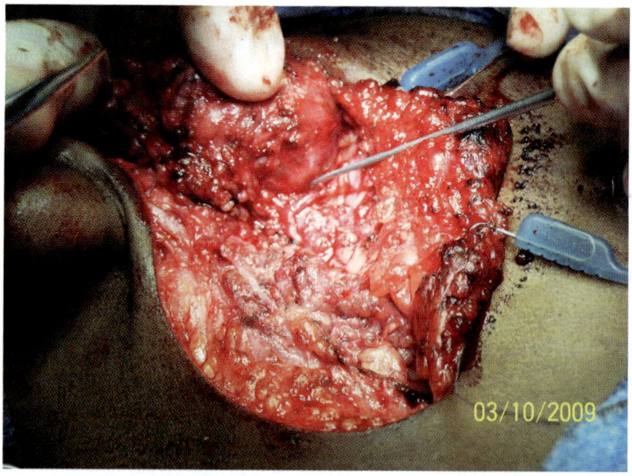


**Fig. 3.** Total parotidectomy with careful dissection around branches of the facial nerve.

In children, true obstructive disease leading to chronic sialadenitis is less frequent than in adults. Obstructive disease in children is frequently associated either with strictures of the salivary ducts or with sialoliths. Strictures may result from trauma, recurrent infection, congenital abnormalities, or neoplasms. Diagnosis is made with sialography with or without sialoendoscopy. Interventional sialoendoscopy has added a new dimension in the treatment of obstructive sialadenitis with early reports demonstrating very encouraging results.[18] Sialoliths are extremely rare in children and most frequently involve the submandibular glands. The average age of presentation is ten years and males are more often affected than females. In cases where the stones are not readily accessible near the ductal orifice, or not amenable to removal via sialoendoscopy, gland excision is indicated.

## AUTOIMMUNE CONDITIONS

### Benign Lymphoepithelial Disease

Benign lymphoepithelial disease in children is less frequent than in adults and typically characterized by unilateral or bilateral enlargement of major or minor salivary glands or lacrimal glands.[19] In children it typically presents after the age of five. Salivary gland enlargement is typically tender to palpation and accompanied by fever. Diagnosis is made by biopsy or fine needle aspiration. In some cases, the enlargement is accompanied by formation of cysts that can either be palpated or discovered on CT or MR imaging. Benign lymphoepithelial cysts represent a clinically and pathologically distinct condition and are frequently associated with HIV infection.[20] Treatment is typically conservative, with observation and antiretroviral therapy in cases of HIV infection. Pure lymphopithelial lesions without cysts typically resolve into adolescence. Surgery is reserved for select cases where cavitary lesions develop that cannot be distinguished from neoplasms. Benign lymphoepithelial lesions may be associated with Sjogren's syndrome and lymphoma.[21]

### Sjogren's Syndrome

Sjogren's syndrome is an autoimmune disease characterized by lymphocytic infiltration of the salivary and lacrimal glands most frequently in association with autoantibodies to nuclear antigens.[22] Inflammation eventually leads to destruction of glandular structures resulting in xerostomia, xerophthalmia, and keratoconjunctivits sicca. The condition is less frequent in children than in adults and the associated clinical manifestations are more variable. Immunologic tests for antinuclear antibodies and antibodies to Sjögren's syndrome antigens A and B (SS-A and SS-B) are present in 50% to 80% of patients.[16] Diagnosis can be made in most cases by minor salivary gland lip biopsy. Treatment of the condition involves mitigating damage caused by the conjunctival and oral dryness. This entails administration of eye lubrication, oral sialogogues, and dental treatment with fluoride. The usage of immunosuppressant medications such as corticosteroids or cytotoxic drugs is handled best by pediatric rheumatologists and reserved usually for cases with severe extrasalivary gland complications such as glomerulonephritis or necrotizing vasculitis.

## GRANULOMATOUS DISEASE

Granulomatous diseases such as mycobacterial disease, sarcoidosis, cat-scratch disease, and actinomycosis can cause chronic sialoadenitis with slow, painless enlargement of the major salivary glands. Localized nodules are often present that must be distinguished from neoplasms.

### Mycobacterial Disease

Primary salivary tuberculosis remains an uncommon entity, however, cervical lymphadenopathy from *Mycobacterium tuberculosis* has become significantly more frequent due to the HIV epidemic. Tuberculosis in the salivary glands is much more common in adults than in children. It is believed to evolve from a focus in the tonsils or gingiva ascending to the major salivary glands by way of the end-excretory ducts. The infection may present in two different forms. One is an acute inflammatory lesion with diffuse surrounding edema. The other is a more chronic, slow growing lesion that may mimic a neoplasm. Constitutional signs and symptoms may or may not be present. Facial nerve involvement is rare. The chest X-ray may be normal, but in some cases may show healed apical granulomatous cavitary lesions. In true tuberculosis of the salivary glands PPD tests should be positive, but the diagnosis is ultimately made by FNA histopathology or bacterial culture. Incisional biopsy can lead to chronically draining skin fistulas. *M. tuberculosis* in the salivary gland is treated with anti-tuberculous triple drug chemotherapy. In cases of medical resistance or uncertain diagnosis, excisional biopsy is recommended.

Atypical, or non-tuberculous, mycobacterial (NTM) disease has become an increasingly important condition in childhood. Periparotid and upper cervical lymph nodes are most frequently affected. The specific organisms most frequently involved include *M. kansasii*, *M. scrofulaceum*, and *M. avium-intracellulare*. These organisms are typically found in soil, domestic and wild animals, milk and other food items. Chest X-ray is most commonly negative. PPD testing is normal or only marginally positive. The initial diagnosis is therefore further suggested by the clinical presentation. The typical age group affected is 16 to 32 months. There is a rapidly enlarging and persistent upper cervical mass that fails to respond to antibiotics. The skin becomes adherent to the underlying mass and develops a characteristic violaceous discoloration. There are minimal systemic symptoms. Traditional culture of NTM often takes six to eight weeks. Diagnosis is therefore difficult, and excisional biopsy with culture and histopathology is the preferred treatment method as incomplete excision or needle drainage may lead to non-healing fistula tracts.[23] However, in cases where lesions are not well encapsulated or invading surrounding important tissues incomplete excision with marsupialization may be the only option. Traditional anti-tuberculous chemotherapy has no role in the treatment of atypical mycobacterium. Prolonged therapy with clarithromycin may be of some benefit especially in cases of incomplete excision.[24]

## Sarcoidosis

Sarcoidosis is a systemic "non-caseating" granulomatous disease which may affect the major salivary glands. More frequently seen in African-American patients, it is also more common in adults. Affected children are typically teenagers. When the salivary glands are involved, the condition may present as bilateral enlargement of the parotids with possible uveoparotid fever (Heerfordt's fever) characterized by swelling of the parotid and lacrimal glands, chorioretinitis, and cranial nerve palsies, most often involving the facial nerve. Systemic symptoms may include fever, malaise, weakness, nausea, and night sweats. Other granulomatous conditions should be excluded. Chest X-ray looking for hilar adenopathy and an acetylcholinesterase (ACE) level will assist with the diagnosis which is ultimately confirmed with tissue biopsy. Treatment is supportive, with steroids reserved for severe systemic involvement.[25]

## Cat-Scratch Disease

Cat-scratch disease (CSD) is a granulomatous lymphadenitis commonly affecting the cervical and peri-parotid lymph nodes caused from cutaneous inoculation of organisms acquired through domestic cat scratch trauma. *Bartonella henselae*, a gram-negative bacillus, is the causative organism. The affected child presents with fever, malaise, and adenopathy, often noted on CT imaging (Fig. 4). The involved nodes frequently grow over one to two weeks and eventually may suppurate. Enlargement may persist for up to three months. Testing for the presence of serum antibodies to *B. henselae* is the preferred method for making the diagnosis.[26] A polymerase chain reaction (PCR) hybridization assay has a higher sensitivity for diagnosis, but is less universally available. Histologic examination of involved tissue will show bacilli that stain positive to Warthin-Starry silver along with reticular cell hyperplasia and granuloma formation. As with atypical mycobacterium, cultures for *B. henselae* requires up to six weeks of incubation. Antibiotics effective against *B. henselae,* such as rifampin, erythromycin, gentamycin,

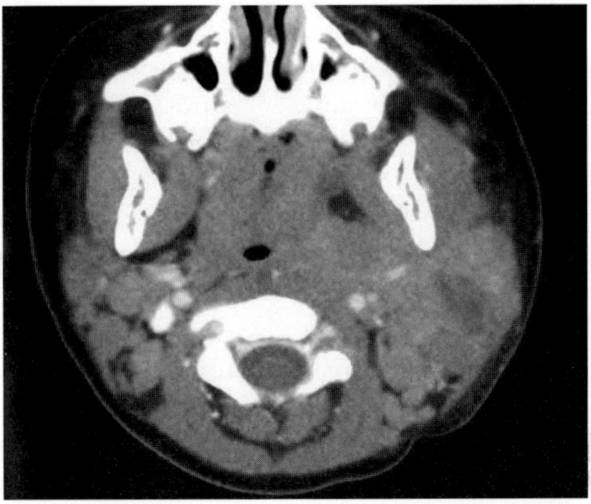

**Fig. 4.** Contrast CT image of child with intraparotid adenopathy secondary to catscratch disease.

azithromycin or ciprofloxacin, are administered to patients who are ill or highly symptomatic.[26] Beta lactam antibiotics are ineffective.

## Actinomycosis

Actinomycosis infection occurs in the cervicofacial region frequently affecting the salivary glands. Infection occurs due to actinomyces, a gram-positive anaerobic non-acid fast bacillus. In most cases infection occurs after trauma or dental extraction. Isolated salivary gland involvement likely occurs by means of retrograde ductal migration. Immune suppression is a predisposing factor. Patients present with a painless, indurated enlargement of the involved salivary gland often mimicking malignant neoplasia.[27] Commonly, multiple draining fistulas develop during the course of the disease. The diagnosis is made from cultures demonstrating gram-positive bacillus containing sulfur granules. Administration of long-term penicillin is the treatment of choice along with occasional abscess drainage.

## CONGENITAL CONDITIONS

### Congenital Cystic Lesions

Congenital cystic lesions of the salivary glands can be classified as branchial cleft anomalies, branchial pouch anomalies, dermoid cysts and congenital ductal retention cysts.

### Branchial Arch Anomalies

Embryological development of the lateral cervicofacial structures in humans is linked with the branchial apparatus system of intrauterine life, where four branchial arches can clearly be identified. Each arch is comprised by a "cleft" of ectodermal origin, and a "pouch" of endodermal origin. Malformation of the branchial apparatus can result in cysts, fistulas, or sinus tracts. Relevant to the salivary glands are malformations of the first branchial arch.[28] Most commonly, the system proposed by Work and Proctor[29] is used to classify fistulas and sinuses of the first cleft. This classification scheme defines two types of fistulas: type I characterized by duplications of the external auditory canal that appear as sinus tracts or swellings in the region of the posterior crease of the pinna, concha or lobule (Fig. 5); and type II characterized by a fistulous tract between the external auditory canal and the parotid region in the upper lateral neck. Some first branchial anomalies can be difficult to categorize by this classification.[30] Repeated incision and drainage and incomplete excisions were frequently seen with first arch anomalies due to misdiagnosis as lymphadenitis.[31] Close and variable association with the facial nerve makes excision of these lesions tedious and sometimes difficult. Complete excision of the lesion while the patient is asymptomatic is the treatment of choice to prevent recurrence (Fig. 6).

First arch branchal pouch anomalies are rare lesions located in the retormandibular area near the middle ear and eustachian tube.[32] Surgical removal through a parotidectomy approach is the definitive treatment.

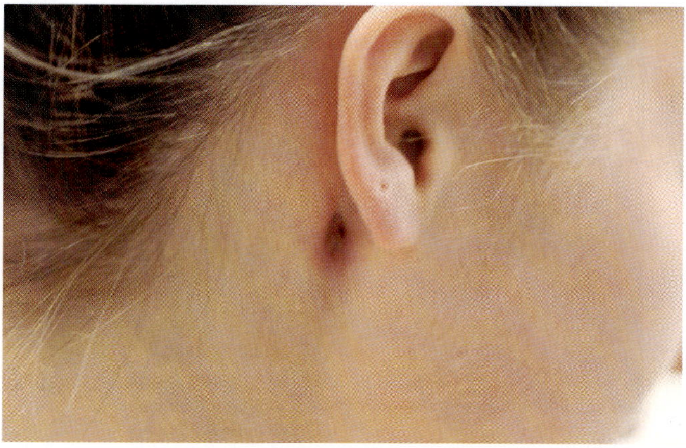

**Fig. 5.** Typical presentation of a first branchial arch, Work type 1 fistula.

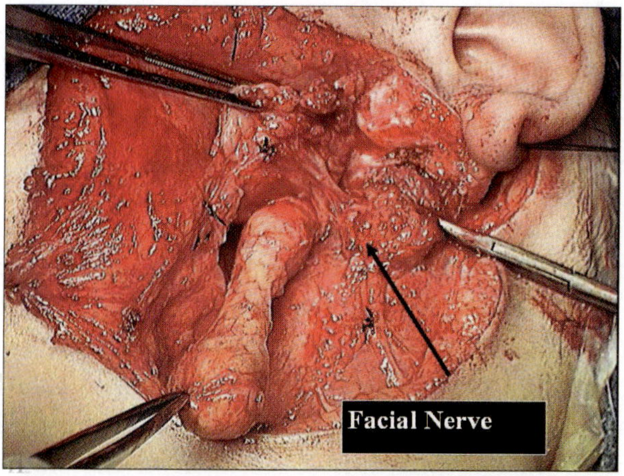


**Fig. 6.** Careful dissection of a first branchial arch anomaly.

## Dermoid Cysts

Dermoid cysts are more commonly encountered in the midline of the neck, away from salivary gland structures,[28] but can rarely occur within the parenchyma of the parotid gland. They are comprised by multiple germ layers forming hair follicles, sweat and sebaceous glands. Total surgical excision is diagnostic and therapeutic.

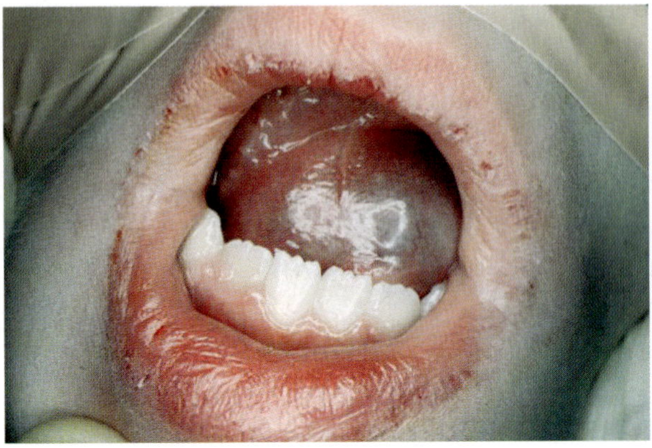

**Fig. 7.** Classic presentation of an intraoral, floor of mouth ranula.

### Congenital Ductal Retention Cysts

Retention ductal cysts of the minor salivary glands are frequently encountered on the palate, tongue, lips, cheeks or the floor of the mouth (Fig. 7). Most are filled with mucous-like material. They are in most cases easily treated with marsupialization. In the floor of the mouth, these lesions are commonly termed "ranulas". A simple ranula results from obstruction of the minor salivary glands in the submucosal layer of the floor of the mouth above the mylohyoid muscle. These are typically unilateral, and are easily treated with marsupialization and in some cases excision. Plunging ranulas extend beyond the floor of the mouth into the neck, making surgical removal more difficult. These lesions result from extravasation of saliva from the sublingual gland into a partially epithelial lined cavity. They can be localized or extensive. Treatment involves complete surgical excision by combined intraoral and external approaches, along with removal of the sublingual glands for more effective long-term outcomes.[33]

## NEOPLASTIC LESIONS

### Hemangiomas

The majority of pediatric salivary gland benign tumors are infantile hemangiomas.[34] These appear shortly after birth and slowly grow over the first year of life. Involution typically occurs by age two. Therefore, treatment is conservative, except for cases where complications occur. These can include extremely rapid growth, ulceration, hemorrhage, infection, or collapse of vital structures. In those instances, the mainstay of medical treatment during the proliferative phase of infantile hemanigoma has included glucocorticoids or interferon-α2a. High dose oral glucocorticoids are effective in halting the growth or even reducing the size of infantile hemangiomas in up to 84% of cases.[35] Recently, propranolol was reported to be effective in treating infantile hemangiomas in a small patient series.[36] The mechanisms of how propranolol functions in hemanigomas have not been studied to date. Despite this, it appears propranolol usage is rapidly becoming a widespread form of medical treatment to the point it may surpass prednisone as a preferred treatment mode.[37] Surgical removal is reserved for the rarest of instances and only when the diagnosis is in question.

## Lymphatic Malformations

Lymphatic malformations (lymphangiomas, cytic hygromas) are benign lesions of lymphatic tissue malformation in the head and neck. They have been classically categorized as cystic, capillary, and cavernous; however they have since been re-classified into macrocystic or microcystic based on their likelihood of response to sclerotherapy.[38] In cases of salivary gland involvement, where the malformation is suprahyoid, these are difficult to treat and carry a 41% complication rate.[39] These lesions are most often present at birth and up to 90% present by the end of the second year of life. They present as soft, asymptomatic, compressible masses that slowly with possible extension into the infrahyoid neck and even into the mediastinum. As lymphatic malformations rarely involute, surgical excision or sclerotherapy are the mainstays of treatment. Salivary gland lymphatic malformations that are microcystic are not responsive to sclerotherapy.[40] Historically, the mainstay of treatment has been surgical removal (Fig. 8). This is an excellent option if complete removal can be achieved without injuring adjacent normal structures. Well-localized parotid or submandibular lymphatic

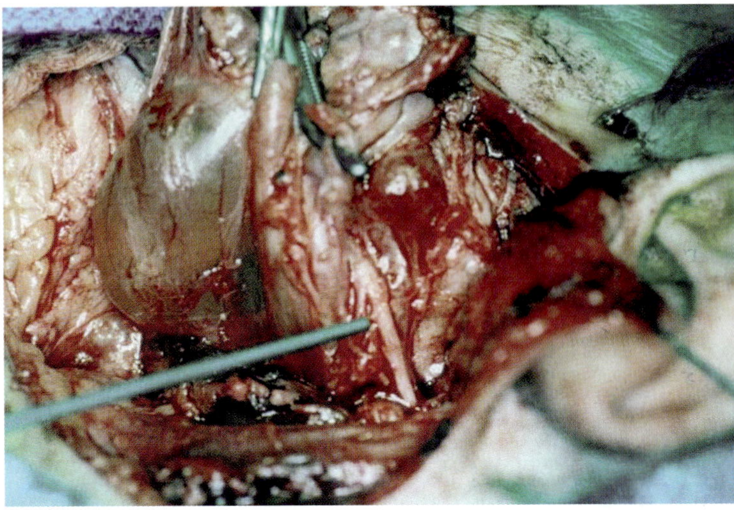

**Fig. 8.** Removal of intraparotid lymphangioma.

malformations can often be excised completely without major complications.[41] However, in cases where there is extensive disease with diffuse infiltration of surrounding normal tissues can make these lesions quite difficult to excise without injuring important structures.[42] Subtotal resection may be the preferred treatment method in those instances, especially if the disease encroaches onto the larynx, pharynx and tongue base.[43] Some have found that the younger a child presents, the more extensive the lymphatic malformation is expected to be with worse prognoses.[44]

## Pleomorphic Adenomas

The majority of firm salivary gland masses in children are malignant. Therefore, histologic confirmation of diagnosis is mandatory in all cases. Of benign epithelial tumors, much like in adults, pleomorphic adenoma is the most common in children. They are rarely seen in younger children, with an overall peak incidence of age ten[34] presenting as firm, discrete, painless, slow-growing masses in the region of the parotid or submandibular glands. Fine needle aspiration can be helpful to diagnose these tumors. The biologic behavior of these in children is no different than in the adult.[45] The treatment of choice is wide surgical excision via parotidectomy with facial nerve preservation. Simple enucleation will lead to recurrence with possible malignant conversion and should never be performed.[45]

Several other benign neoplasms have been described in small numbers within the salivary glands including neurolemmoma, teratoma, xanthoma, and nodular fascitis. Because of the high rate of malignancy for pediatric salivary gland solid tumors, as mentioned, histologic excisional biopsy of any solid persistent mass is essential.

## CONCLUSION

In conclusion, a plethora of benign pathology can be found in the pediatric salivary glands with inflammatory, autoimmune, granulomatous, congenital, or neoplastic conditions possible. The evaluation should focus on the onset, duration, magnitude and location of symptoms. Further work-up and management is dependent on each individual lesion. For solid, persistent masses, malignancy must be ruled out.

## REFERENCES

1. Morgan DW, Pearman K, Raafat F, Oates J, Campbell J. Salivary disease in childhood. *Ear Nose Throat J* 1989;68:155–159.
2. White AK. Salivary gland disease in infancy and childhood: non-malignant lesions. *J Otolaryngol* 1992;21:422–428.
3. Crelin E. *Functional Anatomy of the Newborn.* New Haven: Yale University Press, 1973.
4. Elluru RG. Principles of salivary gland secretion. In: Cummings CW, Haughey BH *et al.*, eds. *Cummings Otolaryngology: Head & Neck Surgery*, 4th Ed. Missouri, USA: Mosby, Inc., 2005, Sec. 2, Chap. 84.
5. Katz P. [Endoscopy of the salivary glands]. *Ann Radiol (Paris)* 1991; 34:110–113.
6. Nahlieli O, Baruchin AM. Sialoendoscopy: three years' experience as a diagnostic and treatment modality. *J Oral Maxillofac Surg* 1997;55: 912–918;discussion 919–920.

7. Marchal F, Dulguerov P. Sialolithiasis management: the state of the art. *Arch Otolaryngol Head Neck Surg* 2003;129:951–956.
8. Hasson O. Sialoendoscopy and sialography: strategies for assessment and treatment of salivary gland obstructions. *J Oral Maxillofac Surg* 2007;65:300–304.
9. Layfield LJ, Tan P, Glasgow BJ. Fine-needle aspiration of salivary gland lesions. Comparison with frozen sections and histologic findings. *Arch Pathol Lab Med* 1987;111:346–353.
10. US Centers for Disease Control and Prevention. Summary of notifiable diseases — United States, 2003. *MMWR* 2005:52:10.
11. Shanley JD. The resurgence of mumps in young adults and adolescents. *Cleve Clin J Med* 2007;74:42–44, 47–48.
12. Strome M. Non-neoplastic salivary gland diseases in children. *Otolaryngol Clin North Am* 1977;10:391–398.
13. Myer C. Salivary gland diseases in children. In: Gates G, ed. *Current Therapy in Otolaryngology — Head and Neck Surgery*. Philadelphia: Mosby, 1990.
14. Leake D, Leake R. Neonatal suppurative parotitis. *Pediatrics* 1970; 46:202–207.
15. Reid E, Douglas F, Crow Y, Hollman A, Gibson J. Autosomal dominant juvenile recurrent parotitis. *J Med Genet* 1998;35:417–419.
16. Hearth-Holmes M, Baethge BA, Abreo F, Wolf RE. Autoimmune exocrinopathy presenting as recurrent parotitis of childhood. *Arch Otolaryngol Head Neck Surg* 1993;119:347–349.
17. Afzelius LE, Walter CG. The surgical treatment of chronic parotitis. *J Laryngol Otol* 1982;96:1131–1135.
18. Papadaki ME, McCain JP, Kim K, Katz RL, Kaban LB, Troulis MJ. Interventional sialoendoscopy: early clinical results. *J Oral Maxillofac Surg* 2008;66:954–962.
19. Batsakis JG. Lymphoepithelial lesion and Sjogren's syndrome. *Ann Otol Rhinol Laryngol* 1987;96:354–355.
20. Dave SP, Pernas FG, Roy S. The benign lymphoepithelial cyst and a classification system for lymphocytic parotid gland enlargement in the pediatric HIV population. *Laryngoscope* 2007;117:106–113.
21. Shaha AR, DiMaio T, Webber C, Thelmo W, Jaffe BM. Benign lymphoepithelial lesions of the parotid. *Am J Surg* 1993;166:403–406.

22. Singer NG, Tomanova-Soltys I, Lowe R. Sjogren's syndrome in childhood. *Curr Rheumatol Rep* 2008;10:147–155.
23. Flint D, Mahadevan M, Barber C, Grayson D, Small R. Cervical lymphadenitis due to non-tuberculous mycobacteria: surgical treatment and review. *Int J Pediatr Otorhinolaryngol* 2000;53:187–194.
24. Tessier MH, Amoric JC, Mechinaud F, Dubesset D, Litoux P, Stalder JF. Clarithromycin for atypical mycobacterial lymphadenitis in non-immunocompromised children. *Lancet* 1994;344:1778.
25. Rice DH. Chronic inflammatory disorders of the salivary glands. *Otolaryngol Clin North Am* 1999;32:813–818.
26. Schutze GE. Diagnosis and treatment of Bartonella henselae infections. *Pediatr Infect Dis J* 2000;19:1185–1187.
27. Varghese BT, Sebastian P, Ramachandran K, Pandey M. Actinomycosis of the parotid masquerading as malignant neoplasm. *BMC Cancer* 2004;4:7.
28. Nicollas R, Guelfucci B, Roman S, Triglia JM. Congenital cysts and fistulas of the neck. *Int J Pediatr Otorhinolaryngol* 2000;55:117–124.
29. Work WP, Proctor CA. The otologist and first branchial cleft anomalies. *Ann Otol Rhinol Laryngol* 1963;72:548–562.
30. Aronsohn RS, Batsakis JG, Rice DH, Work WP. Anomalies of the first branchial cleft. *Arch Otolaryngol* 1976;102:737–740.
31. Choi SS, Zalzal GH. Branchial anomalies: a review of 52 cases. *Laryngoscope* 1995;105:909–913.
32. Myer C, Cotton RT. Salivary gland disease in children: a review. Part 2: congenital lesions and neoplastic disease. *Clin Pediatr (Phila)* 1986;25: 353–357.
33. Batsakis JG, McClatchey KD. Cervical ranulas. *Ann Otol Rhinol Laryngol* 1988;97:561–562.
34. Schuller DE, McCabe BF. Salivary gland neoplasms in children. *Otolaryngol Clin North Am* 1977;10:399–412.
35. Bennett ML, Fleischer AB, Jr, Chamlin SL, Frieden IJ. Oral corticosteroid use is effective for cutaneous hemangiomas: an evidence-based evaluation. *Arch Dermatol* 2001;137:1208–1213.
36. Leaute-Labreze C, Dumas de la Roque E, Hubiche T, Boralevi F, Thambo JB, Taieb A. Propranolol for severe hemangiomas of infancy. *N Engl J Med* 2008;358:2649–2651.

37. Siegfried EC, Keenan WJ, Al-Jureidini S. More on propranolol for hemangiomas of infancy. *N Engl J Med* 2008;359:2846; author reply 2846–2847.
38. Smith RJ, Burke DK, Sato Y, Poust RI, Kimura K, Bauman NM. OK-432 therapy for lymphangiomas. *Arch Otolaryngol Head Neck Surg* 1996;122:1195–1199.
39. de Serres LM, Sie KC, Richardson MA. Lymphatic malformations of the head and neck. A proposal for staging. *Arch Otolaryngol Head Neck Surg* 1995;121:577–582.
40. Giguere CM, Bauman NM, Smith RJ. New treatment options for lymphangioma in infants and children. *Ann Otol Rhinol Laryngol* 2002;111:1066–1075.
41. Kennedy TL, Whitaker M, Pellitteri P, Wood WE. Cystic hygroma/lymphangioma: a rational approach to management. *Laryngoscope* 2001;111:1929–1937.
42. Padwa BL, Hayward PG, Ferraro NF, Mulliken JB. Cervicofacial lymphatic malformation: clinical course, surgical intervention, and pathogenesis of skeletal hypertrophy. *Plast Reconstr Surg* 1995;95:951–960.
43. Riechelmann H, Muehlfay G, Keck T, Mattfeldt T, Rettinger G. Total, subtotal, and partial surgical removal of cervicofacial lymphangiomas. *Arch Otolaryngol Head Neck Surg* 1999;125:643–648.
44. Raveh E, de Jong AL, Taylor GP, Forte V. Prognostic factors in the treatment of lymphatic malformations. *Arch Otolaryngol Head Neck Surg* 1997;123:1061–1065.
45. Garcia-Perla A, Munoz-Ramos M, Infante-Cossio P, Mayorga-Jimenez F, Gutierrez-Perez JL. Pleomorphic adenoma of the parotid in childhood. *J Craniomaxillofac Surg* 2002;30:242–245.

15

# Pediatric Ear, Nose, and Throat Malignancies

*Maie A. St. John, Ontario D. Lau and Elliot Abemayor*

## INTRODUCTION

The differential diagnosis in a child presenting with a head or neck mass includes inflammatory, congenital and neoplastic lesions. A detailed history and physical examination is useful in delineating the nature of the mass. Important information to solicit from the history include: age, family history, onset and duration of symptoms, and any systemic signs of disease such as fever or weight loss.

Overwhelmingly, the majority of pediatric neck masses are due to inflammatory or congenital disease.

However, it should not be forgotten that 10% to 20% of all pediatric head and neck masses are malignant.[1] A firm, painless mass that has grown quickly or has been present for several weeks, a history of unilateral symptoms or cranial nerve palsies increase the concern for malignancy.[2]

Self-evidently, when malignancy is suspected, imaging studies as well as a plan for obtaining a tissue diagnosis should not be delayed. Often a plain chest X-ray (CXR) will detect a pulmonary or mediastinal lesion that is a source for cervical or supraclavicular adenopathy. Ultrasound (US) is used frequently in the pediatric population as it does not involve ionizing radiation and can easily distinguish solid from cystic masses. US is particularly helpful in delineating parotid and thyroid masses.[3] Computed tomography (CT) and magnetic resonance imaging (MRI) enable visualization of soft tissue structures and delineate the anatomic boundaries and extent of invasion of head and neck masses.[2]

Biopsy is needed for lesions suspicious for malignancy based on history and physical. Fine needle aspiration (FNA) has advantages over surgical biopsy, including lower cost, and a decreased chance of tumor seeding.[4,5] Biopsy of deeper masses that may be less accessible is often aided by the use of US or CT guidance. Contrary to popular misconception, there is a great deal to be learned from pediatric FNA's and this modality is still the preferred first step in evaluating neck masses.[6]

Only if the FNA is inconclusive, or if a lymphoid tumor is suspected and there is a significant chance of malignancy, there should be a low threshold for proceeding with open biopsy.[2]

In this chapter, we review the most common pediatric head and neck malignancies: thyroid carcinoma, salivary gland cancers, skull base tumors, rhabdomyosarcoma, and nasopharyngeal carcinoma. We provide an overview of the relevant physiology, state-of-the-art diagnostic techniques, operative interventions, adjunctive therapies, and recommendations for follow-up.

## PEDIATRIC THYROID CARCINOMA

### Incidence

Pediatric thyroid carcinoma is uncommon, comprising less than 3% of all childhood malignancies and only 10% of all thyroid carcinomas.[7–9] Although uncommon, sporadic differentiated thyroid carcinoma (DTC) is the most common endocrine malignancy in children and includes papillary and follicular types.[10,11] The peak incidence occurs in children from ten to 18 years of age, and the incidence in females is twice that in males.[12,13] Males are more likely to have distant metastases at presentation.[14,15] In late adolescence, the incidence of DTC increases and the female:male ratio becomes more pronounced. The incidence of DTC varies by race and gender, with higher rates seen in white and Hispanic females, as compared with black females and males of any race.[16]

The most common presentation for pediatric thyroid carcinoma is a painless neck mass presenting in the lower central or lateral neck. Regional lymphatic spread is present in approximately 50% of patients at the time of diagnosis.[11,17]

The incidence of thyroid nodules in children is 1%–1.5% based on clinical examination.[18] However, as compared to adults, pediatric thyroid masses have a more than fourfold incidence of malignancies. Studies report the incidence of carcinoma in solitary thyroid nodules of pediatric patients to range between 15%–30%.[18] Within the gland itself, thyroid cancer usually presents as a solitary nodule. When present in young children (less than ten years old), and children with a history of head and neck radiation or iodine deficiency, the chance that a nodule will be malignant is even higher.[19] The incidence of well-differentiated thyroid carcinomas in childhood is slightly higher (85%–90%) than in adults with a different distribution of the histologic subtypes of papillary thyroid carcinoma including most notably follicular and follicular-solid growth patterns.[20]

Unlike adults, differentiated thyroid cancer in children frequently presents with metastases (60%–80% nodal and 10%–20% distant). The prevalence of distant metastases, most commonly in lung, is also higher in children, with an incidence of 20%–30%.[21,22] Interestingly, however, the presence of metastasis does not seem to negatively impact the overall survival. Children with metastatic disease have an overall survival of 95% at ten years, whereas half of adult patients with distant metastasis die within five years. The favorable prognosis reflects the fact that most young patients have well differentiated tumor types, few have bone metastasis, and tumors respond well to radioactive iodine therapy.[22,23]

## Risk Factors

Risk factors for developing thyroid carcinoma include genetic predisposition, dysfunctional iodine metabolism, treatment for a prior malignancy, and prior ionizing radiation exposure. The latency period for developing thyroid cancer after radiation exposure ranges from four to six years.[11] The thyroid is one of the most frequent sites of secondary neoplasm in children who receive radiation therapy for other malignancies.[18]

Thyroid cancer constitutes 9% of secondary malignancies, as a complication after the treatment for a primary malignancy.[24] Hodgkin's lymphoma is the most common primary malignancy associated with subsequent thyroid cancer. Children treated for cancer before age ten are at highest risk.[25] The incidence of thyroid cancer increases linearly with radiation doses up to 30 Gy, and declines with higher doses, which is believed to be due to the cytotoxic effects of high-dose radiation.[26]

## Initial Evaluation

When a thyroid nodule is identified in a child, the possibility of thyroid carcinoma needs to be excluded. Serum thyrotropin stimulating hormone (TSH) and calcitonin should be measured. Calcitonin levels are useful in making a diagnosis of medullary thyroid cancer, which accounts for 3%–5% of thyroid cancers.[23] If the TSH is suppressed, a radionucleotide scan may identify a hyperfunctioning nodule.

As part of the initial work-up, a thyroid and neck ultrasound should be obtained. Ultrasound characteristics suggestive of malignancy include indistinct margins and microcalcifications.[27] Ultrasound can also determine the intrathyroidal location of a nodule, identify additional nodules, and assess if there is lymph-node involvement.[23,27,28]

Ultrasonography alone cannot reliably distinguish between benign and malignant lesions. US-guided FNA is indicated for all thyroid lesions greater than 0.5 cm. FNA is considered the most accurate and cost-effective means to evaluate if a thyroid nodule is malignant.[23,27] Patients with aspirates suggesting malignancy, proceed to surgery. Difficulty arises when the FNA is "indeterminate." In children less than ten years of age or those patients at higher risk for malignancy (ionizing radiation exposure, family history of thyroid cancer), prompt surgical removal is recommended.[21,23,29]

### Subtypes of Thyroid Carcinoma in Children

As in adults, the three major types of thyroid cancer in children are papillary, follicular, and medullary carcinoma. Papillary carcinoma is the most common type of thyroid malignancy in children. These tumors are multicentric and spread via lymphatics to regional nodes. Follicular carcinoma is more aggressive than papillary, but less common. These carcinomas metastasize hematogeneously and tend to spread to bone, liver, and lung. Medullary thyroid carcinoma is made up of parafollicular C cells and constitutes 2%–5% of thyroid tumors. Medullary thyroid carcinomas may arise spontaneously or in association with MEN IIA or MEN IIB or FMTC syndrome.[11,30,31]

### Thyroid Cancer Staging

There are multiple staging systems for DTC. The ATA Taskforce advocates the use of the American Joint Committee on Cancer classification system, which is based on TNM criteria. This system is useful in describing the extent of disease and predicting disease mortality.[27] Thyroid cancer patients younger than 45 years of age (and thus, all children) are classified as stage I (any T, any N, M0) or II (any T, any N, M1). For children, the metastasis-age-completeness of resection-invasion-size (MACIS) scheme has been shown to be helpful in determining the risk of recurrence, provided a lower cutoff score is used than for adults.[23,32]

### Thyroid Cancer Biology

The molecular genetics of childhood DTC appear to be different from profiles reported for adults. In children with DTC, gene rearrangements are more common than point mutations.[33] In papillary carcinoma, ret/PTC (Rearranged in Transformation/Papillary Thyroid Carcinomas) rearrangements have a higher prevalence in children than in adults.[34] Mutations in the RAS proto-oncogene have also been associated with thyroid cancer, but most commonly with the follicular variant. RAS proto-oncogene mutations are found in approximately 20% of papillary tumors and 20% of follicular tumors.[35] In MTC, somatic gene rearrangement of the RET proto-oncogene results in a gain of function of the tyrosine-kinase receptor and an increased risk of developing thyroid cancer as well as Hirschsprung's disease.[36] RET genetic translocations can be detected in 35% of papillary thyroid cancers.[37]

## Management

The low incidence of childhood thyroid cancer (1% of all childhood malignancies) in combination with the indolent nature of the disease make it problematic to determine the optimum treatment strategies. Treating children with DTC is a challenge, given that patients frequently present with metastases yet rarely die of disease.

To date, there has not been a single randomized trial comparing total thyroidectomy and postoperative $I^{131}$ to thyroid lobectomy and thyroid suppression. It is unlikely with the small number of children with differentiated thyroid cancer that such a study will be accomplished. All available data are retrospective, but examination of large series of patients from multiple institutions has led most clinicians to advocate total thyroidectomy and adjuvant radioiodine therapy as the minimal standard treatment. The primary goal of surgical therapy is removal of all gross disease with preservation of all vital structures including recurrent laryngeal nerves and parathyroid glands. The extent of lymph-node dissection during initial surgery remains controversial, but preoperative ultrasound and techniques such as sentinel lymph-node biopsy will likely allow for a more directed approach. Elective neck dissection is not advocated in the management of pediatric thyroid carcinoma, whereas therapeutic neck dissection is indicated.

Total thyroidectomy facilitates the use of postoperative radioactive iodine to detect occult metastases as well as its use as ablative treatment of recurrent disease; reducing the morbidity of reoperative neck surgery. Hormonal replacement with L-thyroxine may, in some cases, suppress residual thyroid function or tumor growth.

The overall survival in non-medullary thyroid cancer is 98%.[38] Children with more advanced local disease, lymph node involvement and distant metastasis have much better outcomes than do adults, but also have a much higher likelihood of recurrence. Recurrence is seen more frequently in children who do not receive initial postoperative iodine therapy and those who have palpable nodes at initial presentation. The time to first recurrence ranges from eight months to 15 years, thereby emphasizing the importance of long-term follow-up.[29]

Standard follow-up surveillance for thyroid cancer has included thyroglobulin levels, chest X-ray, and radioiodine scans. In addition, some surgeons include routine neck ultrasound examinations. Data from MD Anderson now recommend a follow-up CXR with an elevation in thyroglobulin.[39] More recently, PET/CT has been identi fied as improving the diagnostic accuracy in a therapeutically relevant way in patients with metastatic thyroid cancer, especially those that are iodine negative.[40]

Advances in understanding the genetics of thyroid cancer continue. Children with DTC clearly have different molecular profiles than do adults. Additional research is needed to elucidate the relationship between specific genes and the biological behavior of thyroid cancer so that treatment can be individualized.

## Surgical Treatment of WDTC

The optimal surgical management of DTC in children has yet to be defined. The surgical approach for children with thyroid cancer was not specifically addressed by the recent ATA guidelines, and remains controversial, reflecting the lack of definitive prospective randomized clinical trials to determine optimal surgical management.[27] The treatment of DTC in children is guided by retrospective data that typically involve small numbers of patients.[23,41]

Interestingly, good long-term outcomes after treatment are seen irrespective of which surgical procedure is performed. Some surgeons perform a thyroid lobectomy maintaining that differentiated thyroid carcinoma in children is an indolent disease and that survival is not clearly related to the extent of gland removal.[42] Others believe that total thyroidectomy is the preferred treatment for thyroid carcinoma due to a high incidence of tumor multifocality and associated bilobar disease in up to 80% of patients. In addition, total thyroidectomy allows for the postoperative administration of radioactive iodine and the use of serial thryoglobulin measurements in follow-up surveillance.[21]

Supporting the role for total thyroidectomy, studies in pediatric patients show a lower recurrence risk after total or near total thyroidectomy compared with lobectomy, an observation that is not surprising as at least 40% of DTC in children is multifocal.[21,41]

In 1998 a multi-institutional analysis of differentiated childhood thyroid cancer was undertaken to define those variables predictive of thyroid cancer progression and to correlate the surgical procedure performed with complications sustained.[39,43] Of the variables examined, only age and residual cervical disease after thyroidectomy had any statistical impact on progression-free survival. The younger the patient and the presence of residual cervical disease were associated with a greater risk of disease progression. At diagnosis, 90% of patients have cervical metastases and 48% have distant metastases. Despite this, the overall survival rate was 100% at ten years. The surgical procedure of choice for these patients was predominantly total or subtotal thyroidectomy (90%) with $I^{131}$ treatment postoperatively.

The largest series of reported childhood cancer patients is from Belarus.[44] This retrospective study reports the long-term follow-up of children with thyroid cancer in the post-Chernobyl era. The tumors were predominantly papillary (94.9%) and the overall survival was 99.5% at five years and 98.8% at ten years. Two-thirds of the patients underwent a total or subtotal thyroidectomy, 33.5% a lobectomy, and 1% a partial lobectomy; 82% had some form of LN dissection. At the time of diagnosis, 2.3% had lung metastasis and 19.7% of tumors were multi-focal. Recurrences occurred in 28% of patients; 9.9% local, and 12% distant. This series suggests that total thyroidectomy, selective LN dissection, and postoperative $I^{131}$ as the optimum treatment strategy for this group of patients.

Few data are available on the optimal approach for treatment of cervical lymph-node disease and dissection in children with thyroid cancer. A multi-institutional analysis by the Children's Cancer Group found that those patients with residual cervical disease after initial operation had a greater risk of disease progression.[43] In performing a cervical lymphadenectomy, one can pursue several courses: one is a conventional nerve/muscle sparing comprehensive lymph node dissection, or a highly selective node dissection guided by sentinel node techniques. In any event, "node plucking" has no place in treating neck disease. The advantages of using sentinel lymph node biopsy in the treatment of thyroid cancer includes a better selection of patients who may benefit from compartment-oriented nodal dissection.

In the most recent set of ATA guidelines, controversy was acknowledged in whether prophylactic or *a priori* central compartment node dissection was mandatory.[23] Notwithstanding this lack of firm guidelines, it is unquestioned that if palpable or ultrasound evidence of nodal disease is present, modified lateral compartment neck dissections should be performed in children with biopsy-proven neck disease, and radical neck dissections avoided.[45]

With respect to complications of surgery, the reported incidence of recurrent nerve injury following total thyroidectomy ranges for 1%–9.5%.[12] Hypoparathyroidism is reported in 6% to 27% of patients of which 12% is permanent.[46] Intraoperative Rapid Parathyroid Hormone (PTH) measurements are useful in determining whether immediate postoperative calcium replacement should be instituted. When performing total thyroidectomy, a greater than 50% fall in PTH levels can help to identify parathyroid gland removal and guide reimplantation as necessary. Risk factors for these postoperative complications include tumor size, positive nodal metastases, multifocality, and undergoing a total thyroidectomy with associated neck dissection of any form.[39]

**Postoperative Radioactive Iodine Treatment**

Radioactive Iodine (RAI) ablation with $I^{131}$ is a mainstay of adjunctive DTC therapy for children and adults. Even after meticulous thyroidectomy, whole body thyroid scans can reveal residual thyroid tissue in the thyroid bed or the presence of metastatic thyroid cancer in cervical lymph nodes and distant sites.[23,29]

RAI is usually given four to six weeks postoperatively with a goal of destroying residual (remnant) cancerous and non-cancerous thyroid tissue. To maximize RAI uptake, the serum TSH level should be high, indicating profound hypothyroidism (30 mIU/ml), which is accomplished by withholding thyroid hormone therapy for at least two weeks. In addition, patients should consume a low iodine diet one to two weeks prior to treatment and should not receive iodinated contrast for imaging studies.[23]

In children, an initial low dose $I^{131}$ scan is routinely performed to determine thyroid bed uptake. If there is greater than 20% uptake, surgical re-exploration to remove residual disease is often undertaken before RAI is administered.[41]

The ATA Taskforce recommends RAI ablation for specific patients with stage I DTC: those with multifocal disease, nodal metastases, extrathyroidal or vascular invasion, or more aggressive histologic subtypes. RAI ablation is also recommended for all stage II patients who are younger than 45 years, most stage II patients older than 45 years, and all patients with stage III or stage IV disease.[23,27]

There is no consensus for RAI dosing in children. Several groups have recommended dosing between 30–150 mCi; whereas other groups recommend dosing based on body weight or surface area.[19] Successful remnant ablation is determined by serial thyroglobulin measurements. In addition, follow-up ultrasound and $I^{131}$ scans are performed six or 12 months after initial therapy. Patients with residual neck disease may undergo repeat RAI treatment. If gross disease is evident by ultrasound or other imaging modality, repeat surgery is undertaken.[47] High-risk patients with lung metastases rarely become disease free regardless of $I^{131}$ therapy, although their disease may remain stable over years.[48]

Although RAI has been used for many years and is well tolerated, there are cumulative dose-related risks with early and late complications. Early complications include gastritis, neck pain from soft tissue swelling, sialadenitis, dental caries, and bone marrow suppression.[27] To prevent late complications, the total cumulative dose of $I^{131}$ should be kept below 600 mCi in children as higher doses are associated with an increased lifetime risk of leukemia and secondary tumors.[23] Higher doses of $I^{131}$ have also been linked with azoospermia and pulmonary fibrosis.[27,41]

**Thyroid Hormone Suppression**

After surgical resection, patients are treated with exogenous thyroid hormone to suppress TSG-mediated stimulation of the thyroid. Equivalent survival rates with all surgical procedures performed may be secondary to the use of hormone suppression with L-thyroxine. Hormonal manipulation at TSH suppressive doses can inhibit normal and neoplastic proliferation, thus preventing cancer progression and relapse.[11]

In low-risk patients, it is not clear if complete suppression of TSH secretion confers benefit. In addition, the long-term impact of supraphysiologic doses of thyroid hormone on bone mineral density is a concern. One scheme, proposed by Baudin *et al.*, initially suppresses TSH to less than 0.1 mU/l and then allows the TSH to rise to 0.5 mU/l once the patient enters remission.[49] These recommendations seem appropriate for children, given data showing that 90% of recurrent PTC develops within ten years after the initial treatment, coupled with the wish to minimize long-term adverse effects of therapy.[23,27]

**Medullary Thyroid Cancer (MTC)**

Medullary thyroid cancer may present as one of several forms: sporadic, familial (without the other associated features of MEN) or part of the multiple endocrine neoplasias (MENI, MEN IIA, MEN IIB). In patients with MEN, MTC is usually the first presenting tumor and is the most common cause of death in these patients.

Surgical resection is the only effective treatment for MTC, thus underscoring the importance of early diagnosis before metastasis.[30] In children with MEN II and familial MTC kindred, presymptomatic detection of the RET proto-oncogene mutation helps in identifying those children who can be treated before malignancy.

The current recommendation for effective treatment is that affected children with MEN IIA undergo total thyroidectomy between ages five to eight, before the tumor spreads beyond the thyroid gland.[31] As MEN IIB tends to be more aggressive, prophylactic thyroidectomy with a central compartment lymph node dissection should be performed at 1 year of age.[50,51] Early detection by DNA mutation analysis and early operative intervention result in a normal life expectancy in these children.[11]

## SALIVARY GLAND MALIGNANCIES

### Introduction

The salivary glands comprise three main pairs of glands: the parotid, the submandibular, and the sublingual. There are also many other small, minor salivary glands throughout the oral cavity, oropharynx, and paranasal sinuses that consist entirely of mucus-secreting cells (minor salivary glands). Neoplasms of salivary glands are rare in children, representing fewer than 10% of all pediatric head and neck malignancies.[52] Approximately 80% of salivary gland neoplasms within major glands are benign. Most salivary gland neoplasms occur in the parotid gland, followed by the submandibular gland.[53] In children, the incidence of benign disease in these glands is lower. The parotid gland is involved in up to 90% of all pediatric salivary gland tumors and 50% of these tumors are malignant.[52] Malignant tumors are generally low grade; however, a malignant tumor in a child younger than age ten is more likely to be a high-grade neoplasm, portending a poor prognosis. Minor salivary gland tumors in the pediatric population tend to arise in the oral cavity, although lesions in the pharynx, larynx, and bronchus have also been reported.[54] As with adults, the majority of *minor* salivary gland tumors are malignant (Tables 1 and 2).

**Table 1. Histologic types and frequencies of pediatric salivary parotid gland neoplasms.**[64]

| | |
|---|---|
| Mucoepidermoid carcinoma | 43.7% |
| Acinic cell carcinoma | 34% |
| Rhabdomyosarcoma | 7.8% |
| Lymphoma | 6.8% |
| Adenocarcinoma | 1.9% |
| Hodgkin's disease | 1.9% |
| Squamous cell carcinoma | 1% |
| Basal cell carcinoma | 1% |
| Adenoid cystic carcinoma | 1% |
| Peripheral neuroectodermal tumor | 1% |

**Table 2. Histologic types and frequencies of pediatric salivary submandibular gland neoplasms.**[64]

| | |
|---|---|
| Acinic cell carcinoma | 30% |
| Adenocarcinoma | 20% |
| Mucoepidermoid carcinoma | 20% |
| Adenoid cystic carcinoma | 10% |
| Intra-ductal carcinoma | 10% |
| Epithelial-myoepithelial carcinoma | 10% |

Salivary gland carcinomas are quite rare in children. Clinical Stage and histologic grade are the main prognostic factors. Children with malignant tumors of all histologic types, have a five-year overall survival rate of 70%, and a 3% chance of developing a second cancer in the following 20 years.[55] Complete excision, with preservation of the facial nerve, is the treatment of choice. A systematic lymph-node dissection is recommended in patients with advanced stage disease and high-grade tumors, perineural invasion, or lymphovascular spread. Long-term follow-up is essential to rule-out late recurrence.

## History and Physical Examination

Physical examination requires palpation of the gland, and a thorough neural assessment of surrounding structures. For oral tumors, bimanual palpation is optimal. This is done with the fingers of one hand examining the intraoral aspect of the gland while the other hand externally manipulates the gland.

The clinical and pathologic features are similar in pediatric and adult populations. The most frequent presentation is an isolated, hard, painless and slow-growing mass in the parotid bed.[56,57] Patients with a submandibular tumor present with a painless swelling or mass in the submandibular triangle. A sudden increase in size may be secondary to infection, hemorrhage, or malignant transformation. In children, as in adults, tumors arise in the parotid gland in 66% of cases, and involve the superficial lobe in 75% of cases.[56] The onset and duration of the lesion may offer insight into the pathologic nature of the problem. A diffuse swelling of the gland is generally associated with inflammatory conditions, whereas a discrete palpable mass may be a neoplasm, inflammatory node, or a stone.

The average duration from the presence of a lump being noticed to definitive diagnosis is 21 months. Clinical features that suggest malignancy are facial nerve involvement, pain, fixation of the mass, involvement of the overlying skin or underlying structures, and associated regional lymphadenopathy.[58] Inflammatory lesions generally do not interfere with facial nerve function. The presence of adenopathy depends on the grade, size, and location of the tumor. Adenopathy is more frequent in submandibular gland malignancies.[59] Distant metastases, especially to the lung, are rare and indicate a poor prognosis.

Minor salivary gland lesions are rare. Benign lesions tend to present as a painless submucosal mass with normal overlying mucosa. A malignant lesion may present as a submucosal mass or an ulcerative lesion. The palate is the most common locale for minor salivary gland neoplasms.[52,60]

## Initial Evaluation

Computed tomography (CT) and magnetic resonance imaging (MRI) have largely replaced sialography. Estimations of the nature of the lesions (benign or malignant) can be obtained, and the extent of the tumor extension and lymph node involvement can be visualized, allowing for preoperative surgical planning.[61] Ultrasound (US) can also be used to distinguish cystic from solid lesions, and in an older child, can be used to assist fine-needle aspiration (FNA). The low cost and avoidance of radiation make this image modality desirable in the pediatric age group.[52]

Despite the reluctance by some clinicians to utilize it in children, FNA is a well established technique for the diagnosis of salivary gland lesions.[62] FNA provides a cytologic specimen for examination. FNA is often difficult to perform in a very young child due to lack of cooperation; however it can be useful in distinguishing between inflammatory, benign, and malignant processes. At times, general anesthesia may be used to obtain adequate samples. The accuracy of FNA varies between 84%–97% in malignant tumors of the salivary gland.[63] The correlation of FNA results to final histopathologic reports varies with the quality of the FNA specimen and the specific disease process affecting the gland.

Open biopsies are occasionally necessary. An excisional biopsy is appropriate when an FNA is non-diagnostic or when there is a high level of concern for a malignancy or minor salivary gland tumors. Excisional biopsies of the parotid gland generally require a superficial parotidectomy with identification and preservation of the facial nerve. Excisional biopsies of lesions within the submandibular gland generally require complete excision of the gland as the biopsy procedure. Incisional biopsies are inappropriate. Incisional biopsies carry the risk of facial nerve injury, tumor spillage, and compromise of the discrete compartments of the neck, all of which may complicate further management.[52]

## Histologic Types of Pediatric Salivary Gland Neoplasms

### Mucoepidermoid Carcinoma (MEC)

MEC is the most common malignancy in the salivary glands and accounts for 50% of malignant salivary gland tumors in children.[53]

MEC is also the most common radiation induced salivary malignancy in children. Only 5% of salivary gland MEC arises during childhood and seldom before the age of ten.[56] MEC is thought to arise from the pluripotent reserve cells of the excretory ducts of the salivary gland that have the potential to differentiate into squamous, columnar, and mucous cells.[65] Tumors consist of a combination of squamous and mucous cells. Histologically, MECs are classified as low-, intermediate-, and high-grade tumors, with most pediatric tumors being low grade.

Low-grade malignancies are often cystic on CT scan. This type of tumor may be mistaken (radiographically or by FNA) for a Whartin's tumor. High-grade MECs tend to be more solid and homogeneous on CT and MRI. Low grade lesions may be treated surgically with wide local resection. High grade neoplasms often require resection of the cervical nodes, radiation, or both.[66] Long-term follow-up is essential to rule out late recurrence.

## Acinic Cell Carcinoma

Acinic cell carcinoma is the second most common salivary carcinoma in children. As with mucoepidermoid carcinoma, the most common presentation is between ten to 16 years of age. On pathologic examination, acinic cell carcinoma consists of nests of cells with basophilic cytoplasm and lymphoid infiltrate into the surrounding stroma.

This tumor is regarded as a low grade malignancy and rarely metastasizes. However, it has a high likelihood of recurrence if it is not excised completely.[52,67]

## Adenoid Cystic Carcinoma

Adenoid cystic carcinoma often demonstrates an indolent course, yet has a relentless tendency for local and perineural invasion. It is associated with a high recurrence rate and relatively poor long-term survival. Distant metastases can occur from one to 20 years after initial diagnosis.[52,68]

### Adenocarcinoma

Adenocarcinoma is observed in early childhood and has a high potential for metastases. In several large series, there was an overall mortality rate of 75%. Therefore, adenocarcinoma in the pediatric population is an aggressive disease and warrants more radical surgical resection and or adjuvant therapy.[52.69]

### Undifferentiated Carcinoma

Undifferentiated carcinoma most commonly occurs in children under the age of ten. It is the only salivary carcinoma reported in the perinatal period. This tumor is highly aggressive and has a poor prognosis despite aggressive treatment protocols.[52,70]

### Management

Generally, nerve-sparing surgery is appropriate for most of the salivary gland malignancies. Exceptions to this rule include high grade tumors or those already presenting with nerve weakness. The treatment of choice for salivary gland malignancies is *en bloc* removal of the tumor with adequate margins. Regardless of grade, it is clear that local and regional recurrence rates are higher in patients with positive or close tumor margins.[53] Superficial parotidectomy may be considered when the tumor is lateral to the facial nerve. Total parotidectomy is recommended when the deep lobe is involved or when there are positive intraparotid lymph nodes. Intraoperative frozen section can be used to guide the extent of resection and prevent under treatment.

The facial nerve should be preserved unless the tumor directly invades the nerve; or if intact nerves limit the complete resection of the tumor.[52] Proper preoperative consideration should be given to facial nerve grafting if facial nerve resection is required. For submandibular neoplasms, dissection of the nodes in the submandibular triangle reduces the risk of recurrence.[71]

The question of prophylactic neck dissection remains controversial. The overall incidence of lymph node metastases in primary parotid carcinomas ranges from 18%–28%.[72] In adults, Spiro *et al.* have proposed a "staging" supraomohyoid neck dissection in patients with high grade tumors and an elective radical neck dissection in patients with undifferentiated or SCCA.[53,73]

Tumor recurrence is most common with adenoid cystic carcinoma (50%), followed by mucoepidermoid carcinoma (38%), and acinic cell carcinoma (20%).[52] The high recurrence rate seen in the pediatric population is likely due to inadequate surgical excision at the initial presentation.

Radiation is generally recommended for high-grade lesions with extra-capsular spread, or when perineural invasion has been identified. In the case of positive margins or microscopic residual disease, radiation is not recommended. A second, more extensive operation should be performed.

Because of the potential for radiation induced sequelae, radiation in children must be used with extreme caution. The use of radiotherapy in children may lead to long-term sequelae in 50% of patients. Potential long-term complications of radiotherapy are facial deformity, trismus, xerostomia, osteoradionecrosis, and secondary tumors.[53]

The role of chemotherapy in the management of salivary gland malignancies is not completely defined but is generally reserved for patients with progressive local or metastatic disease that is not amenable to surgery or radiation therapy. The choice of agents is not clear as it is hampered by the lack of large clinical trials.

## SKULL BASE MALIGNANCIES

### Incidence

Pediatric skull base lesions form a distinctive group from their adult counterparts. Epidemiologically, skull base lesions are less likely to affect children. Demographically, males (69%) are affected more than females because the pediatric population has a lower incidence of meningiomas but higher incidence of benign nerve sheath tumors.[74,75]

## Anatomical Considerations

Anatomically the skull base is divided into three fossae: anterior, middle, and posterior. More than half of reported skull base tumors in children are benign. Approximately 50% of malignant lesions at the skull base are sarcomas.[76] Most series report a predilection for the anterior cranial fossa: 62% (42%–75%) in the anterior cranial base; 25%(15%–45%) in the middle cranial base; and 13% (0%–42%) in the posterior cranial base.[75–79]

Differing anatomy and involvement of growth centers in children can affect the approach to surgery. For example, anterior skull base approaches in children are hindered by the shallow anterior fossa floor and the under pneumatized sinuses. Operations involving a maxillotomy may damage tooth buds. More successful complete resection has been reported than in adults due to the better defined tissue planes in children. Given the higher rate of complete resection and the high incidence of benign tumors, children with skull base lesions tend to have a better prognosis than adults.[75]

## Tumors of the Anterior Cranial Base in Children

The most common lesions of the anterior cranial base in children are esthesioneuroblastomas and benign lesions such as encephaloceles and fibrous dysplasia. In contrary, the most common adult anterior cranial base neoplasms include nasal or paranasal malignancies and meningiomas.[80]

## Surgical Approaches to the Anterior Cranial Base

Surgical approaches to the anterior cranial base include transfacial, anterior craniofacial, craniotomy with orbital and/or zygomatic osteotomy, and transsphenoidal (Table 3).[76] Transfacial approaches can be further subdivided into: transoral, transpalatal, lateral rhinotomy, Le Fort I osteotomy and midfacial degloving.[81] These approaches are frequently used with modification in the pediatric population.

Table 3. Different surgical approaches to the anterior cranial base.[80]

| Approaches | Advantages | Disadvantages |
|---|---|---|
| Transoral labial–mandibulotomy | — Adequate exposure | — Destruction of central incisors<br>— Potential damage to tooth buds in patients less than 6 years old |
| Transpalatal | — Excellent exposure of midline nasopharyngeal centered lesions | — Large amount of soft tissue need to be retracted, restricting exposure of upper clival and sphenoid regions<br>— Possible palatal fistula |
| Le Fort I osteotomy | — Low likehood of affecting facial growth | — Potential damage to tooth buds<br>— Possible epiphora |
| Midfacial degloving | — Good anterior exposure<br>— No facial scar | — Hypoesthesia in area supplied by infraorbital nerve<br>— Possible oroantral fistula and epiphora<br>— Poor superior exposure |
| Anterior craniofacial Approach — bifrontal craniotomy with a transfacial approach | — Excellent exposure to the anterior cranial base, nasal cavities and sinuses | — Formal craniotomy required |
| Trans-nasal, trans-facial | — No need for frontal craniotomy and frontal lobe retraction<br>— Decreased dural defects<br>— Adequate exposure to cribriform plate, dura, and anterior skull base | |

## Esthesioneuroblastomas

Esthesioneuroblastomas or olfactory neuroblastomas are neuroectodermal tumors believed to originate from the mitotically active basal layer of the olfactory epithelium, normally located within the superior one third of the nasal septum, cribriform plate, and superior turbinates.[82] Esthesioneuroblastomas have a bimodal age distribution with 20% of patients affected in their second decade. 30% present with regional and distant metastases to cervical lymph nodes, bone and lung.[83] Hyam *et al.* categorized esthesioneuroblastomas into four grades depending on their degree of pleomorphism, calcification, necrosis and the number of mitoses.[84] Histological grade was identified as the most significant prognostic factor in a series of 49 patients with esthesioneuroblastomas.[85]

*Staging*: There is no universally accepted staging system; commonly used ones include the Kadish system and the Dulguerov-Calcaterra UCLA TNM system (Tables 4 and 5).

Five-year survival rates in patients with Stage A, B, and C disease have been reported to be 75%, 60%, and 41%, respectively.[87]

The TNM system first proposed by Dulguerov and Calcaterra based on both CT and MR data is more useful in-delineating tumor extent.[88]

**Table 4. Kadish Staging System.**[86]

| | |
|---|---|
| **Stage A**: | the tumor is limited to the nasal cavity. |
| **Stage B**: | it is localized to the nasal cavity and paranasal sinuses. |
| **Stage C**: | it extends beyond the nasal cavity and paranasal sinuses. |

**Table 5. Dulguerov-Calcaterra UCLA TNM system.**[88]

| | |
|---|---|
| **T1** | — Tumor involving the nasal cavity and/or paranasal sinuses (excluding sphenoid), sparing the most superior ethmoidal cells. |
| **T2** | — Tumor involving the nasal cavity and/or paranasal sinuses (including the sphenoid), with extension to or erosion of the cribriform plate. |
| **T3** | — Tumor extending into the orbit or protruding into the anterior cranial fossa, without dural invasion. |
| **T4** | — Tumor involving the brain. |
| **N0** | — No cervical lymph node metastasis. |
| **N1** | — Any form of cervical lymph node metastasis. |
| **M0** | — No metastasis. |
| **M1** | — Distant metastasis. |

### Treatment

Due to the rarity of esthesioneuroblastomas, there is no consensus for standard treatment. Craniofacial resection is the "gold standard" by which any other treatment is compared.[89] In select cases where the tumor can be accessed and removed in its entirety form below, a trans-nasal, trans-facial, microscope assisted anterior skull base approach can be used, obviating the need for a frontal craniectomy. In adults, some groups have vigorously advocated an endoscopic approach to these tumors. Postoperative radiotherapy is usually administered except for lesions with negative resection margins. Chemotherapy is often recommended as an adjunct therapy for high grade tumors.[80]

## TUMORS OF THE MIDDLE CRANIAL BASE IN CHILDREN

Pediatric tumors of the middle cranial base are subdivided into three anatomic locales: central (sphenoid sinus/sella turcica), paracentral (cavernous sinus), and lateral (sphenoid wing/infratemporal fossa).[90] The patient's presenting symptoms are directly related to tumor's anatomical location.

### Central

Most patients present with endocrine dysfunction: pituitary and hypothalamic abnormalities such as panhypopituitarism, precocious puberty, secondary amenorrhea, and diabetes inspidus. Visual deficits are also prevalent, due to mass effect on the optic nerve and chiasm.[90]

### Paracentral

Patients often demonstrate cranial neuropathies, suffering intractable facial pain and dysesthesia. The deficits are often due to mass effect on: the optic nerve in the orbital apex; third through sixth cranial nerves; temporal and frontal lobes; and the cavernous carotid artery.[90]

### Lateral

Patients may develop facial asymmetries and oropharyngeal obstruction due to effects on the trigeminal nerve, lateral orbit, and infratemporal fossa.[90]

### Histological Subtypes

Multiple histological subtypes comprise the neoplasms of the middle cranial base in children. Pituitary adenomas, craniopharyngiomas, hemangiomas, giant cell tumors, malignant fibrous histiocytomas, optic nerve gliomas, osteoblastomas, and juvenile nasopharyngeal angiofibromas have all been reported.[81,91]

### Approaches

(1) Frontotemporal with orbital and/or zygomatic osteotomy.
(2) Temporal with zygomatic osteotomy and/or anterior petrosectomy.
(3) Preauricular infratemporal with or without mandibular dislocation or resection.
(4) Transsphenoidal.[92]

### Rhabdomyosarcoma (RMS)

By far, rhabdomyosarcoma is the most commonly diagnosed soft tissue sarcoma in children younger than 15 years of age at skull base or any other subsites; 65% of cases are diagnosed in children younger than six years of age. The annual incidence is estimated to be four to seven per million children.[93]

Thirty-five percent of RMS is found in the head and neck. The most frequently affected site is the orbit (20–40%), followed by parameningeal sites (middle ear, nasal cavity, paranasal sinuses, nasopharynx, and infratemporal fossa), and other sites (scalp, oral cavity, pharynx and neck).[93] Parameningeal involvement is a poor prognostic factor due to the anatomic proximity to the central nervous system.

RMS is one of the differential diagnoses for small, round, blue cell tumors of childhood. Light microscopy, immunohistochemistry and cytogenetic testing help in diagnosing and subtyping RMS:

(1) Embryonal (85%): spindle-shaped cells with a stroma-rich appearance. This subtype is commonly found in the orbit of young children. A variant of embryonal RMS is botryoid RMS, characterized by a protruding "grape-like" appearance.[83,93]
(2) Alveolar (10%): consists of small, round, densely packed cells lined up along spaces reminiscent of pulmonary alveoli.[83,93]
(3) Pleomorphic.
(4) Mixed.

## Presentation and Evaluation

The presenting symptoms in children with RMS vary depending upon the anatomical site of the primary tumor. Most commonly, children present with a painless, enlarging mass. Involvement of the orbit produces proptosis and rarely ophthalmoplgia. Parameningeal involvement leads to nasal, aural, and sinus obstruction symptoms with or without bloody discharge.[93] Evaluation involves mapping the extent of the primary tumor and ruling out metastatic spread. CT and MRI complement each other in determining the exact anatomical boundary of the primary tumor. Complete blood count, serum electrolytes, liver function tests, chest CT, and bone marrow biopsy are important in checking for metastases to common sites of tumor spread such as the lungs, bone, and bone marrow.

## Staging

Surgery is an integral part of a clinical grouping (CG) system developed by the Intergroup Rhabdomyosarcoma Study (IRS). This CG system divides patients into four groups depending on the amount

**Table 6. Clinical group stage system for rhabdomyosarcoma.**[95]

| | |
|---|---|
| **Group 1** | Localized disease, completely excised, no microscopic residual. |
| **A** | Confined to site of origin, completely resected. |
| **B** | Infiltrating beyond site of origin, completely resected. |
| **Group 2** | Total gross resection. |
| **A** | Gross total resection, but with microscopic residual disease. |
| **B** | Regional disease with involved lymph nodes, completely resected without microscopic residual. |
| **C** | Microscopic local and/or nodal residual. |
| **Group 3** | Incomplete resection or biopsy with gross residual. |
| **Group 4** | Distant metastases. |

of tumor left after surgery and the degree of tumor spread at the time of diagnosis (Table 6).[93]

However, this CG system fails to take into account the diverging surgical options at different centers, and other prognostic factors such as tumor size and site.[94]

IRS-IV thus introduced a pretreatment tumor-nodes-metastasis (TNM) staging system modified by site of origin (Table 7).[95]

### Treatment

Resectable RMS is best treated by surgical excision without causing severe functional or aesthetic deformity in the patient. Otherwise, multiagent neoadjuvant chemotherapy and radiotherapy are used in cases of unresectable disease or residual disease after incomplete excision.[93] Significant strides have been made since the inception of IRS-I. Cure rates now approach 70% for new cases of RMS.[93]

## Nasopharyngeal Cancer

Nasopharyngeal cancer (NPC) is one of the few epithelial cancers that presents in childhood. While NPC accounts for 80% to 95% of all adult nasopharyngeal tumors, in children it only accounts for 20%.[83] Adolescents in their second decade are most commonly

Table 7. TNM staging of rhabdomyosarcoma.[95]

| Stage | Sites | Tumor (T) | Size | Node (N) | Metastases (M) |
|---|---|---|---|---|---|
| I | Orbit, head and neck (excluding parameningeal) | T1 or T2 | a or b | N0, N1, or Nx | M0 |
| II | Cranial parameningeal | T1 or T2 | a | N0 or Nx | M0 |
| III | Cranial parameningeal | T1 or T2 | a | N1 | M0 |
| | | | b | N0, N1, or Nx | |
| IV | All | T1 or T2 | a or b | N0 or N1 | M1 |

T = Tumor.
T1 Confined to anatomic site of origin, (a) ≤5 cm in diameter in size, (b) >5 cm in diameter in size.
T2 Extension and/or fixation to surrounding tissue, (a) ≤5 cm in diameter in size, (b) >5 cm in diameter in size.
N = Regional nodes.
N0 Not clinically involved.
N1 Clinically involved.
Nx Clinical status unknown.
M = Metastases.
M0 No distant metastasis.
M1 Distant metastasis present.

affected, with a male predilection (M:F 2–3:1).[96,97] Similar to its adult counterpart, undifferentiated NPC in children is endemic in Southern China. Genetic predisposition includes HLA A2 Bsin2 haplotype, B17 type.[98] EBV infection is implicated in oncogenesis, in addition to other environmental factors such as ingestion of Cantonese-style salted fish during childhood.[98]

## Presentation

Children with NPC can present with: a neck mass (70%–90%), nasal obstruction/epistaxis (50–70%), auditory symptoms (tinnitus, hearing loss, otalgia 30%–45%), headache (27%–32%), cranial neuropathy (26–32%) and trismus (4.5%).[96,97]

## Histopathology

The World Health Organization (WHO) has classified NPC into three subtypes:

Type I: keratinizing squamous-cell carcinoma, characterized by keratin production.
Type II: non-keratinizing epidermoid carcinoma; further divided into type IIa with cellular pleiomorphism and type IIb with lymphoid infiltration.
Type III: undifferentiated carcinoma, also known as lymphoepithelioma, characterized by non-malignant lymphoid infiltration.

Most children (>90%), even those from non-endemic areas, present with type III disease.[96,97]

## Diagnosis and Staging

In addition to CT and MRI of the head and neck, chest CT, bone scans, and liver ultrasonography are recommended to check for distant metastases.[96] Bone marrow biopsy should be performed in advanced disease. Spinal puncture to obtain cerebrospinal fluid for cytological analysis should also be considered in cases of skull base involvement. The AJCC TNM system is commonly used for staging NPC (Table 8).

## Treatment and Prognosis

The optimal treatment strategies for children with NPC have been extrapolated from adult data. First line treatment consists of radiotherapy to the nasopharynx and bilateral cervical nodal basins with or without neoadjuvant or concomitant chemotherapy. The role of surgery is limited generally to biopsy of the primary site, or curative neck dissection for persistent cervical lymphadenopathy after chemoradiation.[96,98] Three- and 5-year survival rates are 80% and 60%, respectively.[97]

**Table 8. American Joint Committee on cancer nasopharyngeal cancer staging classification T stage extent of primary tumor.**

T1 Confined to nasopharynx.
T2 Extends to oropharynx or nasal cavity.
2a Without parapharyngeal extension.
2b With parapharyngeal extension.
T3 Invades bones or paranasal sinuses.
T4 Involvement of cranial nerves, intracranial contents, infratemporal fossa, hypopharynx, or orbit.

**N stage lymph-node disease**

N0 No lymph-node metastases
N1 Unilateral lymph node(s) ≤6 cm
N2 Bilateral lymph nodes ≤6 cm
N3 Metastases in lymph nodes
3a Greater than 6 cm
3b With extension to the supraclavicular fossa

**M stage distant metastases**

M0 Absent
M1 Present

**Stage group T stage N stage M stage**

I T1 N0 M0
IIA T2a N0 M0
IIB T2b N0 M0
T1–T2b N1 M0
III T3 N0–1 M0
T1–T3 N2 M0
IVA T4 N0–2 M0
IVB T1–4 N3 M0
IVC T1–4 N0–3 M1

The majority of children (>80%) present with at least stage III disease.[96–98]

Twenty to fifty percent of treated patients develop recurrent or metastatic disease, mostly within one to two years after initial diagnosis. The most common sites of distant metastases are the lungs and bone.[96,97] Reirradiation can achieve five-year survival rates of 40% in selected patients.[99–101]

## REFERENCES

1. Park YW. Evaluation of neck masses in children. *Am Fam Physician* 1995 June;51(8):1904–1912.
2. Dickson PV, Davidoff AM. Malignant neoplasms of the head and neck. *Semin Pediatr Surg* 2006 May; 15(2):92–98.
3. Turkington JR, Paterson A, Sweeney LE, *et al.* Neck masses in children. *Br J Radiol* 2005 Jan;78(925):75–85.
4. Liu ES, Bernstein JM, Sculerati N, *et al.* Fine needle aspiration biopsy of pediatric head and neck masses. *Int J Pediatr Otorhinolaryngol* 2001 Aug 20;60(2):135–140.
5. van de Schoot L, Aronson DC, Behrendt H, *et al.* The role of fine-needle aspiration cytology in children with persistent or suspicious lymphadenopathy. *J Pediatr Surg* 2001 Jan;36(1):7–11.
6. Rapkiewicz A, Thuy Le B, Simsir A, Cangiarella J, Levine P. Spectrum of head and neck lesions diagnosed by fine-needle aspiration cytology in the pediatric population. *Cancer* 2007 Aug 25;111(4):242–251.
7. Donnellan KA, Carron JD, Bigler SA, *et al.* Metastatic insular thyroid carcinoma in the pediatric patient. *AM J Otolaryngol* 2009 Jan-Feb; 30(1):61–64. Epub 2008 July 9.
8. Goepfert H, Dichtel WJ, Samaan NA. Thyroid cancer in children and teenagers. *NA Arch Otolaryngol* 1984 Feb;110(2):72–75.
9. Buckwalter JA, Gurll NJ, Thomas CG Jr. Cancer of the thyroid in youth. *World J Surg* 1981 Jan;5(1):15–25.
10. Ries LAG, Melbert D, Krapcho M, *et al.* 1975–2004. Bethesda: National Cancer Institute, 2007.
11. Safford SD, Skinner MA. Thyroid and parathyroid disease in children. *Semin Pediatr Surg* 2006 May;15(2):85–91.
12. Collini P, Massimino M, Leite SF, *et al.* Papillary thyroid carcinoma of childhood and adolescence: a 30-year experience at the Istituto Nazional Tumori in Milan. *Pediatr Blood Cancer* 2006 Mar;46(3): 300–306.
13. Palmer BA, Zarroug AE, Poley RN, *et al.* Papillary thyroid carcinoma in children: risk factors and complications of disease recurrence. *J Pediatr Surg* 2005 Aug;40(8):1284–1288.

14. Vassilopoulou-Sellin R, Goepfert H, Raney B, *et al.* Differentiated thyroid cancer in children and adolescents: clinical outcome and mortality after long-term follow-up. *Head Neck* 1998 Sep;20(6): 549–555.
15. Farahati J, Bucsky P, Parlowsky T, *et al.* Characteristics of differentiated thyroid carcinoma in children and adolescents with respect to age, gender and histology. *Cancer* 1997 Dec 1;80(11):2156–2162.
16. Howe HL, WU X, Ries LA, *et al.* Annual report to the nation on the status of cancer, 1975–2003, featuring cancer among U.S. Hispanic/Latino Populations. *Cancer* 2006 Oct 15;107(8):1711–1742.
17. Millman B, Pellitteri PK. Thyroid carcinoma in children and adolescents. *Arch Otolaryngol Head Neck Surg* 1995 Nov;121(11): 1261–1264.
18. Josefson J, Zimmerman D. Thyroid nodules and cancers in children. *Pediatr Endocrinol Rev* 2008 Sep;6(1):14–23.
19. Powers PA, Dinauer CA, Tuttle RM, *et al.* Tumor size and extent of disease at diagnosis predict the response to initial therapy for papillary thyroid carcinoma in children and adolescents. *J Pediatr Endocrinol Metab* 2003 Jun;16(5):693–702.
20. Tronko MD, Howe GR, Bogdanova TI, *et al.* A cohort study of thyroid cancer and other thyroid disease after the chernobyl accident: thyroid cancer in ukraine detected during first screening. *J Natl Cancer Inst* 2006 Jul 5;98(13):897–903.
21. Welch Dinauer CA, Tuttle RM, Robie DK, *et al.* Clinical features associated with metastasis and recurrence of differentiated thyroid cancer in children, adolescents and young adults. *Clin Endocrinol (Oxf)* 1998 Nov;49(5):619–628.
22. Chaukar DA, Rangarajan V, Nair N, *et al.* Pediatric thyroid cancer. *J Surg Oncol* 2005 Nov 1;92(2):130–133.
23. Dinauer CA, Breuer C, Rivkees SA. Differentiated thyroid cancer in children: diagnosis and management. *Curr Opin Oncol* 2008 Jan;20(1): 59–65.
24. Smith MB, Xue H, Strong L, *et al.* Forty-year experience with second malignancies after treatment of childhood cancer: analysis of outcome following the development of the second malignancy. *J Pediatr Surg* 1993 Oct;28(10):1342–1348; discussion 1348–1349.

25. Maule M, Scélo G, Pastore G, *et al.* Risk of second malignant neoplasms after childhood leukemia and lymphoma: an international study. *J Natl Cancer Inst* 2007 May 16;99(10):790–800.
26. Davies SM. Subsequent malignant neoplasms in survivors of childhood cancer: childhood cancer survivor study (CCSS) studies. *Pediatr Blood Cancer.* 2007 Jun 15;48(7):727–730.
27. Cooper DS, Doherty GM, Haugen BR, *et al.* Management guidelines for patients with thyroid nodules and differentiated thyroid cancer. *Thyroid* 2006 Feb;16(2):109–142.
28. Corrias A, Einaudi S, Chiorboli E, *et al.* Accuracy of fine needle aspiration biopsy of thyroid nodules in detecting malignancy in childhood: comparison with conventional clinical, laboratory and imaging approaches. *J Clin Endocrinol Metab* 2001 Oct;86(10): 4644–4648.
29. Hung W, Sarlis NJ, Current controversies in the management of pediatric patients with well-differentiated nonmedullary thyroid cancer: a review. *Thyroid* 2002 Aug;12(8):683–702.
30. Skinner MA. Management of hereditary thyroid cancer in children. *Surg Oncol* 2003 Aug;12(2):101–104.
31. Skinner MA, Moley JA, Dilley WG, *et al.* Prophylactic thyroidectomy in multiple endocrine neoplasia type 2A. *N Engl J Med* 2005 Sep 15; 353(11):1105–1113.
32. Powers PA, Dinauer CA, Tuttle RM, *et al.* The MACIS score predicts the clinical course of papillary thyroid carcinoma in children and adolescents. *J Pediatr Endocrinol Metab* 2004 Mar;17(3):339–343.
33. Yamashita S, Saenko V. Mechanisms of disease: molecular genetics of childhood thyroid cancers. *Nat Clin Pract Endocrinol Metab* 2007 May;3(5):422–429.
34. Fenton CL, Lukes Y, Nicholson D, *et al.* The RET/PTC mutations are common in sporadic papillary thyroid carcinoma of children and young adults. J Clin Endocrinol Metab 2000 Mar;85(3):1170–1175.
35. Lemoine NR, Mayall ES, Wyllie FS, *et al.* Activated RAS oncogenes in human thyroid cancers. *Cancer Res* 1988 Aug 15;48(16):4459–4463.
36. Asai N, Jijiwa M, Enomoto A, *et al.* RET receptor signaling: dysfunction in thyroid cancer and hirschsprung's disease. *Pathol Int* 2006 Apr; 56(4):164–172.

37. Bongarzone I, Butti MG, Coronelli S, *et al.* Frequent activation of RET protooncogene by fusion with a new activating gene in papillary thyroid carcinomas. *Cancer Res* 1994 Jun 1;54(11):2979–2985.
38. Grigsby PW, Gal-or A, Michalski JM, *et al.* Childhood and adolescent thyroid carcinoma. *Cancer* 2002 Aug 15;95(4):724–729.
39. Gingalewski CA, Newman KD. Seminars: controversies in the management of pediatric thyroid malignancy. *J Surg Oncol* 2006 Dec 15;94(8):748–752.
40. Palmedo H, Bucerius J, Joe A, *et al.* Integrated PET/CT in differentiated thyroid cancer: diagnostic accuracy and impact on patient management. *J Nucl Med* 2006 Apr;47(4):616–624.
41. Parisi MT, Mankoff D. Differentiated pediatric thyroid cancer: correlates with adult disease, controversies in treatment. *Semin Nucl Med* 2007 Sep;37(5):340–356.
42. Zimmerman D, Hay ID, Gough IR, *et al.* Papillary thyroid carcinoma in children and adults: long-term follow-up of 1039 patients conservatively treated at one institution during three decades. *Surgery* 1988 Dec;104(6):1157–1166.
43. Newman KD, Black T, Heller G, *et al.* Differentiated thyroid cancer: determinants of disease progression in patients <21 years of age at diagnosis: a report from the surgical discipline committee of the children's cancer group. *Ann Surg* 1998 Apr;227(4):533–541.
44. Demidchik YE, Demidchik EP, Reiners C, *et al.* Comprehensive clinical assessment of 740 cases of surgically treated thyroid cancer in children of belarus. *Ann Surg* 2006 Apr;243(4):525–532.
45. Savio R, Gosnell J, Palazzo FF, *et al.* The role of a more extensive surgical approach in the initial multimodality management of papillary thyroid cancer in children. *J Pediatr Surg* 2005 Nov;40(11):1696–1700.
46. de Roy van Zuidewijn DB, Songun I, Kievit J, *et al.* Complications of thyroid surgery. *Ann Surg Oncol* 1995 Jan;2(1):56–60.
47. Palmer BA, Zarroug AE, Poley RN, *et al.* Papillary thyroid carcinoma in children: risk factors and complications of disease recurrence. *J Pediatr Surg* 2005 Aug;40(8):1284–1288.
48. Okada T, Sasaki F, Takahashi H, *et al.* Management of childhood and adolescent thyroid carcinoma: long-term follow-up and clinical characteristics. *Eur J Pediatr Surg* 2006 Feb;16(1):8–13.

49. Baudin E, Do Cao C, Cailleux AF, *et al.* Positive predictive value of serum thyroglobulin levels, measured during the first year of follow-up after thyroid hormone withdrawal, in thyroid cancer patients. *J Clin Endocrinol Metab* 2003 Mar;88(3):1107–1111.
50. Skinner MA, DeBenedetti MK, Moley JF, *et al.* Medullary thyroid carcinoma in children with multiple endocrine neoplasia types 2A and 2B. *J Pediatr Surg* 1996 Jan;31(1):177–181; discussion 181–182.
51. American Thyroid Association Guidelines Task Force, Kloos RT, Eng C, Evans DB, Francis GL, Gagel RF, Gharib H, Moley JF, Pacini F, Ringel MD, Schlumberger M, Wells SA Jr. Medullary thyroid cancer: management guidelines of the American Thyroid Association. *Thyroid* 2009 Jun;19(6):565–612.
52. Mehta D, Willging JP. Pediatric salivary gland lesions. *Semin Pediatr Surg* 2006 May;15(2):76–84.
53. Rahbar R, Grimmer JF, Vargas SO, *et al.* Mucoepidermoid carcinoma of the parotid gland in children: a 10-year experience. *Arch Otolaryngol Head Neck Surg* 2006 Apr;132(4):375–380.
54. De Campora E, Croce A, Bicciolo G, *et al.* Adenoid-cystic carcinoma (cylindroma) of the pyriform sinus in pediatric age. *Int J Pediatr Otorhinolaryngol* 1987 Dec;14(2–3):235–242.
55. Neglia JP, Friedman DL, Yasui Y, *et al.* Second malignant neoplasms in five-year survivors of childhood cancer: childhood cancer survivor study. *J Natl Cancer Inst* 2001 Apr 18;93(8):618–629.
56. Védrine PO, Coffinet L, Temam S, *et al.* Mucoepidermoid carcinoma of salivary glands in the pediatric age group: 18 clinical cases, including 11 second malignant neoplasms. *Head Neck* 2006 Sep;28(9): 827–833.
57. Thorvaldsson SE, Beahrs OH, Woolner LB, *et al.* Mucoepidermoid tumors of the major salivary glands. *AM J Surg* 1970 Oct;120(4): 432–438.
58. Bentz BG, Hughes CA, Lüdemann JP, *et al.* Masses of the salivary gland region in children. *Arch Otolaryngol Head Neck Surg* 2000 Dec;126(12):1435–1439.
59. Levitt SH, McHugh RB, Gomez-Marin O, *et al.* Clinical staging system for cancer of the salivary gland: a retrospective study. *Cancer* 1981 Jun 1;47(11):2712–2724.

60. Brigger MT, Pearson SE. Management of parapharyngeal minor salivary neoplasms in children: a case report and review. *Int J Pediatr Otorhinolaryngol* 2006 Jan;70(1):143–146.
61. Garcia CJ, Flores PA, Arch JD, *et al.* Ultrasonography in the study of salivary gland lesions in children. *Pediatr Radiol* 1998 June;28(6): 418–425.
62. Amedee RG, Dhurandhar NR, Fine needle aspiration biopsy. *Laryngoscope* 2001 Sep;111(9):1551–1557.
63. Zbaren P, Schar C, Hotz MA, *et al.* Value of fine-needle aspiration cytology of parotid gland masses. *Laryngoscope* 2001 Nov;111(11 Pt 1): 1989–1992.
64. Shapiro NL, Bhattacharyya N, Clinical characteristics and survival for major salivary gland malignancies in children. *Otolaryngol Head Neck Surg* 2006 Apr;134(4):631–634.
65. Batsakis JG. Salivary gland neoplasia: an outcome of modified morphogenesis and cytodifferentiation. *Oral Surg Oral Med Oral Pathol* 1980 Mar;49(3):229–232.
66. Hicks J, Flaitz C. Mucoepidermoid carcinoma of salivary glands in children and adolescents: assessment of proliferation markers. *Oral Oncol* 2000 Sep;36(5):454–460.
67. Sato T, Kamata SE, Kawabata K, *et al.* Acinic cell carcinoma of the parotid gland in a child. *Pediatr Surg Int* 2005 May;21(5):377–380.
68. Bull PD. Salivary gland neoplasia in childhood. *Int J Pediatr Otorhinolaryngol* 1999 Oct 5;49(Suppl 1):S235–S238.
69. Ogata H, Ebihara S, Mukai K. Salivary gland neoplasms in children. *Jpn J Clin Oncol* 1994 Apr;24(2):88–93.
70. Batsakis JG, Luna MA. Undifferentiated carcinomas of salivary glands. *Ann Otol Rhinol Laryngol* 1991 Jan;100(1):82–84. Review.
71. Luna MA, Batsakis JG, el-Nagger AK. Salivary gland tumors in children. *Ann Otol Rhinol Laryngol* 1991 Oct;100(10):869–871. Review.
72. Rodríguez-Cuevas S, Labastida S, Baena L, *et al.* Risk of nodal metastases from malignant salivary gland tumors related to tumor size and grade of malignancy. *Eur Arch Otorhinolaryngol* 1995;252(3):139–142.
73. Spiro RH, Armstrong J, Harrison L, *et al.* Carcinoma of major salivary glands. recent trends. *Arch Otolaryngol Head Neck Surg* 1989 Mar;115(3):316–321.

74. Rickert CH, Paulus W. Epidemiology of central nervous system tumors in childhood and adolescence based on the new WHO classification. *Childs Nerv Syst* 2001;17:503–511.
75. Teo C, Dornhoffer J, Hanna E, *et al.* Application of skull base techniques to pediatric neurosurgery. *Childs Nerv Syst* 1999;15:103–109.
76. Mandonnet E, Kolb F, Tran Ba Huy P, *et al.* Spectrum of skull base tumors in children and adolescents: a series of 42 patients and review of the literature. *Childs Nerv Syst* 2008;24:699–706.
77. Brockmeyer D, Gruber DP, Haller J, *et al.* Pediatric skull base surgery. 2. experience and outcomes in 55 patients. *Pediatr Neurosurg* 2003;38:9–15.
78. Gil Z, Constantini S, Spektor S, *et al.* Skull base approaches in the pediatric population. *Head Neck* 2005;27:682–689.
79. Hanbali F, Tabrizi P, Lang FF, *et al.* Tumors of the skull base in children and adolescents. *J Neurosurg* 2004;100:169–178.
80. Tsai EC, Santoreneos S, Rutka JT. Tumors of the skull base in children: review of tumor types and management strategies. *Neurosurg Focus* 2002;12(5):1–13.
81. Lewark TM, Allen GC, Chowdhury K, *et al.* Le Fort I osteotomy and skull base tumors: a pediatric experience. *Arch Otolaryngol Head Neck Surg* 2000;126:1004–1008.
82. Barnes L, Kapadia SB. The biology and pathology of selected skull base tumors. *J Neurooncol* 1994;20:213–240.
83. Borge MF, *et al.* Tumores otorrinolaringológicos: *An Pediatr* 2003; 58(5):456–463.
84. Hyams VJ, Batsakis JG, Michaels L. Olfactory neuroblastoma. In: Hyams VJ, Batsakis JG, Michaels L, eds. *Tumors of the Upper Respiratory Tract and Ear.* Washington: Armed Forces Institute of Pathology, 1988; pp. 240–248.
85. Morita A, Ebersold MJ, Olsen KD, *et al.* Esthesioneuroblastoma: Prognosis and management. *Neurosurgery* 1993;32:706–715.
86. Kadish S, Goodman M, Wang CC. Olfactory neuroblastoma. A clinical analysis of 17 cases. *Cancer* 1976;37:1571–1576.
87. Elkon D, Hightower SI, Lim ML, *et al.* Esthesioneuroblastoma. *Cancer* 1979;44:1087–1094.
88. Dulguerov P, Calcaterra T. Esthesioneuroblastoma. The UCLA experience 1970–1990. *Layngoscope* 1992 Aug;102(8):843–849.

89. Levine PA. Would Dr. Ogura approve of endoscopic resection of esthesioneuroblastomas? An analysis of endoscopic resection data versus that of craniofacial resection. *Laryngoscope* 2009 Jan;119(1):3–7.
90. Morita A, Sekhar LN. Skull base tumors. In: Bernstein M, Berger MS, eds. *Neuro-Oncology: The Essentials*. New York: Thieme Medical Publishers, 2000, pp. 419–433.
91. Low Y, Foo CL, Seow WT. Childhood temporal bone osteoblastoma: a case report. *J Pediatr Surg* 2000;35:1127–1129.
92. Kennedy JD, Haines SJ. Review of skull base surgery approaches: with special reference to pediatric patients. *J Neurooncol* 1994;20:291–312.
93. Dagher R, Helman L. Rhabdomyosarcoma: an overview. *Oncologist* 1999;4:34–44.
94. Pappo AS, Shapiro DN, Crist WM. Rhabdomyosarcoma. Biology and treatment. *Pediatr Clin North Am* 1997;44:953–972.
95. Crist WM, Anderson JR, Meza JL, *et al.* Intergroup rhabdomyosarcoma study-IV: results for patients with nonmetastatic disease. *J Clin Oncol* Jun 2001;19(12):3091–3102.
96. Ayan I, Kaytan E, Ayan N. Childhood nasopharyngeal carcinoma: from biology to treatment. *Lancet Oncology* 2003;4:3–21.
97. Hong JD, Liao YP, Yuan J, *et al.* Clinical and prognostic analysis of nasopharyngeal carcinoma in 44 children and adolescents. *Zhong Nan Da Xue Xue Bao Yi Xue Ban* 2008 Aug;33(8):723–726.
98. Cvitkovic E. Bachouchi M, Armand JP. Nasopharyngeal carcinoma: biology, natural history and therapeutic implications. *Hematol Oncol Clin North Am* 1991;5:821–823.
99. Vokes EE, Liebowitz DN, Weichselbaum RR. Nasopharyngeal carcinoma. *Lancet* 1997;350:1087–1091.
100. Jenkin RDT, Anderson JR, Jereb B, *et al.* Nasopharyngeal carcinoma — a retrospective review of patients less than thirty years of age: a report of children's cancer study group. *Cancer* 1981;47:360–366.
101. Uzel Ö, Yörük SÖ, Sahinler I, *et al.* Nasopharyngeal carcinoma in childhood: long term results of 32 patients. *Radiother Oncol* 2001;58:137–141.

# PLASTICS

# 16

# Craniofacial Anomalies

*Prabhat K. Bhama and Kathleen C. Y. Sie*

## INTRODUCTION

Children with craniofacial anomalies have anatomic malformations of the cranium, cranial base, mandible, and face. This chapter is structured to provide an overview of the otolaryngologic management of issues in this population, the spectrum of craniofacial disorders commonly encountered in pediatric otolaryngology, and a brief review of head and neck embryology. We focus on the systematic assessment and management of these patients.

### Multidisciplinary Approach

When dealing with patients who have craniofacial disorders, it is essential to take a multidisciplinary team-based approach. Since these patients may have a complex series of issues, it is the standard of care to involve appropriate specialists. These specialists may include: audiology, neurosurgery, nursing, nutrition, oral-maxillofacial surgery, orthodontics, otolaryngology, pediatrics, plastic surgery, psychology, social work, and speech pathology. The team approach ensures that all of the patient's issues are identified and addressed.

**Systematic Assessment**

Every patient with a craniofacial anomaly should undergo a complete history and physical examination. The otolaryngologist should elicit a clinical history regarding airway, feeding and hearing. A complete head and neck exam should be performed on each patient.

## OTOLARYNGOLOGIC MANAGEMENT

### Airway

Hypoplasia of the midface and/or mandible in craniofacial disorders results in crowding of the nasal airways, nasopharynx, oral cavity, and oropharynx. The impact of craniofacial anomalies on the patency of the airway may range from simple nasal obstruction to acute life-threatening airway obstruction, requiring emergent management. Unfortunately, a universally accepted set of guidelines for airway management in these patients does not exist. Interventions may range from positioning to tracheotomy.

There are several anatomic causes of airway obstruction in these patients, as highlighted below.[1] When evaluating the patient, it is essential to assess the degree of airway compromise during normal awake activity, crying, eating, and sleeping[2] to identify the site(s) and degree of airway obstruction.

*Etiologies*

I. Nose
   a. Congenital pyriform aperture stenosis
   b. Septal deviation
   c. Narrow nasal passages
II. Nasopharynx
   a. Choanal atresia
   b. Adenoid hypertrophy
   c. Retruded midface
III. Shortened anterior skull base
IV. Oropharynx/hypopharynx/larynx

a. Palatine tonsil hypertrophy
b. Pendulous uvula
c. Elongated soft palate with poor tone
d. Retrognathia
e. Glossoptosis
f. Malformation of cartilaginous support structures

*Source*: Adapted from Keskin and Jackson (2005).[1]

These etiologies of airway obstruction can be aggravated by other airway disorders, such as laryngomalacia, tracheoesophageal fistula, and diaphragmatic hernia.[3] Thus, when assessing the airway, the clinician should always consider the possibility of synchronous lesions. Patients may also have diseases of the central nervous system or cardiovascular system that exacerbate the consequences of the anatomic airway obstruction.

## Management of the Airway

Management strategies for the airway can be classified into three temporal categories (acute, subacute, and chronic) based upon the urgency of the situation. In any case, it is important to keep in mind that the neonate is an obligate nasal breather, and that airway obstruction in children can be very dynamic.

### *Acute*

I. Positioning
    a. Prone positioning
    b. Jaw-thrust maneuver
    c. Extend head at the neck while supine
II. Appliances
    a. Nasopharyngeal airway
    b. Oral airway
    c. Laryngeal mask airway
    d. Continuous positive airway pressure (CPAP)

e. Bilevel positive airway pressure (BiPAP)

III. Endotracheal intubation

IV. Tracheostomy

*Subacute*

I. Topical vasoconstrictive therapy (i.e. oxymetazoline)

II. Positioning

III. Nasopharyngeal airway

IV. Tongue-lip adhesion

V. Tracheostomy

VI. Mandibular advancement

*Chronic*

I. Positioning (see above)

II. Nasopharyngeal airway

III. Midface advancement

IV. Tracheostomy

Some of the strategies for acute management of the airway can also be used on a chronic basis. For instance, the prone position may be used in the acute setting, or on more chronically to help displace the tongue anteriorly by the effects of gravity. For instance, patients with Robin Sequence will often benefit from chronic prone positioning.[4] The prone position helps keep the base of tongue from obstructing the oropharyngeal airway.

The jaw-thrust maneuver is also a commonly used technique in the setting of acute airway obstruction. It works mainly by relieving oropharyngeal obstruction at the base of tongue. It can be used in conjunction with bag-masking to help ventilate a patient temporarily. Tongue-lip adhesion is also a measure that can be used to help pull the tongue anteriorly. Extending the head at the neck while in the supine position brings the airway more anteriorly, thus facilitating a more ideal view of the glottis, and allows for more efficient bag-mask ventilation.

**Surgical Intervention on the Airway**

I. Choanal atresia repair
II. Uvulopalatopharyngoplasty
III. Tonsillectomy and adenoidectomy
IV. Tongue-lip adhesion — if positioning is not able to alleviate symptoms, and the primary airway obstruction is localized to the tongue base
V. Genioglossus advancement
VI. Hyoid suspension
VII. Mandibular distraction osteogenesis — for those who fail tongue-lip adhesion and have isolated tongue-base obstruction
VIII. Tracheostomy — for patients with multiple sites of upper airway obstruction, or one site of airway obstruction refractory to more conservative treatments
IX. Midface (LeFort) advancement

**Feeding**

Because of the intricate interplay between the craniofacial structures, mastication, and deglutition, patients with craniofacial disorders often suffer from feeding problems. Patients may present with difficulties with sucking, nasal regurgitation, bronchial aspiration and coordinating breathing during feeding. Management options for feeding problems include:

I. Tube feeding (nasogastric) — this can increase the risk of gastroesophageal reflux.[5]
II. Speech/oral therapy[6]
   a. Stimulation of sucking with a pacifier
   b. Massage of the tongue
   c. Manual support of the jaw
   d. Long and soft bottle nipple with 1-mm hole
   e. Rhythmic movements of the nipple in the oral cavity during sucking
III. Caloric supplementation

## Surgical Intervention to Improve Caloric Intake

I. Management of the airway (as above)
II. Gastrostomy tube — in cases with severe dysphagia, and chronic use of nasogastric tube refractory to more conservative treatments

## Ears and Hearing

### *Hearing*

It is important to classify the type of hearing loss as conductive or sensorineural. Conductive hearing loss involves loss of hearing secondary to changes in the external or middle ears. Sensorineural hearing loss is caused by pathology in the inner ear and/or cochlear nerve as it courses to the brainstem.

I. Conductive hearing loss
   a. External auditory canal atresia/stenosis
   b. Ankylosis/ossicular abnormalities
   c. Hypoplastic middle ear cavity
   d. Otitis media and associated complications
   e. Middle ear mass
II. Sensorineural hearing loss
   a. Neoplasia on the auditory or vestibular nerve
   b. Cochlear dysfunction

### *Eustachian tube dysfunction*

Many patients with craniofacial anomalies will have otitis media with effusion resulting in hearing loss secondary to two main etiologies: impaired opening of the Eustachian tube, and defective velopharyngeal valving. This results in accumulation of fluid in the middle ear, which diminishes the amplification function of the ossicular chain. This results in a conductive hearing loss. Additionally, fluid stasis provides a favorable medium for the growth of bacteria, which may lead to otitis media. Children with chronic otitis media are predisposed to having tympanic membrane (TM) perforation, TM retraction pockets, and possibly cholesteatoma. Chronic hearing loss may affect speech and language development, and accordingly, cognitive function.

### Management of the Ears and Hearing

I. Characterize the hearing loss (conductive, sensorineural, mixed)
II. Monitor speech and language development
III. Management of otitis media with effusion
   a. Antibiotics
   b. Nasal steroids
IV. Radiographic evaluation with high resolution computed tomography of the temporal bones
   a. For persistent conductive hearing loss despite normal middle ear function
   b. For mixed or sensorineural hearing loss
V. Amplification
   a. Ear-level hearing aids for sensorineural or mixed hearing loss
   b. Bone conduction hearing aid for conductive hearing loss or for patients unable to accommodate an ear-level hearing aid

### Surgical Intervention for the Ears and Hearing

I. Myringotomy with tube placement
II. Consideration of adenoidectomy (not in patients with cleft palate)
III. Middle ear exploration or ossicular chain reconstruction
IV. Bone anchored hearing aid (BAHA) for patients less than five years of age, unable to accommodate ear-level hearing aids
V. Aural atresia repair if favorable candidate based upon audiogram and CT

## COMMON SYNDROMES

This section focuses on some of the more common syndromes dealt with by the pediatric otolaryngologist. We will first discuss specific craniofacial anomalies and then focus on syndromes involving oral clefting. Prior to describing specific disease states, several definitions are in order.

1. *Malformation* — a structural defect of an organ or a region of the body secondary to an error in development
2. *Anomaly* — a deviation from normal anatomy
3. *Syndrome* — a series of anomalies linked to a single etiology (i.e. mutation, chromosomal deletion/addition)
4. *Sequence* — a series of anomalies, of which all or some are caused by one of the other anomalies[7]

We will now present selected syndromes associated with craniofacial anomalies. While this list is not comprehensive, the idea is to present some of the more commonly encountered syndromes and illustrate guidelines for management.

**Craniofacial Anomalies**

I. Craniosynostoses syndromes
   a. Incidence — 1/1800 births
   b. Pathophysiology — caused by premature closure of one or more cranial sutures, impairing growth in the direction perpendicular to that suture line and causing compensatory growth parallel to the suture. Craniosynostosis can be isolated, or part of a larger syndrome.
   c. Specific types, and sutures involved
      i. Scaphocephaly (sagittal), most common
      ii. Trigonocephaly (metopic)
      iii. Plagiocephaly (unilateral coronal/lambdoidal) — must be distinguished from positional plagiocephaly.
      iv. Brachycephaly (bilateral coronal)
      v. Acrocephaly (sagittal, coronal, lambdoid)
      vi. Cloverleaf/kleeblattschädel
      vii. Turricephaly (frontoparietal)
   d. Management overview — surgical treatment is indicated to prevent intracranial hypertension, and for cosmesis. It consists primarily of releasing the affected sutures.

A. Apert's syndrome (acrocephalosyndactyly)
   i. Incidence — 1/160,000 live births, autosomal dominant
   ii. Diagnosis — bicoronal synostosis, maxillary hypoplasia, syndactyly ± exorbitism, hypertelorism, antimongoloid slant[8]
   iii. Pathophysiology — mutation in gene for fibroblast growth factor receptor 2 (FGFR2)[9]
   iv. Management overview
      a. Three stages:
         1. Craniosynostosis release
         2. Midface advancement
         3. Correction of hypertelorism

B. Crouzon's syndrome (craniofacial dysostosis)
   i. Incidence — 1/25,000 live births, autosomal dominant
   ii. Diagnosis — bicoronal synostosis, proptosis, midface hypoplasia
   iii. Pathophysiology — mutations in fibroblast growth factor receptor 2 or 3[10]
   iv. Management overview — similar to Apert's syndrome

II. Down syndrome (trisomy 21)
   a. Incidence — 1/600 births[11]
   b. Diagnosis
      i. Brachycephaly, structurally normal brain, midface hypoplasia, flat nasal bridge ± small oral cavity, protrusion of the tongue, atlantoaxial instability, hypoplastic paranasal sinuses, hypertrophic nasosinal mucosa, narrow hard palate
      ii. Possible soft tissue abnormalities: upsloping palpebral fissures, epicanthal folds
      iii. Possible otologic malformations: hypoplastic and low-set ears, stenotic external auditory canals, conductive hearing loss, endolymphatic hydrops, Eustachian tube dysfunction
      iv. Possible airway malformations: narrow nasopharynx, adenotonsillar hypertrophy, hypotonia and hyperplasia of the soft palate, laryngomalacia and tracheomalacia

c. Pathophysiology — duplication of chromosome 21 leading to trisomy
d. Management overview
    i. Airway:
        1. Oxygen/CPAP
        2. Tonsillectomy and adenoidectomy
        3. Tongue reduction
        4. Maxillomandibular advancement
    ii. Ears:
        1. Early hearing assessment with diagnostic auditory brainstem responses (ABR)
        2. Myringotomy with tympanostomy tube placement
        3. Canalplasty
    iii. Communication:
        1. Speech therapy assessment
        2. Sign language instruction

III. Goldenhar syndrome (oculoauriculovertebral spectrum)
a. Incidence — 1/3500 to 5600 live births
b. Diagnosis
    i. OMENS classification[12]
        1. O: Orbital distortion
        2. M: Mandibular hypoplasia
        3. E: Ear anomaly
        4. N: Nerve involvement
        5. S: Soft-tissue deficiency
    ii. Preauricular appendages and fistulas, microtia, aural atresia
    iii. Epibulbar dermoids or lipodermoid, coloboma, *or* other eye anomalies such as anophthalmia, microphthalmia, cataracts, astigmatism, blepharophimosis, or antimongoloid slanting of palpebral fissures
    iv. Unilateral macrostomia (lateral facial cleft)
    v. Unilateral facial hypoplasia, prominent forehead, hypoplasia of zygoma, maxillarymandibular hypoplasia
    vi. Vertebral anomalies[13]

c. Pathophysiology — abnormal development of first and second branchial arches, first branchial cleft, and primordial of temporal bone[13]
d. Management overview (see management guidelines above for overview) — staged reconstruction and strict follow-up. Unique treatment concepts with Goldenhar syndrome — approximately 22% of patients will need tracheostomy.[14] Extirpation of dermoids and pre-auricular tags is often warranted.[15] Ophthalmology consultation by age three months for repair of epibulbar limbal dermoids is important.[16]

IV. Pierre Robin Sequence (Robin syndrome/complex/anomaly)[17]
a. Incidence — 1/8500 to 1/20,000 births
b. Diagnosis — micrognathia, glossoptosis, airway compromise, cleft of the secondary palate, >80% of these patients may have an associated syndrome,[18] e.g. Stickler, velocardiofacial, fetal alcohol syndrome
c. Pathophysiology — micrognathia → elevation of tongue → crowding of nasopharynx and cleft of the secondary palate → feeding problems
d. Management overview (see management guidelines above for overview). Unique treatment concepts with Pierre Robin Sequence includes endoscopic evaluation of the airway. Surgical management is often necessary.[19] Early management of the airway can improve feeding because it relieves the upper airway obstruction that may be the cause of feeding problems in patients with isolated Robin Sequence[20]

V. Treacher Collins syndrome (mandibulofacial dysostosis)
a. Incidence — 1/50,000 live births
b. Diagnosis — midface hypoplasia, micrognathia, microtia, conductive hearing loss, cleft palate, coloboma of the lower eyelids, antimongoloid slanting of the palpebral fissures ± choanal atresia; physical features are bilateral and symmetric[21]
c. Pathophysiology — pathological growth of the first and second branchial arches secondary to insufficient neural crest cells

d. Management overview (see management guidelines above for overview).[21] Unique treatment concepts with Treacher Collins syndrome — anatomical assessment: craniofacial CT scan from top of skull through entirety of cervical spine with 3D reformats, with attention to the petrous temporal bone. Staged reconstruction of craniofacial skeleton:
   1. Zygomatic and orbital
   2. Maxillomandibular
   3. Nasal
   4. Soft tissue reconstruction

VI. Fetal alcohol syndrome
   a. Incidence — 0.5–2/1000 live births
   b. Diagnosis[22]
      i. Narrow forehead, short palpebral fissures, small nose and midface, long and thin vermillion border of upper lip with deficient philtrum, misalignment of dentition
      ii. Hearing disorders (both conductive and sensorineural), vestibular injury resulting in postural instability, otosclerosis, narrow external auditory canals, prominent or deformed pinnae
   c. Pathophysiology — consumption of alcohol during pregnancy results in teratogenic effects by altering development of cranial neural crest cells
   d. Management overview (see management guidelines above for overview), management of malocclusion by dentist is important in these patients. Behavioral and developmental support is also important.

*Clefting syndromes* (Table 1)

I. Cleft lip and palate
   a. Diagnosis
      i. Submucous cleft palate — diastasis of soft palate musculature with intact mucosa
      ii. Cleft of primary palate — cleft of palate anterior to incisive foramen

**Table 1. General timing of surgical treatments for oral clefting.**

| Procedure | Timing |
|---|---|
| Cleft lip repair | 3 months |
| Consider tympanostomy tube placement | |
| Palatoplasty | 9–18 months |
| Consider tympanostomy tube placement | |
| Surgical treatment of velopharyngeal insufficiency (if indicated) | >3 years of age |
| Alveolar bone grafting | 9–11 years |
| Nasal reconstruction | 12–18 years |
| Orthognathic surgery | 16 years |

iii. Cleft of secondary palate — cleft of palate posterior to incisive foramen
    1. Midline
    2. Typically associated with more serious pathology

iv. Lip:
    1. Unilateral
        a. Complete — full-thickness through entire height of lip and through nasal floor
        b. Incomplete — partial thickness through lip only
    2. Bilateral
        a. Complete — complete detachment of premaxilla from the each maxilla
        b. Incomplete — continuity of the maxilla with mild or no protrusion of the premaxilla
    3. Microform — diastasis of central orbicularis oris without cleft

b. Pathophysiology
    i. The primary palate and lip form at approximately four to eight weeks of intrauterine life via fusion of the median nasal prominences
    ii. The secondary palate begins to form at approximately eight weeks, following formation of the primary palate via fusion of the maxillary processes

c. Unique issues
   i. Feeding — most patients will have trouble feeding secondary to impaired suckling that results because of inability to seal off the oropharynx from the nasopharynx. This will also result in nasal regurgitation of feeds. Patients will often fail to gain weight adequately.[23]
   ii. Ears and hearing — these patients have otitis media with effusion and their complications secondary to two main etiologies:
      1. Impaired opening of the Eustachian tube.
      2. Defective velopharyngeal valving.
d. Management
   i. Feeding
      1. Prosthetic feeding appliance/obturator
      2. Compressible feeder
      3. Use of soft rubber nipples with cross-cuts
   ii. Ears/hearing (see management guidelines above for overview)

## EMBRYOLOGY/ANATOMY

### The Branchial Apparatus

Normal anatomical development of the head and neck is largely dependent on the successful remodeling of a series of structures in the human embryo known as branchial arches, clefts, and pouches. The branchial structures are evident at five weeks gestational age and are located at the site of the future face and neck. The branchial arches are fingerlike projects separated by branchial clefts. The medial surfaces of the clefts are known as the pharyngeal pouches.

Ectoderm lines the surfaces of the branchial arches and clefts, whereas tissue within the arches is composed of mesoderm. The pharyngeal pouches are lined with endoderm. The branchial arches will subsequently develop into structures composed of muscle or bone, and the pharyngeal pouches will develop into glandular structures, or will be associated with the gastrointestinal tract. Table 2 describes the embryologic precursors and their adult derivatives.

**Table 2. Derivatives, innervation, and pathology associated with branchial arches and pharyngeal pouches.**

| Arch or pouch | Innervation | Bony/cartilaginous derivatives | Muscular derivatives | Pouch derivatives | Cleft derivatives |
|---|---|---|---|---|---|
| 1 | Trigeminal nerve | (Meckel's cartilage) → ramus and body of the mandible, sphenomandibluar ligament, anterior malleolar ligament, malleus (except manubrium), incus (except long process) | Muscles of mastication, tensor tympani, tensor veli palatini, anterior belly of digastric, mylohyoid | Epithelial lining of middle ear, tympanic membrane | External auditory canal |
| 2 | Facial nerve | (Reichert's cartilage) → stylohyoid ligament, styloid process, manubrim of malleus, long process of incus, stapes suprastructure, portion of body of the hyoid and lesser cornu of hyoid | Muscles of facial expression, posterior belly of digastric, stylohyoid, stapedius muscles | Palatine tonsil | |

*(Continued)*

Table 2. (*Continued*)

| Arch or pouch | Innervation | Bony/cartilaginous derivatives | Muscular derivatives | Pouch derivatives | Cleft derivatives |
|---|---|---|---|---|---|
| 3 | Glossopharyngeal nerve | Body and greater cornu of hyoid | Stylopharyngeus muscle | Inferior parathyroid, thymus | |
| 4–6 | Vagus nerve | Thyroid, cricoid, arytenoid, corniculate, and cuneiform cartilages | Superior, middle, inferior constrictor muscles, striated muscle from the upper half of the esophagus, extrinsic muscles of the larynx, cricothyroid, intrinsic muscles of the larynx that move the arytenoid and true/false vocal cords | Superior thyroid gland, thyroid C cells | |

## REFERENCES

1. Keskin M, Jackson IT. Airway management in craniofacial anomalies. *Eur J Plast Surg* 2005;28:253–258.
2. Sher A. Mechanisms of airway obstruction in Robin sequence: implications for treatment. *Cleft Palate Craniofac J* 1992;29:224–231.
3. Holinger L, Weiss K. Diagnosis and management of airway obstruction in craniofacial anomalies. *Otolaryngol Clin North Am* 1981;14: 1005–1017.
4. Perkins J, Sie K, Milczuk H, Richardson M. Airway management in children with craniofacial anomalies. *Cleft Palate Craniofac J* 1997;34: 135–140.
5. Gomes G, Pisani J, Macedo E, Campos A. The nasogastric feeding tube as a risk factor for aspiration and aspiration pneumonia. *Curr Opin Clin Nutr Metab Care* 2003;6:327–333.
6. Marques I, de Sousa T, Carneiro A, Peres S, Barbieri M, Bettiol H. Robin sequence: a single treatment protocol. *J Pediatr (Rio J)* 2005;81:14–22.
7. Shprintzen R. The implications of the diagnosis of Robin sequence. *Cleft Palate Craniofac J* 1992;29:205–209.
8. Cohen MJ, Kreiborg S. A clinical study of the craniofacial features in Apert syndrome. *Int J Oral Maxillofac Surg* 1996;25:45–53.
9. Lajeunie E, Catala M, Renier D. Craniosynostosis: from a clinical description to an understanding of bone formation of the skull. *Childs Nerv Syst* 1999;15:676–680.
10. Meyers G, Orlow S, Munro I, Przylepa K, Jabs E. Fibroblast growth factor receptor 3 (FGFR3) transmembrane mutation in Crouzon syndrome with acanthosis nigricans. *Nat Genet* 1995;11:462–464.
11. Venail F, Gardiner Q, Mondain M. ENT and speech disorders in children with Down's syndrome: an overview of pathophysiology, clinical features, treatments, and current management. *Clin Pediatr (Phila)* 2004;43:783–791.
12. Tewfik T, Manoukian J. The syndromial child. In: Bailey BJ, Johnson JT, Newlands SD, eds. *Head and Neck Surgery — Otolaryngology*. Philadelphia: Lippincott, Williams and Wilkins, 2006, pp. 1371–1387.
13. Kokavec R. Goldenhar syndrome with various clinical manifestations. *Cleft Palate Craniofac J* 2006;43:628–634.

14. Sculerati N, Gottlieb M, Zimbler M, Chibbaro P, McCarthy J. Airway management in children with major craniofacial anomalies. *Laryngoscope* 1998;108:1806–1812.
15. Sommer F, Pillunat L. Epibulbar dermoids — clinical features and therapeutic methods. *Klin Monatsbl Augenheilkd* 2004;221:872–877.
16. Panda A, Ghose S, Khokhar S, Das H. Surgical outcomes of Epibulbar dermoids. *J Pediatr Ophthalmol Strabismus* 2002;39:20–25.
17. Breugem C, Mink van der Molen A. What is 'Pierre Robin sequence'? *J Plast Reconstr Aesthet Surg* 2008;oct 31 [Epub ahead of print].
18. Shprintzen R. Pierre Robin, micrognathia, and airway obstruction: the dependency of treatment on accurate diagnosis. *Int Anesthesiol Clin* 1988;26:64–71.
19. Schaefer R, Stadler J, 3rd, Gosain A. To distract or not to distract: an algorithm for airway management in isolated Pierre Robin sequence. *Plast Reconstr Surg* 2004;113:1113–1125.
20. Lidsky M, Lander T, Sidman J. Resolving feeding difficulties with early airway intervention in Pierre Robin Sequence. *Laryngoscope* 2008; 118:120–123.
21. Posnick J, Ruiz R. Treacher Collins syndrome: current evaluation, treatment, and future directions. *Cleft Palate Craniofac J* 2000;37:434.
22. Sant'Anna L, Tosello D. Fetal alcohol syndrome and developing craniofacial and dental structures — a review. *Orthod Craniofac Res* 2006; 9:172–185.
23. Paradise J, McWilliams B. Simplified feeder for infants with cleft palate. *Pediatrics* 1974;53:566–568.

17

# Pediatric Ear, Nose, and Throat Trauma

*T. J. O-Lee and Peter J. Koltai*

## INTRODUCTION

Trauma is the leading cause of death of children in the United States. Each year, 15,000 children die and approximately 100,000 become permanently disabled due to trauma related injuries. Medical care rendered for these injuries are valued greater than US$15 billion annually.[1] Despite these staggering numbers, pediatric ear, nose, and throat (ENT) trauma are relatively rare. The majority of head and neck injuries consist of soft tissue trauma, in the forms of laceration, contusion, or abrasion.[2] Bony injuries occur even less frequently. Pediatric maxillofacial injuries account for approximately 5% of all facial fractures, with reported incidence ranging between 1.5% and 15%.[3–7] Children under five years have a significantly lower risk ranging from 1% to 1.5%.[8] With increasing age, the incidence of facial fracture also increases, ultimately reaching the pattern and frequency of adult trauma victims around late adolescence.[8]

For the purposes of this chapter, we will consider soft tissue injuries separately from the bony injuries. Although not mutually exclusive, these two types of injuries do require different treatment algorithms to achieve the most effective results.

## FACIAL SOFT TISSUE INJURIES

Soft tissue injuries to the face is perhaps the most commonly encountered ENT trauma in pediatric patients. Some general guidelines in their treatment include:

1. Judicious cleaning of laceration wounds, carefully removing all foreign bodies that may be embedded in the tissue. This process should take place after the wound is adequately anesthetized to minimize secondary trauma to the child and ensure thorough exploration of the wound.
2. Carefully re-aligning tissue prior to starting repair. Meticulous preservation of tissue will often make re-alignment more accurate.
3. Tissue should be closed in layers when possible. This would both increase the strength of the repair and also increase the accuracy of skin approximation. Absorbable sutures should be used whenever possible to avoid the trauma of suture removal for the child.

### Special Circumstances

*Oropharyngeal injuries*

Although relatively rare, oropharyngeal injuries are very alarming for physicians due to dramatic blood loss and the possibility of carotid injuries.[9] The most common scenario that leads to this type of trauma is a child playing or running while holding a stick-like foreign body in the mouth. Once injured, the rich vasculatures of the oropharynx tend to produce bleeding that causes panic for family members. Fortunately, these episodes are usually self-limiting and are often stopped by the time the child reaches the emergency room. Injuries limited to the medial portion of the palate and pharynx can usually be treated with prophylactic antibiotics to prevent retropharyngeal or parapharyngeal abscesses.[10] The injury site seldom requires repair since the rich vasculature often allows for rapid healing.[11] Injuries to the lateral pharynx, especially those lateral to the tonsils, have the potential for carotid injuries. An immediate CT angiogram to ascertain the status of the great vessels can detect obvious injuries such as dissection or aneurysm.[12] In cases where the injury tract is close to the great vessels but no obvious defects are detected on CT, overnight in-hospital observation is a prudent course of action since delayed onset of neurological deficits have been reported. Theses neurological symptoms are often highly reversible if detection is made quickly and treatment for cerebral ischemia is rendered in a timely fashion.

*Bites*

Animal or human bites often result in large avulsions of soft tissue. The wounds should be thoroughly irrigated with sterile saline prior to closure to decrease the bacterial load. Prophylactic antibiotic is indicated and amoxicillin-clavulanate is often used as a first line drug to cover oral flora. In children with penicillin allergy, clindamycin or azithromycin are often substituted.[13]

*Facial nerve*

Facial nerve function needs to be assessed at the earliest possible opportunity in all facial soft tissue injuries. Initial function preservation may be a favorable outcome predictor if facial paralysis occurs later and allows for additional confidence in conservative management. If immediate paralysis is observed, early exploration may allow for easier identification of severed ends of the nerve. In general, if the injury is medial to a vertical line drawn from the lateral canthus, facial nerve exploration is not required.[2] The smaller caliber of terminal branches and high frequency of overlapping innervations make exploration both difficult and unnecessary. If the nerve injury is lateral to the lateral canthal line, however, prompt exploration and repair may yield significant benefit is restoring facial nerve function.

*Tissue loss*

Any significant tissue loss in a wound presents a challenge to the surgeon. In the immediate period after the injury, it may not be possible to distinguish viable and non-viable tissue. After a thorough cleaning of the wound, a moist dressing to preserve tissue viability is a reasonable course of action in wounds where tissue loss prohibits immediate closure. After a period of 24 to 48 hours, once the margins of viable tissue is declared, the use of advancement or various local flaps can be considered. Skin graft is also an option; however, the limited tissue thickness, poor color match and donor site morbidities make grafting less desirable. Vacuum assisted wound dressing (Wound VAC) has shown remarkable results in many instances and should be considered in large wounds.

## BONY INJURIES

Great advances have been made in the management of pediatric facial fractures during the recent decades. The specific techniques used for reconstruction in children must accommodate their developing anatomy, rapid healing, immature psychology and potential for deformity as a consequence of altered facial growth.[8] The prevalence of CT scans makes accurate diagnosis of facial fractures possible in most instances.[14,15] Rigid internal fixation has been successfully adapted from adults to pediatric cases although with careful modification. Open reduction and rigid internal fixation is indicated for severely displaced fractures. Primary bone grafting is preferred over secondary reconstruction. Alloplastic materials should be avoided when possible.[16]

Associated injuries are a common feature of childhood maxillofacial trauma. Neurologic and orthopedic injuries were seen in 30% of children with facial fractures, which reinforce the importance of a complete initial assessment of a child with facial trauma and highlights the dilemma with regard to the timing of the reconstruction because of the rapid healing of bony injuries in children.[8]

### Etiology

To understand the cause of pediatric facial fractures, two separate issues need to be addressed: (1) the traumatic event that results in injury to a child's face and (2) the unique anatomic features of the pediatric facial skeleton that predispose it to a pattern of injuries observed.[8]

Falls, motor vehicle accidents (MVA), and sports-related injuries are the most frequent causes of facial fractures in children.[17] Falls are low-velocity injuries that commonly affect young children below the age of six.[17] While prevalent, falls rarely produce serious injuries. On the other extreme, MVA's produce high-velocity forces that often cause devastating injuries. MVA's are the leading cause of death in children after the perinatal period and the incidence of MVA-related maxillofacial injuries increases with age.[18] Improved vehicle safety features (padded dash boards, collapsible steering columns, airbags, child safety seats) and enforcement of safety belt laws have led to a significant decrease in the incidence and severity of MVA-related facial fractures.[19–21] Most sports-related facial fractures occur in children ten to 14 years of age. As motor skills improve from childhood to adolescence, corresponding increases in activity level and outdoor exposure are seen and thus make older children more susceptible to sports-related traumatic injuries.[22]

A young child's face has characteristics that make fractures less likely to happen. Facial soft tissue of children is relatively thicker, which protects the underlying bony framework. The bony structures are soft and elastic and their relatively thickness and strength are not weakened by paranasal sinuses. In addition, immature bone has greater elasticity that is caused by thin cortical plates and a greater proportion of cancellous bone. This elasticity is also the reason that greenstick fractures occur more frequently in children. The presence of unerupted teeth in the maxilla and mandible are the final features that make pediatric faces more resistant to fracture.[23]

## Facial Growth

At birth, the ratio between cranial volume and facial volume is 8:1, whereas in adults, this ratio is 2.5:1. Eighty percent of cranial growth occurs during the first years of life. Only after the first two years of life will the rate of facial growth begin to exceed that of skull growth.

The orbit and the brain are near the completion of growth by age seven; however, lower facial growth continues into the early 20's. The consequence of the retruded position of the face relative to the skull is an important reason for the lower incidence of midface and mandibular fractures and higher incidence of orbital roof and cranial injuries in young children. Fractures below the orbits generally occur after the age of seven and are not associated with cranial injuries, whereas orbital roof and cranial injuries are most commonly seen in children less than five years old.[24]

The possibilities of growth disturbances after facial fractures need to be considered in treatment planning. Injuries to certain vulnerable sites, such as the nasal septum, head of the condyle, and the multiple suture sites of the midface, may adversely affect future facial growth.[8] Growth potential may serve to improve long-term results with compensatory condylar growth after condylar fractures. Children with deciduous and mixed dentition also demonstrate some capacity for spontaneous occlusal readjustment as deciduous teeth are shed and permanent dentition erupts.[17]

## Sites of Injury

Nasal fractures are by far the most common facial bone injuries in children followed by dentoalveolar injuries. Theses fractures are usually treated in the outpatient setting without surgical intervention. Exact statistics regarding incidence and treatment are difficult to obtain since records are typically not as well kept as those in the hospitals.[23]

Fractures of the mandible are the most common facial fractures requiring hospitalization. They account for 30%–50% of all pediatric facial fractures when nasal fractures are excluded.[23,25,26] Because pediatric condyles are highly vascularized and the thin necks are poorly resistant to impact forces, the most vulnerable part of the pediatric mandible is the condyle. More than 50% of pediatric mandibular fractures involve one of the condyles whereas only 30% of adult cases show condylar involvement.[27] As the patients mature, the frequency of symphyseal, body and ramus fractures increases.

Midfacial fractures are rare in children. Usually resulting from high-impact, high velocity forces such as MVA's. Orbital fractures are the most common, accounting for 20%–25% of pediatric fractures. Zygomaticomalar complex (ZMC) fractures are seen in 10%–15%, and LeFort maxillaryfractures are seen in 5%–10%. Orbital roof fractures occur in very young children whose frontal sinuses are still under-developed. These are often associated with skull injuries.[3–5]

## Management

### *Nasal fractures*

The initial examination of a child with nasal fracture may be very limited by midfacial swelling. Several days are required for the swelling to subside before the true extent of the deformity can be appreciated. On the other hand, immediate intranasal examination is important to detect the presence of septal hematoma. Unilateral nasal obstruction is the hallmark of septal hematoma and can be observed on anterior rhinoscopy as an obvious purple bulge on one side of the nose. The bulge is compressible with a cotton tip applicator and does not shrink with topical vasoconstriction. A septal hematoma requires immediate evacuation upon detection. An untreated hematoma can become a thick, fibrotic and obstructive septum. And if the hematoma becomes infected, the resulting loss of cartilage can cause a saddle nose deformity.[16]

In cases of nasal fracture without septal hematoma, the patient is asked to return three to four days after injury, when a more accurate examination is possible. If a cosmetic deformity or a fixed nasal obstruction is detected, then definitive surgical management is undertaken. Closed reduction of the bony fracture can be performed with intranasal instrumentation and bimanual external manipulation. If significant dislocations are present or if the injury is more than two weeks old, then open reduction may be necessary.

*Mandible fracture*

Clinical signs of mandibular fractures may include displacement of the fragments, mobility, swelling, mucosal tears, limited mouth opening, malocclusion, and pain. Clinical suspicion of a fracture is confirmed by either a panorex X-ray, a complete mandible series, or by CT scans. CT's are especially helpful in condylar fractures to help determine three-dimensional displacement of the condyles.

Immobilization is difficult before two years of age because of incomplete eruption of the deciduous teeth; however, later growth and remodeling frequently compensate for less-than-ideal post-injury alignment. The primary teeth, which have firm roots between two and five years of age, can be used for splints and arch bars. Deciduous roots are resorbed between six and 12 years of age; hence arch bars may need extra support from circum-mandibular wiring and piriform aperture suspension. Permanent teeth are safe anchors for fixation after 13 years of age.[16]

The central question in the management of pediatric condylar fracture is whether the patient needs immobilization. Although minimally invasive endoscopic open reduction with internal fixation (ORIF) is gaining popularity in the management of adult condylar fractures, most authors still advocate conservative management when it comes to pediatric cases.[17,28] If the patient has normal occlusion and normal mandibular movement, only a soft diet and movement exercises are necessary. However, if open bite deformities with retrusion of the mandible and movement limitation are present, then a brief period of immobilization, lasting two to three weeks, followed by the use of guiding elastics can yield normal function in the end.[16]

Displaced symphysis fractures can be treated by ORIF through an intraoral incision after age six, after the permanent incisors have erupted.[17] ORIF in parasymphyseal fractures is possible once the buds of the canines have moved up from the mandibular border after age nine. In body fractures, the inferior mandibular border can be plated, when the buds of the permanent premolar and molar have migrated superiorly toward the alveolus.

Frequent postoperative follow-up are necessary to detect and treat early complications such as infection, malocclusion, malunion or nonunion. Late complications such as damage to permanent teeth, temporomandibular joint (TMJ) dysfunction, or midface deformity with facial asymmetry also need attention and possible treatments.

*Nasoethmoid complex fractures*

In nasoethmoid fractures, the medial canthal ligament integrity must be assessed. This is done by inserting a hemostat into the nose toward the medial orbital rim. The child should be anesthetized for this examination. Mobility of the underlying fragments suggests that the bone with its canthal attachment has been displaced and that reconstruction of the nasal maxillary buttress and possibly transnasal wiring is necessary.[16] Measurement of soft-tissue intercanthal distance is difficult since ethnic, racial and gender variations can significantly impact its values. Nevertheless, the average intercanthal distance at four years of age is approximately 25 mm; by age 12, 28 mm; and by adulthood, 30 mm. One can easily see that near adult intercanthal distance is achieved at a very early age; hence an easy mistake is to set the intercanthal distance too wide. Intercanthal distances 5 mm more than the average values tend to be indicative of and 10 mm confirms the diagnosis of displaced fractures of the nasoethmoidal complex. Attempts should be made to narrow the distance between the eyes excessively and project the nose of a child.

*Zygomaticomalar complex fractures*

ZMC fractures parallel the pneumatization of the maxillary sinus and are uncommon before the age of five years. Surgical correction of ZMC fractures is indicated when bony displacement is present. Adequate exposure is essential in such correction and in achieved by a process called triangulation.[8] Three key sites need to be directly visualized: (1) the frontozygomatic suture, (2) the infraorbital rim, and (3) the anterior zygomaticomaxillary buttress. Access can be achieved via the lateral upper eyelid incision, the lower eyelid infraciliary or transconjuctival incision, and the transoral buccal sulcus incision.[8] Contrary to adults, one-point fixation at the frontozygomatic suture may suffice in children, because of shorter lever arm forces from the frontozygomatic suture to the infraorbital rim.

*Orbital floor fractures*

The treatment of isolated blowout fractures is symptom dependent. If persistent enophthalmos, extraocular muscle restriction, or pain on movement of the eye is present, then surgical exploration is indicated. Large fractures are also routinely explored as are fractures that on CT have obvious muscle entrapment. Absorbable gelatin film is usually sufficient for reconstructing small defects of the floor; however, large disruption are best repaired with calvarial bone grafts.

*Orbital roof fractures*

Pediatric orbital roof fractures are different than those of adults. They occur more frequently due to the lack of frontal sinus penumatization. Children have a craniofacial ratio of 8:1 at birth, compared to 2:1 in adults, thus expose more of their cranium and skull base to potential injuries. Most orbital roof fractures, particularly those that are non-displaced or with fragments displaced superiorly (blow-out fractures) can be safely observed in the acute setting. Treatments should be directed by the presence of symptoms, such as extraocular muscle entrapment, enophthalmos, exophthalmos, diplopia, vision changes or dystopia. Large blow-in fractures have a higher chance for late onset complications; therefore surgical thresholds should be lower. Depending on the extent and location of the orbital roof fracture, various approaches are available to access the area of interest. Cooperation between neurosurgery, ophthalmology, and head and neck surgery are essential to optimize the care for these patients.

*Temporal bone fractures*

Temporal bone fractures are not uncommon after blunt head trauma in the pediatric population. The most common presenting symptoms include otorrhea, hearing loss, and facial paralysis. Diagnostic signs include hemotympanum, bruising of the mastoid soft tissue (Battle's sign), and persistent clear drainage from the ear canal.[29] High resolution CT scans are the current gold standard for the diagnosis of these fractures. Traditionally, temporal bone fractures are divided based on the direction of the fracture line.[29] Arbitrary delineations made between longitudinal, transverse, and oblique fractures have become less useful since details of temporal bone are now visible on the high resolution CT scan. Detailed examination of facial nerve, cochlea, semicircular canals, and ossicles on the CT images allow clinicians to predict possible injuries to the specific structures.

In the assessment and treatment of temporal bone fractures, elements to consider include:

1. Facial nerve integrity. Facial nerve paralysis is a relatively rare complication of temporal bone fracture, with an incidence of approximately 4%.[30–32] The timing of facial paralysis onset has profound prognostic value and can direct future therapy. It is therefore of utmost importance for the initial evaluator to take judicious inventory of facial nerve function. Due to frequently associated facial swelling, altered mental status, and injuries to other parts of the body, facial nerve status is often neglected by first responders and emergency department personnel. The ENT surgeon must therefore evaluate all branches of the nerve carefully, documenting responses to grimaces in addition to voluntary movements. All branches need to be assessed since swelling can make one branch appear paralyzed when the nerve trunk is actually functioning. Immediate onset of total paralysis coupled with CT evidence of facial nerve injury makes a strong case for nerve decompression. Otherwise, observation often yields return of function in majority of cases.[29]

2. CSF leak. This can occur with frequency of 20%–25% for pediatric patients.[33–35] While the presentation may be alarming, great majority of these injuries will heal spontaneously with conservative treatment, including bed rest and head elevation. Systemic antibiotic use is controversial but antibiotic ear drops are often utilized. In cases where brain herniation or large tegmen defects are detected on CT, prompt surgical interventions may be indicated.[36,37]
3. Hearing. This test will require patient participation and is not as critical in the acute setting. However, prior to discharging the patient from the hospital, it is important to determine if hearing is subjectively normal for the patient. If not, a formal audiogram after discharge is indicated.[31,37] In patients with conductive or mixed hearing loss, a middle ear exploration to investigate possible ossicular disruption should be offered.

## CONCLUSION

Children of all ages can be afflicted by ENT trauma, often resulting in functional and cosmetic deficits. A thorough understanding of pediatric skull and facial growth enables us to focus our search for subtle fractures in the most age-appropriate locations. Soft tissue injuries can often point out the possible locations of fracture and should be carefully treated. Anticipation of mandibular growth facilitates repair because most injuries can be treated with intermaxillary fixation. Unerupted dentition requires careful selection of fixation methods and cautious screw placement if rigid fixation is ultimately required. The modern rigid plating systems have greatly enhanced surgeons' ability to reconstruct facial fractures in a three-dimensional fashion. Temporal bone fractures have a special set of considerations that need to be addressed in a timely fashion. Depending on the site of injury, a multidisciplinary team approach can ensure that injuries to organs systems around the face are cared for in an optimal manner.

## REFERENCES

1. Rowe IM, Fonkalsrud EW, O'Neil JA, *et al.* The injured child. In: Rowe MI, O'Neill Jr JA, Grosfeld JL *et al.*, eds. *Essentials of Pediatric Surgery*. St. Louis: Mosby, 1995.
2. Hogg NJV, Horswell BB. Soft tissue pediatric facial trauma: a review. *J Can Dent Assoc* 2006;72(6):549–552.
3. Gussack GS, Lutterman A, Rodgers K, *et al.* Pediatric maxillofacial trauma: unique features in diagnosis and treatment. *Laryngoscope* 1987;97:925–930.
4. Kaban LB. Diagnosis and treatment of fractures of the facial bones in children 1943–1993. *J Oral Maxillofac Surg* 1993;51:722–729.
5. Koltai PJ, Rabkin D, Hoehn J. Rigid fixation of facial fractures in children. *J Craniomaxillofac Trauma* 1995;1:32–42.
6. McGraw BL, Cole RR. Pediatric maxillofacial trauma. *Arch Otolaryngol Head Neck Surg* 1990;116:41–45.
7. Rowe NL. Fractures of the facial skeleton in children. *J Oral Surg* 1967;26:505–515.
8. Koltai PJ, Rabkin D. Management of facial trauma in children. *Pediatr Clin North Am* 1996;43:1253–1275.
9. Marom T, Russo E, Ben-Yehuda Y, *et al.* Oropharyngeal injuries in children. 2007;23(12):914–918.
10. Law RC, Fouque CA, Waddell A, *el al.* Lesson of the week: penetrating intra-oral trauma in children. *BMJ* 1997;314:50–51.
11. Domarus HV, Poeschel W. Impalement injuries of the palate. *Plast Reconstr Surg* 1983;72:656–658.
12. Pierrot S, Bernardeschi D, Morrisseau-Durand MP, *et al.* Dissection of the internal carotid artery following trauma of the soft palate in children. *Ann Otol Rhinol Laryngol* 2006;115(5):323–329.
13. Stefanopoulos PK, Tarantzopoulou AD. Facial bite wounds: management update. *Int J Oral Maxillofac Surg* 2005;34(5):464–472.
14. Holland AJ, Broome C, Steinberg A, Cass DT. Facial fractures in children. *Pediatr Emerg Care* 2001;17:157–160.
15. Posnick JC, Wells M, Pron GE. Pediatric facial fractures: evolving patterns of treatment. *J Oral Maxillofac Surg* 1993;51:836–844.
16. Koltai PJ. Pediatric facial fractures. In: Bailey BJ, ed. *Atlas of Head and Neck Surgery — Otolaryngology*, 2nd Ed. Philadelphia: Lippincott, 2001.

17. Zimmermann CE, Troulis MJ, Kaban LB. Pediatric facial fractures: recent advances in prevention, diagnosis and management. *Int J Oral Maxillofac Surg* 2006;35:2–13.
18. Statistics NCfH. *National Vital Statistics Report* 2001;49:16–29.
19. Adam CD, Januszkiewcz JS, Judson J. Changing patterns of severe craniomaxillofacial trauma in Auckland over eight years. *Aust N Z J Surg* 2000;70:401–404.
20. Reath DB, Kirby J, Lynch M, Maull KI. Injury and cost comparison of restrained and unrestrained motor vehicle crash victims. *J Trauma* 1989;29:1173–1176.
21. Tyroch AH, Kaups KL, Sue LP, ODonnell-Nicol S. Pediatric retraint use in otor vehicle collisions: reduction of deaths without contribution to injury. *Arch Surg* 2000;135:1173–1176.
22. Iizuka T, Thoren H, Annino DJ *et al.* Midfacial fractures in pediatric patients. Frequency, characteristics and causes. *Arch Otolaryngol Head Neck Surg* 1995;121:1355–1371.
23. Koltai PJ. Maxillofacial injuries in children. In: Smith JD, Bumstead R, eds. *Pediatric Facial Plastic and Reconstructive Surgery.* New York: Raven Press, 1993.
24. McGraw BL, Cole RR. Pediatric maxillofacial trauma. Age-related variations in injury. *Arch Otolaryngol Head Neck Surg* 1990;116:41–45.
25. Hardt N, Gottsauner A. The treatment of mandibular fractures in children. *J Craniomaxillofac Surg* 1993;21:214–219.
26. Thoren H, Iizuka T, Hallikainen D, *et al.* Different patterns of mandibular fractures in children: an analysis of 220 fractures in 157 patients. *J Craniomaxillofac Surg* 1992;20:292–296.
27. Kaban LB, Mulliken JB, Murray JE. Facial fractures in children: an analysis of 122 fractures in 109 patients. *Plast Reconstr Surg* 1977;59:15–20.
28. Troulis MJ, Kaban LB. Endoscopic approach to the ramus/condyle unit: clinical applications. *J Oral Maxillofac Surg* 2001;59:503–509.
29. Lee D, Honrado C, Har-El G, *et al.* Pediatric temporal bone fractures. Laryngoscope 1998;108(6):816–821.
30. Nicol JW, Johnstone AJ. Temporal bone fractures in children: a review of 34 cases. *J Accid Emerg Med* 1994;11:218–222.

31. Williams WT, Ghorayeb BY, Yeakley JW. Pediatric temporal bone fractures. *Laryngoscope* 1992;102:600–603.
32. McGuirt WF, Stool SE. Temporal bone fractures in children: a review with emphasis on long-term sequelae. *Clin Pediatr (Phila)* 1992;31:12–18.
33. Mitchell DP, Stone P. Temporal bone tractures in children. *Can J Otolaryngol* 1973;2:156–162.
34. Shapiro RS. Temporal bone fractures in children. *Otolaryngol Head Neck Surg* 1979;87:323–329.
35. Liu-Shindo M, Hawkins DB. Basilar skull fractures in children. *Int J Pediatr Otorhinolaryngol* 1989;17:109–117.
36. Caldicott WJH, North JB, Simpson DA. Traumatic cerebrospinal fluid fistulas in children. *J Neurosurg* 1973;38:1–9.
37. McGuirt WF, Stool SE. Cerebrospinal fluid fistula: the identification and management in pediatric temporal bone fractures. *Laryngoscope* 1995;105:359–364.

# SPECIALIZED CHAPTERS

# 18

# The EXIT Procedure

*Richard W. Hong, Samuel H. Wald and Daniel DeUgarte*

## OVERVIEW

The *Ex Utero* Intrapartum Treatment (EXIT) procedure is a technique that utilizes placental life support during partial cesarean section delivery to allow time so that a fetal airway can be established in a safe and controlled manner. The EXIT procedure was initially developed to remove tracheal clips placed *in utero* to plug and grow the lung in infants with congenital diaphragmatic hernia. The technique has been adapted to infants with the prenatal diagnosis of a possible airway obstruction to help prevent cardiorespiratory failure during delivery. In order for placental life support to be sustained, the uterus must be relaxed and well-perfused. Thus, the EXIT procedure requires a coordinated multidisciplinary effort between the obstetrician, obstetric anesthesiologist, surgeon, and neonatology team. The EXIT procedure involves two patients — mother and child — and the well-being of both must be taken into consideration when considering the procedure.

## PATIENT IDENTIFICATION AND SELECTION

*Patient identification*

- The diagnosis of possible airway obstruction is made with prenatal ultrasound. Patients should be referred to a maternal-fetal medicine (MFM) specialist at a fetal care center with pediatric subspecialty services.

*Indications for "EXIT to airway"*

- Airway obstruction can be causes by extrinsic or intrinsic obstruction.
    - Extrinsic airway compression can be caused by a neck mass. The most common neck masses are lymphatic malformations and cervical teratomas. Teratomas are more likely to required surgical intervention to establish an airway.[1] Other sources of extrinsic airway compression include hemangioma, goiter, neuroblastoma, ranula, and laryngocele.[2]
    - Intrinsic airway obstruction can be caused by the atresia or stenosis of the larynx or trachea. Other etiologists include laryngeal cysts and webs. Congenital high airway obstruction syndrome (CHAOS) can be seen with severe intrinsic airway obstruction that prevents egress of lung fluid from the tracheobronchial tree. It is characterized by the presence of large echogenic lungs, flattened diaphragms, dilated airways distal to the obstruction, and ascites/hydrops.
- Other indications for EXIT include mediastinal masses and lung masses (e.g. congenital cystic adenomatoid malformation or bronchopulmonary sequestration).

*Imaging (US, MRI) and interpretation*

- Prenatal diagnosis is usually made with ultrasound. Fetal magnetic resonance imaging (MRI) can be useful in predicting the etiology and extent of airway obstruction and help with operative planning.

*Case discussion*

- The discussion should include representatives from all relevant services, namely obstetrics (maternal-fetal medicine), neonatology, pediatric and obstetric anesthesiology, and necessary surgical services.

- The group should consider the appropriateness of an EXIT procedure (versus conventional vaginal or cesarean delivery) given the fetal disease, expert opinions, and data from the current literature. The odds of an acceptable fetal outcome should be weighed against the risks to the mother.

*Informed consent*

- Consent for an "EXIT to airway" procedure should be obtained by the surgical team after discussing the risks and benefits of the procedure for both her and the unborn child.

## MULTIDISCIPLINARY PREPARATIONS

*Establishing roles and lines of communication*

- The *team leader* coordinates and directs the team during the EXIT procedure, delegating responsibilities as needed. This individual should be familiar with the role of each member of the team. (In our practice, this is a pediatric anesthesiologist.)
- The *pediatric anesthesiologist* prepares the operating room for the specific needs of the neonate. This individual may be the primary person involved in monitoring of a partially or completely delivered neonate, dosage and delivery of resuscitation medications, and establishment of a definitive non-surgical airway.
- The *pediatric surgeon* is ultimately responsible for establishing an airway and should be prepared to perform rigid bronchoscopy or surgical intervention as required.
- The *maternal anesthesiologist* prepares and provides general anesthesia for the mother and obtains feedback from the obstetrician to maintain optimal uterine conditions throughout the EXIT procedure. This person also coordinates anesthetic choices which may affect the fetus with the pediatric anesthesiologist and neonatologist.
- The *maternal-fetal medicine obstetrician* delivers the fetus via carefully coordinated uterotomy, communicates uterine conditions back to maternal anesthesiologist, and monitors the fetus via ultrasound and electronic fetal heart rate monitors.

- The *OB circulating nurse and scrub tech* assist the obstetrician in surgical management of the mother and delivery of the fetus.
- The *surgery circulator and scrub tech* assist the pediatric anesthesiologist, surgeon, and otolaryngologist in airway management and other necessary measures for the neonate.
- The *neonatology* team (neonatologist, NICU nurses, and respiratory technician) communicate with the pediatric anesthesiologist and surgeon to care for the neonate after airway management.
- Depending on the indication, an "ECMO team" may be available for support of the neonate via an extracorporeal membrane oxygenation device.

*Schematic diagram of operating room setup*

- All personnel and equipment should be available prior to initiating the EXIT procedure. The schematic diagram below provides a sample OR layout.

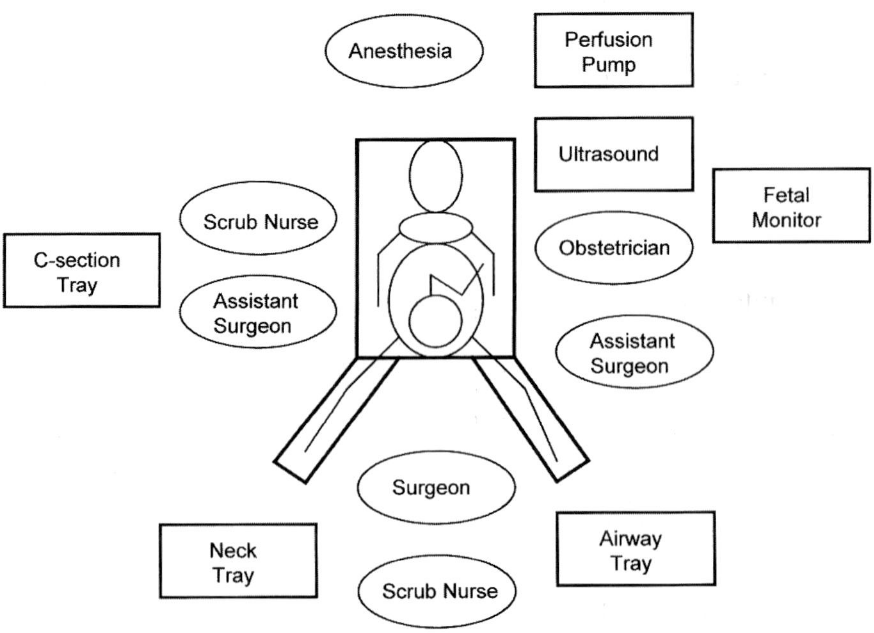

*Fetal management algorithm*

- A case-specific management algorithm should be agreed upon by all team members and made known to the entire care team prior to the procedure. (See sample flowchart under the section "Establishing an airway.")

*Operating room coordination*

- EXIT procedures require advanced planning and elective scheduling to insure that all members of the team are available. The procedure is best performed in a large operating room to accommodate all necessary personnel and equipment.

## OR SET-UP

*Surgical equipment*

- Bronchoscopy supplies, including rigid bronchoscopes (2.5 and 3.0 mm).
- Glidewires (in case retrograde passage of endotracheal tube is performed).
- Surgical tray for neonatal tracheostomy, including tracheostomy tubes.
- Surgical tray for neck mass dissection (in case excision is required).

*Pediatric anesthesia equipment*

- Monitoring.
    - Pulse oximeter and foil (sterile) to block light.
    - EKG.
    - Neonatal non-invasive blood pressure cuff.
    - Pediatric stethoscope (sterile).
- Airway equipment.
    - Pediatric laryngoscope handle.
    - Miller 00, Miller 0, Miller 1 laryngoscope blades.

- 30, 40, 50 mm oral airways.
- 2.0, 2.5, 3.0, 3.5, 4.0 mm PVC endotracheal tubes.
- 3.0, 3.5 mm armored endotracheal tubes.
- 2.2 mm tube exchanger.
- #1, #2 pediatric masks.
- #1, #1.5 pediatric laryngeal mask airways.
- 2.2–2.5 mm, 2.8 mm pediatric fiberoptic bronchoscope.

*Neonatal resuscitation supplies*

- Umbilical artery catheterization kit.
- Umbilical vein catheterization kit.
- Intravenous access supplies, albumin, normal saline.
- Atropine (20 mcg/kg) prefilled sterile syringe.
- Epinephrine (10 mcg/kg) prefilled sterile syringe.
- Infant warmer/isolette for post-delivery.

*Maternal anesthesia equipment*

- Standard adult anesthetic supplies for general anesthesia with rapid-sequence intubation.
- Supplies on-hand for maternal difficult airway management.
- Maternal resuscitation drugs (particularly pressor infusions) as well as uterotonic and uterine relaxant medications.
- Preparations for possible maternal blood transfusion.
- Large-bore intravenous access, preferably through two separate veins.

*Obstetrical equipment*

- Special uterine stapler for hemostasis during hysterotomy in the relaxed uterus (e.g. Auto Suture Premium Poly CS-57 disposable 0.140 inch; Norwalk, CT).
- External and internal fetal heart rate monitoring equipment available prior to and through delivery.
- Obstetric ultrasound machine with suitable probes and sterile sleeves.
- Standard cesarean section surgical supplies.
- Stay sutures on-hand to improve surgical exposure after hysterotomy.

- Rapid fluid infuser primed with several liters of Lactated Ringer's and soft sterile tubing appropriate for intrauterine placement.
- Drapes and suction devices suitable for collecting large volumes of effluent (amniotic fluid, blood, and infused Lactated Ringer's).

## PERIOPERATIVE CARE (CHRONOLOGICAL, STEP-BY-STEP SEQUENCE)

*Induction*

- All members of multidisciplinary team should be immediately present, as the progression from induction of anesthesia to delivery and fetal management can quickly change from what was planned.
- Standard maternal surgical precautions should be taken, including reflux prophylaxis for the appropriately NPO patient, supine positioning with left uterine displacement on an OR table capable of lithotomy position for the patient, and sequential compression devices (SCD's).
- All monitors and lines should be placed prior to induction of maternal anesthesia with rapid-sequence intubation (unless an awake fiberoptic intubation is indicated).
- Train of four (TOF) monitoring for use of maintenance non-depolarizing muscle relaxants is advised.
- For gastric decompression, an orogastric (not nasogastric) tube is recommended unless otherwise contraindicated.
- Maternal anesthetics and opioid analgesics should be provided as needed, after discussion of the potential for placental cross-over. Placental cross-over may be desired for fetal anesthesia or may be undesired for fetal respiratory depression, depending on the circumstances and chosen management algorithm.
- IV antibiotics should be given to the mother prior to surgical incision.
- The mother should be placed in lithotomy position to improve access to the maternal abdomen for fetal management.

- Perform surgical preparation with antiseptic and then drape with large-capacity effluent bag and suction.

*Pre-hysterotomy*

- Maintain high oxygen concentrations (>50%) to the mother.
- The obstetrician will connect sterile tubing on the field to rapid fluid infuser managed by the maternal anesthesiologist.
- Maternal low transverse abdominal incision is made for uterine exposure.
- Prepare a secondary monitor for fetal pulse oximetry, positioned so that screen is visible to all. Confirm that the pulse oximetry cable is sterile and of adequate length to reach onto surgical field.
- Intraoperative sonography with a sterile sleeve over probe will precisely locate the fetus and placental margins to avoid. Consider ultrasound-guided transuterine intramuscular anesthetics to fetus.
- Begin high-dose (e.g 1.5–3 MAC) inhalational agents for uterine relaxation. Titrate to maintain uterine relaxation as determined by the obstetrician. Consider agents with faster onset/offset (e.g. desflurane, sevoflurane) to achieve optimal relaxation immediately before anticipated uterine incision to minimize undesired hemodynamic effects on mother (and their consequences to uteroplacental perfusion).
- Provide additional uterine relaxants (e.g. nitroglycerin) as needed per the obstetrician's assessment of uterine tone.

*Post-hysterotomy/partial delivery*

- Hysterotomy should be an incision based on the exposure needed and the placental location, with the incision made more than 3 cm from placental margin. An initial 2 cm uterine incision is made with electrocautery and then extended in opposite directions using a uterine stapler device (e.g. Auto Suture Premium Poly CS-57 disposable 0.140 inch surgical stapler) for a 6–8 cm transverse hysterotomy. Stay sutures (e.g. 2–0 Vicryl SH) may be placed above and below the middle of this incision. Control wound-edge bleeding with full-thickness figure-of-eight stitches (e.g. 2–0 Vicryl SH sutures).

- Partially deliver the fetus. Only the head, torso and one arm (preferably right arm for possible IV placement pre-ductal $O_2$ saturation measured by pulse oximetry) should be delivered initially, and a vacuum device can be used to assist with delivery of the fetal head through the small uterine incision.
- Maximize fetal oxygenation at this critical juncture. Utilize pressors (e.g. phenylephrine, ephedrine, dopamine) to the mother to maintain uteroplacental perfusion. Minimize umbilical cord manipulation. Place sterile tubing connected to rapid fluid infuser and titrate body-temperature Lactated Ringer's solution to maintain fetal warmth and uterine distension (which aids in preventing early placental separation). Maximize uterine relaxation with medications (e.g. nitroglycerin, inhalation anesthesia).
- Fetal heart rate monitoring should reflect fetal well-being and can be assessed by ultrasound, sterile fetal scalp electrode, fetal pulse oximetry, and/or formal intraoperative fetal transthoracic echocardiography by pediatric cardiologist.
- Monitoring fetal oxygenation can be done by clinical observations of surrogate measures (e.g. color, fetal heart rate) as well as fetal pulse oximetry. The latter is not always attempted or successful due to signal quality, but generally the minimum $O_2$ saturation is 40%, the ideal $O_2$ saturation pre-intubation is 60%–70%, and the ideal $O_2$ saturation post-intubation is 85%.
- Neonatal anesthesia may be administered via the intramuscular (IM) route (e.g. fentanyl 10–20 mcg/kg and/or vecuronium 0.2 mg/kg)

*Establishing an airway*

- Direct laryngoscopy and insertion of endotracheal tube should be attempted. Rigid or flexible bronchoscopy can be utilized if initial attempts are unsuccessful. A tube exchanger or glidewire can then be introduced to guide an endotracheal tube into position.
- If non-surgical methods fail, a tracheotomy can be performed and retrograde passage of a glidewire can be attempted. If

endotracheal tube placement is unsuccessful, tracheostomy is indicated. Tracheostomy may required for mobilization, partial or complete excision, or drainage of an obstructing mass.

- If all else fails, extracorporal membrane oxygenation (ECMO) can be considered. ECMO requires advanced planning and coordination and is more relevant to obstructing mediastinal and lung masses.[3]
- Flowchart for airway management
    - The flowchart below provides a sample algorithm for establishing an airway during an EXIT procedure. After an airway is established, the tube position should be confirmed with flexible bronchoscopy. Once confirmed, the umbilical cord can be clamped and the infant delivered.
    - The EXIT procedure should be aborted if there is evidence of placental separation.

Attempt Direct Laryngoscopy and Intubation

↓ Fail

Attempt Rigid Bronchoscopy and Intubation

↓ Fail

Consider Video-Assisted Laryngoscopy
or Fiberoptic Intubation

↓ Fail

Surgical Airway:
1. Tracheotomy with Retrograde Intubation
2. Tracheostomy
3. Excise or Decompress Mass to Allow for Tracheostomy

↓ Fail

ECMO (Extracorporeal Membrane Oxygenation)

*Post-delivery*

- Uterine tone should be established. Start an oxytocin infusion (30 U in 1 L of LR, wide open), discontinue any nitroglycerin infusion being used, switch to low-dose inhalational agents to promote uterine tone (~ 0.5 MAC) in a balanced anesthetic with nitrous oxide, opioids, benzodiazepines, and propofol at the anesthesiologist's discretion. Uterotonic medications should be given as needed to restore uterine tone, including Pitocin (oxytocin) 5–10 U IVP, Methergine (methylergonovine) 200 mcg IM, Hemabate (prostaglandin F2-alpha) 250 mcg IM, and Cytotec (misoprostol) 400 mcg PR or SL or IU given per the obstetrician's assessment.
- Maternal paralysis need not be maintained after delivery and can be reversed at the end of case.
- The mother should be recovered in a post-anesthesia care unit (PACU) with standard postoperative cesarean recovery and pain management orders.

## POSSIBLE PITFALLS AND WORDS OF WISDOM

*Maintaining placental life support*

- The mean duration reported for EXIT procedures is 30 minutes.[4] However, placental life support has been maintained for over one hour. It is important to have all equipment and supplies immediately available.
- It is also essential to maintain uterine relaxation and prevent cord compression by infusion of warm Lactated Ringer's solution into the uterus.
- The EXIT procedure should be aborted if there is placental abruption, maternal hemorrhage, or fetal bradycardia or arrest.[5]

*Reducing risks with planning*

- It is practically impossible to perform an EXIT procedure emergently. The necessary equipment, facilities and specialists preclude rapid mobilization.

- In advance, consider a risk/benefit analysis of the delay needed to mobilize versus immediate delivery under emergency conditions such as fetal distress and imminent delivery.
- Establish protocols before prospective patients are identified.
- Initiate early discussion and planning as early in the pregnancy as possible.
- Choose a realistic date for a scheduled EXIT procedure. Viability and morbidity are related to gestational age, but the later the date, the higher the likelihood that unexpected events will force an expedited, non-EXIT delivery.
- Maintain a contact list/e-mail group (with back-ups) for all specialists.
- Designate a supervising "team leader" who is not directly involved procedurally and thus not preoccupied by just one aspect of the EXIT procedure. With various sub-specialists working toward related but separate goals, oversight and intraoperative communication are necessary.
- Create equipment checklists and a schematic diagram of the OR layout during an initial "dry-run" done in the chosen operating room with representatives from each discipline present to enable them to voice their opinions in advance.

*Limiting OR traffic to essential personnel*

- An EXIT procedure tends to attract a crowd of curious onlookers. For academic purposes, consider video recording or a video feed to another room as alternatives.
- The number of essential personnel and amount of equipment usually limits the free space in the operating room.
- Increased OR traffic may increase infectious risks to the mother and neonate.

## REFERENCES

1. Steigman SA, Nemes L, Barnewolt, Estroff JA, Valim C, Jenning RW, Fauza DO. Differential risk for neonatal surgical airway intervention in prenatally diagnosed neck masses. *J Pediatr Surg* 2009;44:76–79.

2. Crombleholme TM, Albanese CT. The fetus with airway obstruction. In: Harrison MR, Evans M, Adzick NS, Holzgreze W, eds. *The Unborn Patient: The Art and Science of Fetal Therapy*. Philadelphia, PA: WB Saunders, 2001, Chap. 24, pp. 357–371.
3. Kunisaki SM, Fauza DO. Barnewolt CE, Estroff JA, Myers LA, Bulich LA, Wong G, Levine D, Wilkins-Haug LE, Benson CB, Jennings RW. *Ex utero* intrapartum treatment with placement on extracorporeal membrane oxygenation for fetal thoracic masses. *J Pediatr surg* 2007; 42:420–425.
4. Bouchard S, Johnson MP, Flake AW, Howell LJ, Myers LB, Adzick S, Crombleholme TM. The EXIT procedure: experience and outcomes in 31 cases. *J Pediatr Surg* 2002;37:418–426.
5. Marwan A, Crombleholme TM. The EXIT procedure: principles, pitfalls, and progress. *Semin Pediatr Surg* 2006;15:107–115.

# 19

# Special Issues in Anesthesia for Pediatric Otolaryngology

*Swati Patel and Keren Ziv*

## INTRODUCTION

Care of pediatric patients in the operating room is unique from that of an adult. Differences in coping skills, anatomy, physiology, pharmacology from adults make providing anesthesia for pediatric patients a challenge. Furthermore, knowledge of developmental differences by age is imperative to a safe perioperative experience. While surgeons and anesthesiologists always work closely together, no other surgical subspecialty is asked to share much of their surgical field and concerns with the anesthesiologists as the otolaryngologist. Therefore, knowledge of indications, techniques, and risks of anesthesia are crucial to successful care of the pediatric patient undergoing head and neck surgery. This chapter will serve as a guide to the anesthetic care and concerns of these patients.

## DEVELOPMENTAL DIFFERENCES AND CONSIDERATIONS FOR PEDIATRIC PATIENTS

Compared to adults, pediatric patients have developmental differences that make anesthetic choices unique. Furthermore, infants

**Table 1. Comparison of neonate and infant characteristics with that of adults.**

| | |
|---|---|
| **Physiological** | |
| | Heart rate-dependent cardiac output |
| | Faster heart rate with lower blood pressure |
| | Faster respiratory rate |
| | Lower functional residual capacity |
| | Lower lung compliance |
| | Greater chest wall compliance |
| | Higher ratio of body surface area to body weight |
| | Higher total body water content |
| **Anatomical** | |
| | Non-compliant left ventricle |
| | Potential residual fetal circulation |
| | Large head and tongue |
| | Narrow nasal passages |
| | Anterior and cephalad larynx |
| | Long epiglottis |
| | Weak intercostal and diaphragmatic muscles |
| **Pharmacological** | |
| | Immature hepatic biotransformation |
| | Decreased protein binding |
| | Rapid induction and recovery |
| | Large volume of distribution for water-soluble drugs |

Adapted from Ref. 1.

and neonates have immature organ systems making their response to drugs and drug metabolism and elimination distinct from that of older children. Understanding organ systems development is therefore crucial to the care of pediatric patients. Table 1 outlines differences that are detailed below.

## Respiratory System

Respiratory control is immature in infants and neonates so that hypercarbia and hypoxia may induce apnea rather than hyperventilation. Infants and neonates have weak intercostals and diaphragmatic musculature (paucity of type 1 fibers) making their ventilation less efficient and predisposing them to fatigue. Infants also have a lower functional residual capacity (FRC) secondary to reduced lung compliance and a very compliant rib cage. This decreased FRC coupled with higher minute ventilation (up to three times higher and even greater with stress, sepsis, etc.) per kilogram of body weight than adults predisposes them to more rapid desaturation from hypoventilation and apneic periods. Furthermore, the decreased FRC predisposes neonates and infants to atelectasis.

Anatomic differences also add to the challenge of caring for pediatric patients. Neonates and infants have proportionately large occiput so that positioning with a shoulder roll is often necessary to maintain adequate "sniffing position" and airway patency. Furthermore, the tongue is larger relative to mouth size adding to the risk for obstruction. The narrowest point of a child's airway is at the level of the cricoid (as opposed to the glottis in adults), making endotracheal tube sizing crucial to avoid injury to the tracheal mucosa and postoperative croup and potential subglottic stenosis. Finally, the epiglottis is long and floppy and the larynx is more anterior and cephalad (at level of C4 versus C6 in adults) making the airway appear more "anterior" on laryngoscopy and potentially more difficult to visualize.

### Cardiovascular System

Cardiovascular responses are also immature. The heart of the neonate has relatively few myocytes and more connective tissue so the myocardium is poorly compliant with a relatively fixed stroke volume; hence, cardiac output is rate dependent. Therefore, anesthetics and medications that depress myocardial function or cause bradycardia should be used with caution in neonates and infants. This immaturity gives the neonate and infant poor tolerance to volume overload and increases in afterload. The vascular tree is less able to respond to hypovolemia with vasoconstriction thus intravascular depletion in neonates and infants is manifested by hypotension without significant tachycardia.[1] They also have a lower catecholamine store predisposing them to catecholamine depletion.

Sick infants and neonates are therefore more prone to bradycardia quickly progressing to potential asystole. In newborns and preterm infants the pulmonary vasculature is very reactive, and hypoxia, hypercarbia and acidosis will quickly increase pulmonary vascular resistance and potential right-to-left shunting of blood through a patent ductus arteriosus or atrial septal defect decreasing pulmonary blood flow worsening hypoxemia and acidosis. Without immediate intervention the worsening hypoxemia will perpetuate this "vicious cycle."

## Renal And Hepatic Function

Renal function is diminished in neonates and infants secondary to immature glomerular and tubular function and relatively low perfusion pressure. Maturation of renal function does not occur until approximately two years of age thus younger patients are less able to handle free water and solute loads so that the excretion of medications (certain antibiotics for example) that rely on glomerular filtration will have a prolonged half-life requiring longer intervals for dosing.[2]

Hepatic function is mature by the age of one year. The ability of the infant to metabolize medications increases as they grow secondary to increasing hepatic blood flow and enhanced metabolic activity. Glycogen stores are proportionately less than adults making them more susceptible to hypoglycemia. Additionally, plasma levels of albumin and other plasma proteins are lower in infants so that there is a greater level of unbound drug (examples include thiopental, bupivicaine and many antibiotics) enhancing potency and potential toxicity.[1]

## Pharmacological Differences

Neonates and infants have proportionately higher total water content (70%–75%) than adults (50%–60%). Total body water content decreases as fat and muscle content increase with age. As a direct result, the volume of distribution for water soluble drugs is disproportionately higher in neonates, infants, and young children, and the dose required is usually higher than in older children and adults.

Responses to anesthetic agents also differ according to patient age. Preterm and full-term newborns require lower concentrations of inhaled anesthetics than do older children or adults. Inhalational agents may cause more depression of cardiac output in infants and may have a more profound effect on baroreflexes. Clearance of narcotics is less rapid and more variable in infants.

### Thermoregulation

Because infants have a larger surface area/weight ratio than adults, thin skin, and very little subcutaneous fat they are more prone to heat loss from cold operating rooms and intravenous fluids. Preterm infants are even more prone to hypothermia. Hypothermia is a serious problem that has been associated with delayed awakening from anesthesia, cardiac irritability and failure, respiratory depression, increased pulmonary vascular resistance, and altered drug responses. Prior to three months of age, the major mechanism for heat production is non-shivering thermogenesis by metabolism of brown fat. This mechanism can be limited in premature infants and in sick neonates who are deficient in fat stores. Cold stress-induced acidosis and increased pulmonary vascular resistance may predispose preterm and newborn infants to reverting to neonatal circulation. With a patent ductus arteriosus, increased pulmonary vascular resistance will force blood to bypass the lungs resulting in decreased oxygenation and ventilation causing further physiologic stress. It is imperative to avoid hypothermia by warming the operating room and fluids, using a warming blanket or radiant heat device during surgery and transporting the patient with adequate protection or a even a warming mattress for the especially susceptible premature patients.

## RISKS OF ANESTHESIA

In the United States, devastating neurologic injury and death in healthy pediatric patients as the result of an anesthetic-related cause is exceedingly rare. Adverse events are also rare and tend to have a higher incidence in children younger than one year and are highest in those less than one month old.[3] This higher risk may be, in part, attributed to physiologic changes and organ system immaturity.

Over the last decades, the standard use of pulse oximetry and capnography has dramatically decreased the number of preventable respiratory complications.[4–6] Newer anesthetic agents (sevoflurane vs. halothane) are associated with less frequent cardiac arrest in infants (see section on anesthetic agents). Despite an overall decrease in the incidence of anesthesia-related complications, the pediatric population continues to have a higher incidence than adults and the risk seems to increase with decreasing age.

A prospective survey from 1978 to 1982 of over 40,000 pediatric patients found an overall complication rate of 4.3% in infants and only 0.5% in patients from age one to 14 years and a nearly ten times higher cardiac arrest rate (1.9%) in the younger age group. They further found that risk increased with advancing ASA status and in emergency surgery.[7] Table 2 shows the preoperative physical status classification according to the American Society of Anesthesiologists. Note that while the ASA physical status classification does not directly translate to operative risk, it does help to assess the degree of "sickness" or "physical state" of the patient prior to selecting the anesthetic or performing surgery. Thus one can,

**Table 2. ASA Physical Status Classification according to the American Society of Anesthesiologists.**

| ASA physical status | Definition |
|---|---|
| I | Normal healthy patient |
| II | Patient with mild systemic disease |
| III | Patient with severe systemic disease |
| IV | Patient with severe systemic disease that is a constant threat to life |
| V | Moribund patient who is not expected to survive without the operation |
| VI | A declared brain-dead patient for organ procurement |
| E | If the procedure is an emergency an E follows the physical status |

Modified from the American Society of Anesthesiologists.

perhaps estimate higher or lower medical risk when factoring anesthetic technique and the extent of surgical trauma.[8,9]

The Pediatric Cardiac Arrest Registry (POCA) a voluntary contribution database examined cases of cardiac arrest at several institutions (75% of which are university-affiliated) for complication trends. Analysis of the data reveals a cardiac arrest incidence of 1.4 in 10,000 cases at these institutions. Respiratory causes of cardiac arrest account for 28% of events with laryngospasm as the primary cause followed by inadequate ventilation or oxygenation.[10] Furthermore, arrest from laryngospasm occurred more often in healthy patients under two years of age and over one third of these cases were associated with upper respiratory infections[5] (see section on upper respiratory infections). Nearly 50% of the cases of cardiac arrest secondary to respiratory causes occurred in patients undergoing ENT surgery. Cardiovascular causes of cardiac arrest (approximately 40% of cases) included hypovolemia, hyperkalemia from massive transfusion or succinylcholine or in patients with congenital heart disease or ASA physical status III to V where the exact cardiovascular cause of cardiac arrest was not determined. The overall mortality following cardiac arrest in this study is 28%, with patients more likely undergoing emergent surgery or ASA physical status III to V.[10]

A recently identified potential risk of apoptosis in neonates caused by medications used to provide sedation, analgesia, and anesthesia has been a topic of much interest. Because this is a time of rapid brain growth this population is particularly vulnerable. Many of the commonly used anesthetic agents such as ketamine, propofol, etomidate, benzodiazepines, and inhaled anesthetic agents have been implicated in increased apoptosis impacting development in laboratory animals.[2,11,12] Interpretation of these animal studies is difficult because the majority of animal studies use drug doses many times higher than those used in clinical practice with much longer exposures than typical in our patients. Furthermore, many did not control for normal vital signs. Finally, the period of rapid brain growth is different in each animal species making the parallel comparison difficult. Further research will reveal the clinical significance of this data in humans so that, at present, there is insufficient evidence to change our clinical practice.

## SPECIFIC CONCERNS FOR THE ANESTHESIOLOGIST

Certain comorbidities afford additional risk with anesthesia or require additional planning. Whether a further work up is initiated by the surgeon or the patient is referred for an evaluation by an anesthesiologist, understanding and recognizing specific anesthetic concerns during the surgical evaluation can help to avoid unnecessary delays and cancellations of procedures.

### Upper Respiratory Infection

The risk of adverse respiratory events increases in patients undergoing general anesthesia with an active URI. Since pediatric patients, especially school aged children, get as many as six to eight respiratory infections a year scheduling elective procedures can be difficult.[13] While some cancellations will occur immediately before surgery in the preoperative suite, many surgeons are faced with phone calls in the days before surgery from parents whose children have new onset URI symptoms. Understanding the risks of proceeding with surgery/anesthesia is important in preventing "over" cancellation as well as the inconvenience, emotional stress, and potential financial burden to the family who arrives for the surgery just to be cancelled by the anesthesiologist.

Numerous studies have shown that the overall risk of adverse respiratory events increases in patients with an active URI in the perioperative period with increases in incidence of laryngospasm, bronchospasm, and postoperative croup and atelectasis. Cohen *et al.* showed a two- to seven-fold increased risk of adverse respiratory events with URI and up to 11-fold if the patient is intubated for the procedure.[14]

Many studies also indicate that the risk of proceeding with surgery and anesthesia in patient with an uncomplicated URI (clear rhinorrhea, dry cough, no or low grade fever and the patient is acting well) while increased, may be acceptable.[15–17] However, other studies would indicate that the procedure itself (airway surgery), the method of airway management (intubation vs. mask general anesthesia) and the age of the patient (higher incidences of laryngospasm seen in children under one year of age) increase the risk to the patient.[15,16] So that a patient having a tonsillectomy with intubation has a higher risk for adverse respiratory events than if undergoing myringotomy tubes with mask general anesthesia.[18]

More "complicated" URI's including malaise, high fever, purulent coryza and signs of lower respiratory symptoms such as wet cough or wheezing may significantly increase risk of complications and may warrant postponement of an elective procedure. The ideal URI free time required to be considered "recovered" is four to six weeks. This is the amount of time required for the lower respiratory tract to recover its mucocilliary function and airway reactivity to normalize. When surveyed, most anesthesiologists were in favor of postponing surgery for at least three to four weeks.[16,17] Other risk factors associated with adverse events include a history of prematurity, a history of reactive airway disease, parental smoking, and surgery involving the airway.[19,20]

The increased risks of anesthesia must be weighed against the risk of postponing surgery and the decision to proceed must include a dialogue between the anesthesiologists, the surgeons and the parents. A thorough history from the parents is crucial. One study showed that a confirmation of a URI by parents was a better predictor of laryngospasm than symptoms alone.[21] In determining whether to proceed with surgery/anesthesia one must consider whether this is a mild URI that is resolving or is it prodromal to a more severe infection? Eliciting a history of URI in other household members may give an indication of severity of potential infection and course. Is this a bacterial infection warranting treatment with antibiotics prior to surgery? Is there a non-infectious allergic component to these symptoms? How often is the child free of infection? Many school-aged children are rarely infection-free for long enough to allow for the full four- to six-week recovery. Figure 1 shows a suggested algorithm for determining whether to proceed with surgery/anesthesia.

Concomitant conditions such as reactive airway disease, obstructive sleep apnea, congenital heart disease may increase risk of perioperative complications in patients with URI and the decision to

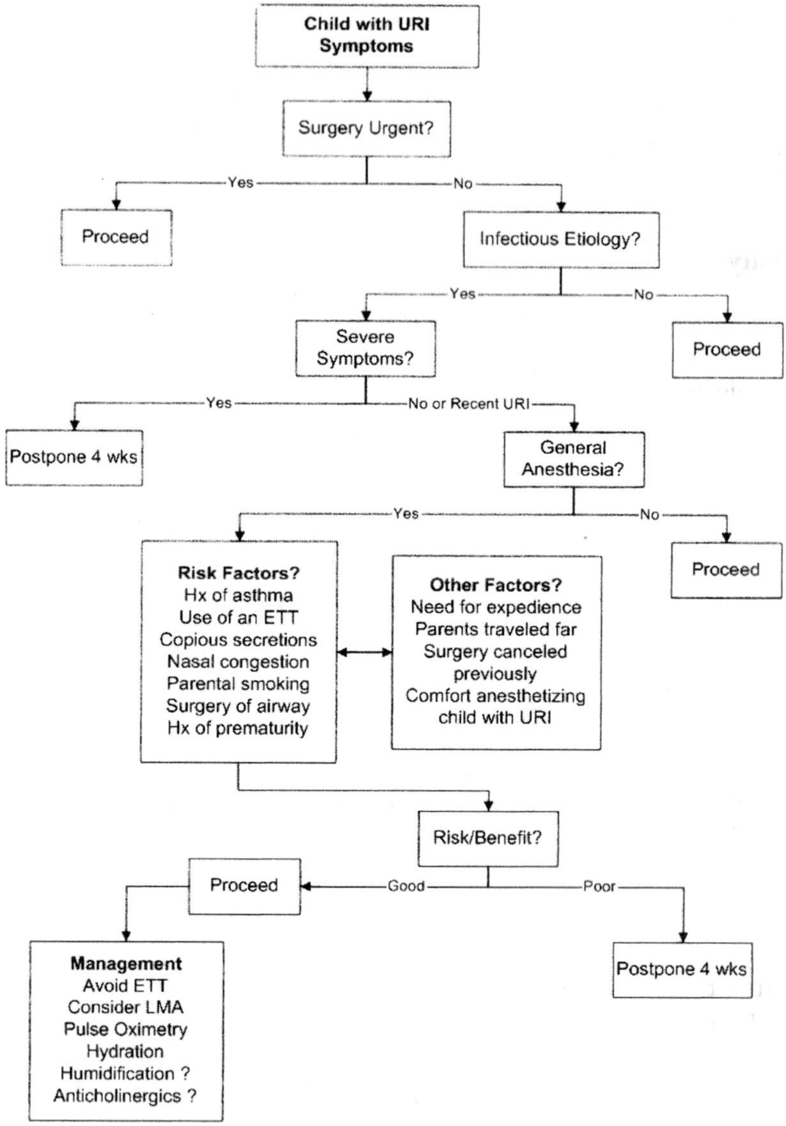


**Fig. 1.** Suggested algorithm for the assessment and anesthetic management of the child with an upper respiratory infection.

From Ref. 13, with permission.

proceed should be considered carefully.[16] Finally, the experience of the anesthesiologist to handle potential complications under anesthesia (laryngospasm, bronchospasm, breath holding, postoperative croup, etc.) should also be considered when deciding to proceed with the surgery.

## Obesity

The rate of pediatric obesity has been increasing in the United States with approximately one third of children being classified as overweight or obese. While the causes of this are beyond the scope of this chapter, the implications of obesity in the perioperative period are significant and warrant discussion. Comorbities associated with obesity in the pediatric patient include many previously considered "adult" issues and as such are often missed in the pediatric population. Clinically significant hypertension exists in 30% of obese pediatric patients and has significant cardiac implications including left ventricular hypertrophy and cardiac hypertrophy if untreated. There is a ten-fold increase in "adult-onset" diabetes (type 2 diabetes) in the pediatric population in the last 20 years.[22] Longstanding hyperlipidemia and fatty liver may also have significant anesthetic implications. Furthermore, there is an increase in incidence of asthma in obese children and an increase in severity of "attacks" in pediatric patients that are obese (see below for perioperative preparation of pts with asthma).

In otolaryngology, obese patients are likely to present for treatment of obstructive sleep apnea (2% of general pediatric population vs. 40% of obese)[23] and longstanding OSA puts the patient at risk for pulmonary hypertension, right-sided heart failure, and systemic hypertension.[24] Pts with OSA, regardless of type of surgery may require more intensive postoperative monitoring including potential need for ICU stay. When evaluating an obese or overweight patient for surgery a high index of suspicion should be maintained and a thorough exam is warranted for the above conditions that will have not only intraoperative anesthetic implications but potential postoperative implications for blood pressure management, blood sugar control and airway support. Preoperative vital signs for blood pressure screening, lab work, and possibly a sleep study, EKG, or ECHO may be indicated. Obese patients are extremely sensitive to central nervous system-depressant drugs and may exhibit prolonged sedation, resedation or apnea so that premedication and postoperative narcotics should be used cautiously. Multimodal pain therapy should be used to minimize the need for narcotics (dosed on ideal body weight). These patients also tend to have difficult intravenous access, may likely have GERD, and are at higher risk for difficulty for mask ventilation and airway management secondary to fatty deposits, all of which increase perioperative risk and require adequate planning.

**Asthma**

Patients with asthma require good preoperative preparation. A through history and physical is imperative. A history of severity including frequency of ER visits, need for steroid therapy, recent exacerbations and meds taken should be elicited and may require consultation with the child's primary care physician. Recent or active upper respiratory infection may exacerbate asthma and elective surgery should be postponed. Furthermore, active wheezing warrants postponement for maximizing therapy. Pulmonary function tests (PFT's) may be useful for assessing the degree of obstructive disease and response to bronchodilators but as results are effort-related they may be of limited use in patients less than five years of age. All daily asthma-related medications (oral and inhalational) should be continued up to the morning of surgery. Patients who take only rescue medications for exacerbations may be encouraged to take their medications for 24 hours preoperatively or at minimum prophylactic nebulized $\beta_2$ agonists such as albuterol may be beneficial just prior to surgery. Patients with a history of bronchospasm are at higher risk for an "attack" under anesthesia secondary to light anesthesia, instrumentation of the airway, etc. Precautions that should be taken will be discussed in the section on anesthesia induction.

## Trisomy 21

Patients with Trisomy 21 or Down Syndrome often present for adenotonsillectomy for obstructive sleep apnea and have characteristic abnormalities of interest to the anesthesiologist.[25] Besides OSA, macroglossia, subglottic stenosis, and atlantoaxial instability contribute to airway challenges of these patients.[26]

Approximately 20% of patients will also have ligamentous laxity of the atlantoaxial joint.[27] This laxity and associated odontoid process immaturity may predispose patients to spinal cord injury with flexion or extension that may be required for laryngoscopy and positioning for surgical intervention for procedures such as tonsillectomy and bronchoscopy. Signs and symptoms of atlantoaxial instability (easy fatigability, difficulty in walking, abnormal gait, neck pain limiting neck mobility, torticollis, incoordination and clumsiness, sensory deficits, spasticity, hyperreflexia) are usually not manifested until after five years of age. Pain and numbness and tingling, while indicative of potential instability, may be difficult to illicit in patients with developmental delay. Laxity of other joints such as fingers, thumb, elbows and knees tends to correlate well with presence of atlantoaxial dislocation.[28] No specific guidelines for preoperative evaluation exist but flexion and extension films and neurology consultation may be warranted if signs or symptoms are present. At minimum, if abnormalities are present, a neutral position should be maintained for intubation and somatosensory evoked potential (SSEP) monitoring of the upper extremities may be considered.[29]

Up to 60% of patients with Trisomy 21 will have congenital heart disease including AV canal defects, VSD, ASD, PDA, and tetrology of fallot and warrants a thorough history and physical and cardiac evaluation (see below).

## Congenital Heart Disease

The perioperative management of the child with congenital heart disease is a special challenge for the anesthesiologist because of the vast array of anatomic variations. Some of these children will require palliative or corrective surgery early in their lives. Many children with congenital heart disease will not require early intervention and some will even have relatively benign lesions that go unrecognized until under a physiologic stress such as surgery and anesthesia.

Most children with significant cardiac disease have regular follow-up evaluations by a cardiologist. If not recent, or if clinical status has changed since the last exam a preoperative visit to the cardiologist may be necessary for complex congenital heart lesions. The evaluation obtained from the cardiologist should address the specific lesion, any surgical repairs, a description of current anatomy, and any interval changes in function. It is important to have available recent ECHO or cardiac catheterization data as the anesthesiologist will need to review the data in planning the anesthetic.

Injury to conduction pathways during repair of certain congenital heart defects can lead to life-threatening cardiac arrhythmias and conduction defects. The incidence of right bundle branch block after tetrology of fallot repair is up to 59% and complete heart block occurs in 1% of patients.[30] Other defects associated with arrhythmias include AV septal defects and transposition of the great arteries.

Therefore a thorough preoperative evaluation should also include an EKG for evaluation of potential conduction disturbances as well as an evaluation of permanent pacemakers should one be present. Interrogation of the pacemaker to determine the type, the mode of cardiac pacing and specific settings is important prior to surgery so that the anesthesiologist can adequately plan its intraoperative management. While rarely necessary with newer pacemakers, a magnet should be available to change the pacemaker to asynchronous mode should electrocautery be utilized. Furthermore, the electrocautery grounding pad should be placed as far away from the pacemaker generator so that the path between the grounding pad and surgical site does not cross the mediastinum.

In patients with certain congenital heart diseases and repaired conditions, endocarditis prophylaxis may be warranted when undergoing adenoidectomy or tonsillectomy; antibiotic prophylaxis is not recommended for bronchoscopy unless the procedure involves incision or biopsy of the respiratory mucosa. For patients with any of the following, endocarditis prophylaxis may be reasonable[31,32] and if there is any question, the patients' cardiologist should be consulted for recommendations prior to the day of surgery.

- Unrepaired cyanotic CHD, including palliative shunts and conduits.
- Completely repaired congenital heart defect with prosthetic material or device, whether placed by surgery or by catheter intervention, during the first six months after the procedure.
- Repaired CHD with residual defects at the site or adjacent to the site of a prosthetic patch or prosthetic device (which inhibit endothelialization).
- Cardiac transplantation recipients who develop cardiac valvulopathy.

Finally, patients with congenital heart defects, even those that are "repaired" may have residual shunts predisposing them to right to left shunting. Care must be taken to avoid even the smallest air bubble in the intravenous fluids which can put the patient at high risk for stroke, myocardial ischemia, etc. If a high index of suspicion exists for residual connection between the venous and arterial circulation, air filters should be used in the intravenous line. Note that most air filters have a high resistance and may make rapid infusion of fluids difficult.

## NIL-PER-OS GUIDELINES

Aspiration pneumonitis is a rare but potentially devastating complication from passive regurgitation of gastric contents. An adequate period of fasting prior to induction of anesthesia is necessary to decrease the risk. As morbidity and mortality due to aspiration of gastric contents is rare[33] and gastric emptying is much faster in infants and children (evidenced by the frequency of feeding in infants of q2–4 hours) the typical "NPO after midnight" instruction given to adults is not appropriate for pediatric patients.

**Table 3. Recommended fasting time (hours).**

| Patient Age | Solids (includes breast milk and formula) | Clear liquids |
|---|---|---|
| Younger than 6 months | 4 | 2 |
| 6–36 months | 6 | 2 |
| Older than 36 months | 8 | 2 |

Adapted from Ref. 99.

Studies have demonstrated similar residual volumes and gastric pH in pediatric patients who receive clear liquids (water, juice without pulp, carbonated beverages, etc.) two to three hours before induction as those in patients that had longer fasting times. In fact, some studies indicate lower residual volumes with shorter fasting times[34] and that the volume of liquid ingested is less important than the type of liquid. These more liberal guidelines (see Table 3) have been adapted in recent years decreasing the incidence of preoperative dehydration (and ensuing intraoperative hypotension and possible difficult IV access), potential hypoglycemia and patient irritability and have significantly increased parental satisfaction.[35] Because of studies that show gastric emptying of breast milk is more rapid than formula, it is unclear whether it should be considered in the same category as formula or as a clear liquid. Therefore, some institutions allow breast milk with the same restrictions as clear liquids and others as a solid.[22,36,37] It is prudent to check with your institutions specific NPO guidelines. Finally, it is important when giving these instructions to parents to emphasize the safety issues involved to maximize compliance and avoid unnecessary delays in the start of the procedure.

## PREOPERATIVE MANAGEMENT

### Family Preparation

Up to 65% of all children undergoing anesthesia and surgery develop intense anxiety and fear in the preoperative period and during induction of anesthesia. This anxiety can be attributed to separation from parents and uncertainty about the anesthesia and surgery and are in part dependent on the child's age. Knowledge of developmental stages and coping mechanisms may help the anesthesiologist and surgeon to anticipate the needs of the patient. Details of anesthetic plan should be explained, as much as possible directly to the patient in age-specific language. A recent study in healthy seven to 17 year old preoperative pediatric patients found that the vast majority of children desired comprehensive information regarding their surgery, anesthesia, how much postoperative pain they will have, and the duration of pain. Furthermore, the more anxious patients were found to desire more information specifically about pain. Finally, they found that children who had previous surgery did not require less perioperative information.[38] This study demonstrates the importance of the preoperative discussion with the patient however, questions from all family members should be addressed as parents who receive comprehensive preoperative information report significantly less anxiety than parents who received minimal information.[39]

Perioperative anxiety has been associated with new onset maladaptive behavior including temper tantrums, nightmares, bed-wetting and attention-seeking.[40] Parental anxiety also increases anxiety in the patient so that planned interventions should address both the parents and patients concerns.[41] Preoperative preparation, including play therapy, operating room tours, printed materials or videos can allay anxiety in both the parents and the patient.[42]

## Premedication

The primary goal of premedication in children is to facilitate a smooth separation from the parents and ease the induction of anesthesia. As separation anxiety develops after the age of seven or eight months, premedication prior to this age is rarely indicated. Premedication may also be helpful for patients who have had previous unpleasant hospital experiences or patients with developmental delay that may make communication or cooperation without sedation difficult. The choice of medications used for anxiolysis is dependent upon the procedure, the patient, the desired effect and duration of effect, and practitioner preference. The routes used for premedication include intravenous, intramuscular, oral, intranasal, rectal and sublingual. Each has obvious benefits and drawbacks. Oral premedication is the most popular route but may be difficult in an upset, uncooperative child or developmentally delayed or severely autistic child. Intramuscular injection may be useful in this situation.

Oral midazolam is the most commonly administered premedication. An oral dose of 0.25–1.0 mg/kg (maximum 20 mg) can provide satisfactory anxiolysis and separation from parents within ten to 15 minutes. Midazolam can also be given IM (0.5 mg/kg), IN (0.2 mg/kg), PR and sublingually. Ketamine (2–6 mg/kg depending on desired effect) in combination with midazolam is another popular premedication and can be given IM or oral routes. Children over seven or eight years of age may not require premedication with adequate preparation. Some may even be willing to allow intravenous access especially if it can be done nearly painlessly. EMLA, a eutectic mixture of local anesthetics can be placed on the skin can provide adequate analgesia for IV start in 60 minutes. EMLA cream is a mixture of lidocaine and prilocaine that penetrates the skin and significantly decreases the pain associated with an intravenous insertion. Because of the risk of methemoglobinemia it should be used with caution in children younger than three months old or in children who are receiving other medications that may also induce methemoglobinemia. Plasma concentrations of lidocaine and prilocaine are well below the toxic level but may be higher in patients with broken skin, when placed in multiple sites or left on for prolonged period of time. EMLA causes vasoconstriction, making intravenous access potentially more challenging in small patients.

An alternative topical anesthetic gaining popularity is Synera®. The Synera® patch, a eutectic mixture of lidocaine and tetracaine impregnated peel and stick patch integrated with an oxygen activated heating component works in as little as 20 minutes. Furthermore, the self-warming element causes vasodilatation rather than vasoconstriction and blanching from EMLA. Clinical trials have shown safety in patients as young as four months of age.[43] Very limited drug absorption and no risk of methemoglobinemia make this topical anesthetic a desirable but costly alternative to EMLA. One can argue that the benefit of vasodilation and the shorter onset of action may make its use cost effective in young patients and patients with a history of difficult access.

Once intravenous access is established IV anxiolysis can be titrated to effect (unlike a single oral dose) — a benefit in patients at risk for airway obstruction or cardiovascular instability but requiring sedation/anxiolysis to separate from the parents.

## INTRAOPERATIVE MANAGEMENT

### Parent Present Induction

Potential benefits from parent present induction include reducing the need for preoperative sedatives and avoiding the fear and anxiety that may occur on separation when premedication is not used. It is especially beneficial for short procedures such as tonsillectomy, myringotomy tubes, etc. where the sedative effects of the premedication can outlast the duration of the procedure and may delay awakening.[44] Parental presence may also be useful for children undergoing repeated procedures. Studies examining the effect of parental presence have shown a decrease in patient anxiety. However, others have shown an increase in anxiety and have shown that the parent's anxiety impacts the child so that highly anxious parents should probably not participate. Another study found that in a patient premedicated with oral midazolam, the presence of a parent for induction had no additional anxiolytic effect for the patient; however, parents who accompanied their children into the operating room had less anxiety and were more satisfied with the process.[25,42,45,46]

Before considering a parent present induction, the parent must be educated to the induction process, including the expected changes in their child's consciousness as they progress through the stages of anesthesia, the changes in breathing pattern and the fact that once the child is asleep, they will be asked to leave and must do so immediately. Allowing a parent into the operating room without this preparation may be counterproductive and may increase the anxiety of the parent, anesthesiologist and patient.

## Intraoperative Monitoring

Because pediatric patients are at risk for respiratory complications and bradycardia with desaturation, strict application of the American Society of Anesthesiology monitoring standards is imperative to early identification.[47] During all anesthetics, the patient's oxygenation, ventilation, circulation shall be continually evaluated. Oxygenation via pulse oximetry and the concentration of inspired oxygen should be continuously monitored. Assessment of ventilation should include qualitative (chest excursion, observation of the reservoir bag, and auscultation of breath sounds) and quantitative (end-tidal $CO_2$ analysis) measurements. Every patient receiving anesthesia should have the electrocardiogram continuously displayed and blood pressure and heart rate determined and evaluated at least every five minutes. Temperature should be monitored when clinically significant changes in body temperature are intended, anticipated or suspected.[48] Patients under 10 kg body weight, being particularly vulnerable to hypothermia, should always be monitored for temperature. Finally, all monitors should have age appropriate alarms set that are audible to the anesthesiologist above the noise of the operating room. The normal range for vital signs at particular ages is defined in Table 4.

**Table 4. Mean vital signs at various ages.**

| Age | Respiratory rate | Heart rate | Systolic | Diastolic |
|---|---|---|---|---|
| Newborn | 40 | 140 | 65 | 45 |
| 12 months | 30 | 120 | 95 | 60 |
| 2 years | 25 | 100 | 100 | 65 |
| 9 years | 20 | 80 | 105 | 65 |

## INDUCTION OF ANESTHESIA

General anesthesia in pediatric patients is most commonly induced via inhalational or intravenous technique. Certain conditions (full stomach or gastroesophageal reflux, blood in the airway, difficult airway, etc.) make intravenous induction the better choice; however, because of an inherent fear of "needles" and "shots" inhalational induction is usually better tolerated by younger patients. Once the monitors are applied, beginning with odorless nitrous oxide and oxygen can allow the introduction and incremental increase of the more pungent sevoflurane (or halothane) until an adequate depth of anesthesia is achieved. Alternatively, if the child is upset or uncooperative, a single breath technique using oxygen (with or without nitrous oxide) and 8% sevoflurane can be used to speed up induction. Since infants have a higher alveolar ventilation and smaller FRC to minute ventilation ratio than adults, a more rapid induction (and emergence) is possible.

Scents (bubble gum, root beer, strawberry, grape, etc.) can be placed inside the mask to disguise the odor of the gas. Distractions such as a story or engaging conversation for older children can also aid in a smooth inhalational induction. Care must be taken to avoid noxious stimulation such as IV start, excessive manipulation of the airway or painful jaw thrust during the excitation phase of induction (characterized by increase in heart rate and possibly blood pressure, irregular respiratory pattern and disconjugate gaze) as airway reflexes are heightened and risk of laryngospasm is increased. Once adequate depth of anesthesia is achieved intravenous access can be established.

In patients with intravenous access induction of anesthesia can be achieved using intravenous agents (see below). Preoxygenation with 100% $FIO_2$ prior to induction of anesthesia is necessary to help prolong time before desaturation with apnea. The advantage of intravenous induction is the rapidity of induction decreasing the time in the excitation stage and the presence of intravenous access if emergency medications are needed.

Finally, patients who are at risk for aspiration (full stomach or gastroesophageal reflux) require a rapid-sequence intravenous induction. Preoxygenation is especially important in these patients as bag mask ventilation is avoided when possible to decrease risk of regurgitation from positive pressure forced air in the stomach. The induction agent and muscle relaxant (succinylcholine 2 mg/kg or high dose rocuronium) of choice are given while cricoid pressure is applied. Manual pressure at the level of cricoid seals the esophagus potentially preventing passive regurgitation. This pressure should not be released until appropriate placement of the endotracheal tube is verified.

Intramuscular injection for induction of anesthesia is also possible with ketamine but is the least desirable method because of the inability to titrate the dose given. It is reserved for special conditions such as combative or developmentally disabled patients that will not allow either inhalational or intravenous induction.

Inadequate anesthesia is a common cause of bronchospasm in susceptible patients. Particularly prior to airway instrumentation, adequate depth of anesthesia must be assured. Supplementation of general anesthesia with topical lidocaine or intravenous lidocaine can help prevent bronchospasm. Potent inhalational anesthetics (sevoflurane, halothane as well as isoflurane, desflurane) can all relieve bronchospasm however, with severe bronchospasm delivery of the inhaled agent or even inhaled bronchodilators may be limited. In such situations, intravenous agents such as propofol can be used. While propofol has no intrinsic bronchodilator effect, increasing depth of anesthesia may ameliorate the bronchospasm caused by light anesthesia. Ketamine acts as a potent bronchodilator and will increase depth of anesthesia and may be a useful induction agent in patients with active wheezing or severe disease.

## ANESTHESIA MAINTENANCE

### Inhalational Agents

Inhalational anesthetics comprise one of the most widely used anesthetic classes in children and adults. Knowledge of the physiologic differences in pediatric patients compared with adults is required in order to utilize these agents effectively. In general, infants and young children have higher alveolar ventilation and greater distribution of cardiac output to vessel rich organs compared with adults, which speeds inhalation inductions. In addition, the minimum alveolar concentration (MAC) of the inhalation agents is higher in infants than in older children and adults, thus resulting in a higher concentration of inhaled anesthetic necessary to anesthetize them. Finally, the myocardium and compensatory mechanisms (i.e. tachycardia, vasoconstriction) in neonates and infants is immature, resulting in increased sensitivity to inhalational anesthetics manifested by myocardial depression and hypotension.

*Nitrous oxide*

Nitrous oxide ($N_2O$, laughing gas) is in wide clinical use in both children and adults. It is odorless, colorless, and has a low blood solubility. This allows it to have rapid induction and recovery, and to augment the uptake of the other inhalational agents when used together. Nitrous oxide is 35 times more soluble than nitrogen in blood. It therefore diffuses into air-containing cavities such as the middle ear more rapidly than nitrogen can exit. Because the middle ear is a fixed cavity, this effect can result in an increase in pressure, resulting in graft disruption during tympanoplasty. Thus nitrous oxide should be avoided during this procedure or if used, discontinued 15 minutes before closure.[49,50] Caution should also be used in patients with previous middle ear reconstruction, as well as during prolonged surgery as nitrous oxide can diffuse into and expand the cuff on the endotracheal tube.

*Halothane*

Halothane is the least expensive volatile anesthetic, and although largely replaced by newer agents, is still in use worldwide, especially in developing nations. Historically, halothane was the most commonly used agent for infants and children, especially during inhalational induction due to its lack of airway irritation, rapidity of induction, and potent bronchodilatory effects. However, several side effects are associated with halothane. These include direct myocardial depression, slowing of the sinoatrial node conduction, and blunting of the baroreceptor function. In infants, with low ventricular compliance and direct reliance on heart rate for cardiac output, halothane must be used with an abundance of caution and careful attention to vital signs.[51] Halothane also sensitizes the myocardium to the arrhythmogenic effects of epinephrine which should be used with caution at the lowest acceptable dosages if administration is needed. Finally, halothane has rarely been associated with postoperative "halothane hepatitis," which is probably related to multiple exposures at short intervals.[52] The incidence is estimated to be one in 35,000 cases. Overall, while halothane is no longer used in many US centers, it continues to be available worldwide and can be safely used with close monitoring and attention to its potential side effects.

### *Sevoflurane*

Sevoflurane has largely replaced halothane in most US pediatric institutions. It is less pungent than halothane and has rapid alveolar uptake which makes it an excellent agent for inhalational inductions. It is also associated with less myocardial depression than halothane and does not exhibit myocardial sensitization to catecholamines.[53] It is an excellent bronchodilator as well, which may be useful in cases of bronchospasm. Sevoflurane is probably the most widely used inhalational anesthetic in short duration pediatric head and neck cases such as PE tubes, adenotonsillectomies, and tracheal examinations, due to the above properties. The low solubility of sevoflurane allows patients a rapid emergence upon its discontinuation. While convenient for timing of cases, this has been associated with a greater incidence of emergence delirium in some pediatric patients, particularly when used without associated narcotics.[54]

### *Isoflurane*

Isoflurane is a nonflammable volatile anesthetic discovered in 1965 and used clinically for many years in children and adults. Unlike sevoflurane, it has a pungent odor and is thus unsuitable for inhalation (mask) inductions. Additionally, time to emergence from isoflurane is longer compared to sevoflurane and desflurane, which also presents a disadvantage to its use in rapid pediatric procedures. During longer cases, isoflurane is a reasonable, less expensive alternative agent for use during the maintenance phase of anesthesia[1,2]

*Desflurane*

Structurally similar to isoflurane, desflurane is the most recent inhalational agent to be used clinically. Despite a similar structure, the substitution of a fluorine atom for a chlorine atom confers upon desflurane profound differences from isoflurane. Most notably is its low solubility causes a very rapid uptake and washout of this agent.[55] Wakeup times from desflurane are approximately 50% faster than from isoflurane. However, its pungency, airway irritation, and ability to stimulate coughing, salivation, and laryngospasm make desflurane unsuitable for inhalational inductions and bronchoscopic procedures. It is also associated with an increased risk of emergence delirium owing to its rapid washout.[54]

**Intravenous Agents**

*Opioids*

Opioid receptors are present throughout the central nervous system and other tissues. The opioids primarily provide analgesia yet can result in moderate sedation as well. There are four major opioid receptor subtypes: mu, kappa, delta, and sigma. The primary clinical effect of mu receptor binding is supraspinal analgesia and respiratory depression. Kappa binding produces sedation and spinal analgesia, delta binding produces analgesic and behavioral effects, while sigma binding is responsible for dysphoria and hallucinations.[2] The properties of each specific opioid are determined by which receptors are activated and with what affinity. Because neonates and children exhibit enhanced responses to opioids compared with adults, close, continuous monitoring of intraoperative and postoperative ventilation and vital signs is imperative.

### *Fentanyl*

Owing to its rapid onset and relatively brief duration, fentanyl is one of the most commonly administered narcotics in infants and children. It is often used as an analgesic as well as an adjunct to sedative agents and inhalational anesthetics. When used in smaller doses (1–3 mcg/kg), the duration of action is 30 to 60 minutes and termination of action results mainly from redistribution. Larger doses of fentanyl (up to 100 mcg/kg) can produce general anesthesia and may result in longer elimination times due to drug accumulation. Thus large doses of fentanyl will result in properties similar to long acting narcotics, and postoperative ventilatory support and monitoring will be necessary. While fentanyl administration generally results in a stable cardiovascular response, it may be associated with bradycardia, especially in neonates who are most dependent on heart rate for cardiac output[56] and may require treatment with atropine or glycopyrrolate.

### *Morphine*

Morphine has been used in adults, children, and neonates as a long acting analgesic and anesthetic adjunct for many years. It must be used with caution, however, in neonates due to decreased clearance of morphine metabolites secondary to reduced hepatic conjugation and renal clearance. At an intravenous dose of 0.05 to 0.1 mg/kg, the half-life of morphine in young children and infants (greater than six months) is approximately three hours. This time may be significantly greater in infants less than six months, critically ill children, or in the presence of renal insufficiency. Histamine release may also occur during morphine administration resulting in skin rash.[1]

### *Hydromorphone*

Another commonly administered opioid, hydromorphone, resembles morphine in its duration of action and may be useful in patients with renal insufficiency due to its less active metabolite, hydromorphone-3-glucuronide. In addition, the side effects commonly observed with morphine (pruritus, rash, nausea) may not occur as frequently with hydromorphone due to decreased histamine release. Like other opioids, ventilatory levels and hemodynamic function must be closely monitored, especially in neonates.

### Other Intravenous Agents

#### *Midazolam*

Midazolam is a short acting benzodiazepine commonly used in children as an anxiolytic premedication or sedative adjunct to other anesthetics. Midazolam has the shortest elimination half-life (approximately two hours) among the benzodiazepines, however, its clearance is significantly less in neonates than in older children (half-life six to 12 hours).[57] Midazolam is rapidly absorbed via intravenous (0.025–0.05 mg/kg), intramuscular (0.1–0.15 mg/kg), oral (0.25–1.0 mg/kg), rectal (0.75–1.0 mg/kg), nasal (0.2 mg/kg), or sublingual (0.2 mg/kg) administration and this, along with its rapid onset of action make it a practical choice for preoperative administration.[58] Caution must be used when midazolam is administered together with narcotics, due to the possibility of enhanced respiratory depression and hypotension. Severe hypotension has been reported in neonates after bolus administration of midazolam especially in the presence of fentanyl.

#### *Propofol*

Propofol is a highly lipophilic anesthetic and thus has rapid distribution, redistribution, hepatic transformation and renal clearance. Propofol is used frequently to induce general anesthesia in children with existing intravenous access, as a sedative for brief and not very stimulating procedures (i.e. MRI), or as a sedative infusion in an ICU setting. Infants and young children require greater doses of propofol than adults because of their larger volume of distribution.[1]

Propofol also possesses antiemetic properties and has been associated with a decreased rate of postoperative nausea and vomiting. Pain on intravenous injection of propofol may be minimized with small doses of lidocaine prior to its injection.

### *Ketamine*

Ketamine is a dissociative agent which provides analgesia and amnesia. Ketamine may be used as a premedication, as a sedative for procedures which do not require general anesthesia, or as analgesia for the insertion of intravenous access or invasive monitoring devices which may be needed prior to the induction of general anesthesia. It can be given intravenous (0.5–1 mg/kg), intramuscular (2–3 mg/kg), rectal (10 mg/kg), oral (6–10 mg/kg), or intranasal (3–6 mg/kg) routes.[1] Ketamine causes increased production of secretions and usually requires the co-administration of an antisialogogue such as glycopyrrolate, this side effect would also make ketamine a poor choice in a child with an active upper respiratory tract infection. The other major undesirable side effect of nightmares or hallucinations can usually be avoided by co-administration of midazolam.

### *Dexmedetomidine*

An alpha-2-adrenergic agonist, dexmetetomidine is the newest agent being used as a sedative in adults and children. It provides sedation without significant respiratory depression and also possesses anxiolytic, analgesic, and sympatholytic qualities. It should be administered via slow intravenous infusion (0.2–0.8 mg/kg) after a loading dose (0.5–1 mg/kg) given over ten minutes. Although the most frequent side effect of dexmedetomidine are hypotension and bradycardia, several recent studies[59] in children have reported adequate procedural sedation with maintenance of blood pressure and heart rate in range limits normal for age. Additional reports have documented the utility of dexmedetomidine in children requiring fiberoptic intubation, undergoing awake craniotomy, and to reduce the incidence of emergence agitation.[60,61]

## MUSCLE RELAXANTS

### Depolarizing Muscle Relaxants

*Succinylcholine*

Succinylcholine is the only depolarizing muscle relaxant currently in use in children and adults. Because it is highly water soluble and infants have a higher volume of distribution than older children and adults, infants require a significantly higher dose of succinylcholine (2–3 mg/kg vs. 1–1.5 mg/kg intravenously). Reliable muscle relaxation and excellent intubation conditions occurs 40 seconds after intravenous administration. Succinylcholine may also be given intramuscularly (5 mg/kg for infants and 4 mg/kg in children older than six months) with muscle relaxation occurring three to four minutes after injection and lasting up to 20 minutes, as opposed to lasting five minutes after intravenous injection.[1]

Because of its potential side effects, succinylcholine has been replaced by intermediate acting non-depolarizing muscle relaxants for many cases that do not require a muscle relaxant with very rapid onset and short duration of action. However, it still remains indicated for use in rapid sequence inductions and for the treatment of laryngospasm, provided there are no contraindications to its use.

Side effects of succinylcholine are unfortunately numerous and consist of the following. Cardiac arrhythmias are possible, including bradycardia and cardiac sinus arrest, particularly after repeated bolus administration. This effect is pronounced in infants and young children and is usually responsive to intravenous atropine.[1] Many providers routinely administer atropine intravenously prior to the first dose of succinylcholine in this population. Succinylcholine is also associated with a potential for hyperkalemia, rhabdomyolysis, masseter spasm, and malignant hyperthermia. As a result of depolarization serum potassium may increase as much as 0.5 mEq/L in normal children; however life-threatening hyperkalemia may occur in conditions which cause a proliferation of extrajunctional potassium receptors such as extensive burns, major denervation injuries, paraplegia, crush injuries, or prolonged immobility.[2] There have been reports of a series of boys under the age of eight years old exhibiting cardiac arrest, rhabdomyolysis, and massive potassium release, presumably due to unrecognized muscular dystrophies. Succinylcholine is also a triggering agent for malignant hyperthermia (see below). It is for these reasons that many pediatric anesthesiologists have abandoned the use of succinylcholine except in cases where an alternative non-depolarizing muscle relaxant is not appropriate (i.e. emergency intubation in a child with a full stomach, laryngospasm).

### Non-Depolarizing Muscle Relaxants

Non-depolarizing muscle relaxants act by binding to the acetylcholine receptor and blocking access to the receptor. Neonates exhibit a variable response to non-depolarizing muscle relaxants as compared to older children and adults. The neuromuscular junction in the neonate is immature which tends to increase sensitivity, while a large volume of distribution dilutes the drug concentration.

A variety of non-depolarizing muscle relaxants are available. The choice of agent depends on the potential side effects, speed of onset, and duration of action. Rocuronium has the fastest onset time with acceptable intubating conditions produced three to four minutes after an intravenous dosage of 1.2 mg/kg, which is almost as rapid as succinylcholine. The duration of action of rocuronium is approximately 60 to 90 minutes and thus may make rocuronium an undesirable choice for short procedures. Vecuronium and cisatracurium are also intermediate-acting non-depolarizing muscle relaxants frequently used in pediatric anesthesia. Cisatracurium excretion does not rely on hepatic or renal function and thus is a good choice in a child with renal or liver disease.

## MALIGNANT HYPERTHERMIA

Malignant hyperthermia (MH) is a rare (1:15,000 in pediatric patients and 1:40,000 in adults) pharmacogenetic condition that results in a hypermetabolic cascade that originates at the level of the skeletal muscle cell following exposure to certain “triggering” anesthetics. Agents known to trigger malignant hyperthermia are the halogenated anesthetic agents (sevoflurane, halothane, desflurane, isoflurane) and succinylcholine.[62] While usually presenting intraoperatively, it can also present in the recovery room. Furthermore, nearly 50% of patients with MH had a previous uneventful anesthetic exposure.[1]

The earliest signs are often masseter muscle rigidity (MMR), tachycardia and hypercarbia many of which are non-specific making diagnosis difficult. Other signs include cyanosis, generalized rigidity and rhabdomyolysis, and hyperthermia (often a late sign).[2] Sympathetic stimulation causes arrhythmias and hypertension. Generalized muscle rigidity may be present, and dark colored urine is secondary to myoglobinuria. Laboratory evaluation reveals a mixed acidosis, hyperkalemia, elevated CK and low mixed venous oxygen saturation. Once MH is suspected the triggering agent should be removed, treatment with dantrolene should be started and supportive measures should also be initiated. Aggressive treatment of hyperkalemia, acidosis, hyperventilation with 100% $FiO_2$ and cooling measures should be taken. Vasopressors may be necessary to maintain adequate perfusion pressure and intravenous fluid resuscitation and diuresis should be considered to prevent renal failure from myoglobinuria.

Autosomal dominant (variable penetrance) inheritance makes eliciting a family history of malignant hyperthermia an important part of the preoperative evaluation. It may also be caused as a mutation of a gene on several chromosomes or may occur sporadically, therefore making occurrence possible in any patient. Furthermore certain disorders such as central-core disease,[63] King Denborough syndrome, and hypokalemic periodic paralysis have a higher incidence of MH.[64] Although newer evidence shows that muscular dystrophies (such as Duchenne's and Becker's) are unlikely to have an increased risk of MH, exposure to volatile anesthetics may be associated with life-threatening rhabdomyolysis and life-threatening hyperkalemia from succinylcholine so they must be used with caution in these patients.[65] Because these X-linked myopathies may not manifest symptoms until later in childhood many pediatric anesthesiologists do not routinely use succinylcholine in younger patients (especially boys), unless specifically indicated.

If a case of MH is suspected or verified, there are physicians on call at the Malignant Hyperthermia Hotline 24 hours a day (MHAUS hotline, 1-800-MH-HYPER). Even with prompt treatment, the mortality from MH may still be as high as 5%–30%.[1,2,62]

## EMERGENCE FROM ANESTHESIA

Whether to extubate a patient while under deep planes of anesthesia or awake depends on many factors. Deep extubation may be preferred in patients with asthma to prevent bronchospasm or for patients that increase in blood pressure and coughing during emergence may be a contraindication. Emergence from anesthesia tends to be smoother with a deep extubation. However, patients that are difficult to mask ventilate (either because of anatomy or because of surgical procedure), were difficult to intubate, have a full stomach, and have significant airway edema or copious secretions or blood in the airway should not be extubated deep but rather, awake with airway reflexes intact. If deep extubation is chosen, emergence from anesthesia should occur in the operating room or in the presence of skilled individuals able to manage potential laryngospasm or reintubation should the need arise.

## SPECIFIC CASES

### Laryngeal Surgery and Rigid Bronchoscopy

Laryngeal surgery and rigid bronchoscopy requires the airway to be shared by the surgeon and the anesthesiologist affording some anesthetic challenges. Providing suitable surgical conditions while maintaining adequate oxygenation and ventilation as well as patient comfort and safety is a challenge for the anesthesiologist. Good communication between the surgeon and anesthesiologist is crucial. Common indications for this procedure including vocal cord disorders, laryngeal webs, larynogomalacia, subglottic stenosis, airway foreign bodies and recurrent papillomatosis all have their own risk considerations for the anesthesiologist.

Different anesthetic techniques have been used successfully and can be divided into two main categories — controlled ventilation and spontaneous ventilation. The spontaneous ventilation technique is preferred when dynamic changes in the airway must be assessed (vocal cord movement or paresis, laryngomalacia or tracheomalacia) or for debridement of laryngeal papillomas and recovery of airway foreign bodies (positive pressure may push the object further into the airway or worsen obstruction).

After induction of anesthesia (inhalational or intravenous), intravenous access should be secured. Once adequate depth of anesthesia is achieved the table can be turned 90 degrees to the surgeon. After suspension laryngoscopy, maintenance of anesthesia can be achieved with inhalational anesthesia and 100% $FiO_2$ (unless laser will be used — see below for discussion on airway fires) by attaching the anesthesia circuit directly to the side port of the bronchoscope or by attaching it to a small endotracheal tube placed in the nasopharynx. When placed in the nasopharynx care must be taken to avoid bleeding which may impede surgical visualization or cause laryngospasm or aspiration of blood. Scavenging of gases can be accomplished by a small suction placed in the mouth. Despite high concentrations of gas, supplemental anesthesia may be needed to maintain adequate depth of anesthesia and can be given intravenously. In lieu of inhalational anesthetics an intravenous infusion of propofol can be utilized to provide an adequate plane of anesthesia. Topical anesthesia (aerosolized lidocaine) provided by the surgeon under direct visualization can aide in maintaining adequate depth of anesthesia and good surgical conditions.

In procedures that do not require spontaneous ventilation, the patient may be intubated by the anesthesiologist (with or without muscle relaxation) and once suspension laryngoscopy is achieved, the endotracheal tube may be removed temporarily while the surgery proceeds. The tube is replaced as necessary for ventilation and oxygenation. While effective, especially in young patients with relatively high oxygen consumption the period of apnea the patient will tolerate may be short requiring frequent interruptions in the procedure. Furthermore, repeated intubations may predispose the patient to airway trauma and edema in excess of that from the surgery. The use of a small diameter cuffed endotracheal tube may, in this case be a good compromise. The surgeon may be able to work around the smaller tube decreasing the number of intubations. Postoperative pain is usually less than that of other procedures and secondary to the nature of surgery, care must be taken to monitor and treat postoperative stridor or airway obstruction (see below for treatment). These patients may require prolonged monitoring in the recovery room or even benefit from ICU admission.

## Tonsillectomy

Tonsillectomy with or without adenoidectomy is a common surgical procedure in pediatric patients. Over the past years obstructive sleep apnea has emerged as an important indication for this procedure. Furthermore, for this indication, surgery is being performed in younger patients than for the indication of recurrent tonsillitis. Anesthesia for tonsillectomy may be induced in a similar fashion as described for bronchoscopy. As many of these patients presenting for surgery have symptoms of obstruction difficulty with bag-mask ventilation and challenging intubation secondary to enlarged tonsils should be anticipated. Similarly, postoperatively, residual blood in the mouth/airway may cause laryngospasm and care should be taken to suction prior to extubation. Furthermore, younger patients may still have symptoms of obstruction immediately postoperatively (secondary to edema) or have residual periodic breathing and appropriate precautions must be taken.

Because the duration of the surgery may be as short as 15 minutes, antiemetics (ondansetron, decadron and possibly metoclopramide), analgesics, and antibiotics should be given immediately upon establishment of intravenous access. Multimodal pain therapy may include Tylenol suppository (30–40 mg/kg) and narcotics (fentanyl 2–4 mcg/kg or morphine 0.1 mg/kg) given early should have little effect on emergence time. Patients with OSA and history of recurrent hypoxemia during preoperative sleep studies may have a heightened sensitivity to the analgesic properties[66] as well as respiratory depressant effects of narcotics[67] so that careful dosing is indicated. Intraoperative maintenance includes nitrous oxide, oxygen and sevoflurane (or halothane) titrated to effect.

Extubation should occur when the patient is fully awake with return of airway reflexes to avoid laryngospasm and aspiration of blood in case of bleeding. Deep extubation has also been used successfully but care must be taken to assure good hemostasis and suctioning of residual blood in the airway. Adequate depth of anesthesia must be ensured to prevent laryngospasm on extubation. A small percentage (4%) of postadenotonsillectomy patients will present with bleeding of the tonsillar bed requiring emergent return to the operating room.[68] Bleeding occurs most commonly on the day of surgery or seven days postoperatively and is associated with significant morbidity if not managed appropriately. Because of the potential for a significant volume of swallowed blood and potential recent meal this patient is considered a full stomach and at a high risk for aspiration of gastric contents on induction of anesthesia. Furthermore, the degree of blood loss is difficult to ascertain so the patient's volume status must be carefully assessed by physical exam and the patient's vital signs. Intravenous access should be established immediately and a sample should be sent for type and screen or cross-match. Euvolemia should be established with a balanced salt solution (lactated ringers or plasmalyte) or normal saline and blood products if the degree of loss warrants it.

Once the patients' hemodynamics are stabilized the patient should be preoxygenated (given 100% $FIO_2$ with tight facemask seal) and a rapid sequence induction with cricoid pressure and the airway should be secured. With ongoing bleeding visualization of the airway may be impaired and large yankauer type suction should be available. Furthermore, edema from the initial surgery and intubation may exist so that a wide array of tube sizes must be available.

It is prudent to have assistance of another airway skilled physician in case of difficulty. Once the airway is secured and surgery for hemostasis is completed, the stomach should be thoroughly suctioned. Suctioning the airway for aspirated blood should be considered. Antiemetic and analgesic therapy should be similar to what is outlined in this section above.

## Epiglottitis

Although the incidence of epiglottis is decreasing with the *Hemophilus influenzae* type B vaccine (1.8 in 10,000)[69] it is still seen in patients that are not immunized and those that are immunocompromised (especially transplant patients).[70] Epiglottitis is associated with high fever, sore throat and dysphagia severe enough to prevent swallowing and cause drooling. Onset is usually rapid and can proceed to airway obstruction rapidly. In face of impending airway failure, intubation should be performed in the operating room in a controlled fashion with surgical support standing by in case of need for emergency tracheostomy. Humidified oxygen and aerosoled therapy with racemic epinephrine may provide slight improvements of symptoms but should be given with caution to avoid agitation of the patient and acute worsening of obstruction. Similarly, once in the operating room induction of anesthesia should be achieved as smoothly as possible with care to maintain spontaneous ventilation (parental presence may assist in keeping the patient calm in the operating room). If IV access is not present inhalational induction with sevoflurane (or halothane) and 100% $O_2$ (maintaining spontaneous ventilation if possible) should be followed by IV placement. Adequate depth of anesthesia must be established before laryngoscopy and intubation to avoid laryngospasm. Because of airway swelling an endotracheal tube a half to one size smaller may be necessary. Using a cuffed endotracheal tube may allow adjustment in the ventilation leak as edema resolves but care must be taken to avoid over-inflation of the cuff causing injury to the tracheal mucosa predisposing the patient to stridor after extubation.[70,71]

**Airway Fires**

With only one in ten to one in 100 operating room fires reported, an estimated 50 to 200 fires occur in the operating room each year in the United States[72] and as many as a fifth of those reported result in serious injury or death. Furthermore certain procedures are considered at higher risk for fire including those where an ignition source (electrocautery) can come in proximity to an oxidizer-enriched atmosphere (see below for definitions of ignition source and oxidizers). Examples of high-risk procedures include tonsillectomy, tracheostomy, laser airway surgery, eye surgery or removal of lesions on the head, neck and face.[73] Numerous case reports exist of airway fires during tracheostomy placement, tonsillectomy and laser airway surgery.[74–78] As described in the case reports airway fires can be a potentially devastating complication of airway surgery causing airway burns and smoke injury, facial burns and even death.

Fire requires three components — an oxidizer, an ignition source, and fuel (also known as a "fire triad").

**Oxidizers** in the operating room include oxygen and nitrous oxide. An oxidizer-enriched atmosphere increases the likelihood of combustion and exists within the breathing system, the patient's airway, and can accumulate under surgical drapes with open oxygen sources or in the presence of an airway "leak" as might be the case with a pediatric patient.

**Ignition sources** that might be used in head and neck surgery include electrocautery devices, laser-heated probes, fiberoptic light cables, defibrillator paddles or pads.

**Fuel sources** include (but are not limited to) endotracheal tubes, gauze, surgical sponges, surgical drapes, gloves, alcohol-containing solutions (prepping solutions), oxygen masks/nasal cannulae, suction catheters, flexible fiberoptic scope/cable coverings, the patient's hair and gowns.

Understanding the potential risk of airway fire, the equipment and conditions that may increase that risk are the responsibility of the entire operating room team. This multidisciplinary effort may include an expanded time out including risk of airway fire, what each member of the team will do to minimize the risk and what action each will take if a fire were to occur.

Efforts include minimizing $FiO_2$ and avoiding nitrous oxide. Using a special FDA approved "laser" endotracheal tubes designed to be resistant to the particular type of laser may reduce, but not eliminate the risk. While these tubes are more resistant to ignition than standard PVC (polyvinylchloride) endotracheal tubes, a prolonged laser strike may still pose a fire hazard.[79] The cuff of the endotracheal tube should be inflated with saline that is methylene blue tinted to alert the surgeon early of cuff puncture. Wet gauze and surgical sponges when laser or electrocautery or diathermy is used, thoroughly allowing prep solutions to dry, and covering hair/face with wet towels are other precautions that may decrease the risk of fire. For surgery utilizing an ignition source within the airway, a cuffed endotracheal tube should be used when clinically appropriate (minimizing leak of oxidizer). Furthermore, entry of the airway (in procedures such as tracheostomy) with ignition sources as electrocautery should be avoided.[80] Finally, the use of the laser's pulse mode provides a significantly decreased risk of laser-induced fire than the continuous mode.

Figure 2 details the algorithm suggested by the American Society of Anesthesiologists for the prevention and treatment of operating room fires.

In case of fire rapid and effective action by the entire team is required. The mnemonic "4 E's" is useful in remembering action that needs to be taken.[81]

- Extract
- Eliminate
- Extinguish
- Evaluate

If a fire were to occur, all combustible materials (fuel sources) should be *extracted* from the airway at once. Simultaneously, oxygen supply (oxidizer) through the tube should be *eliminated* by

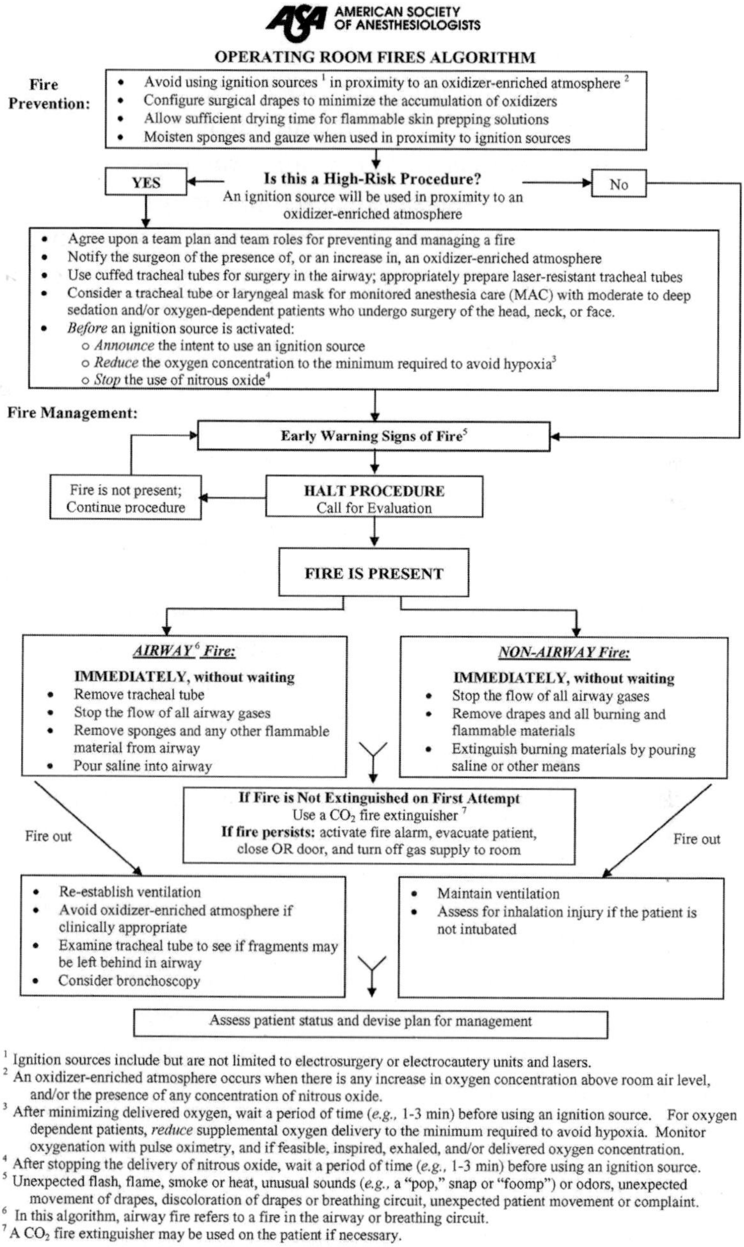


**Fig. 2.** Algorithm suggested by the American Society of Anesthesiologists for the prevention and treatment of operating room fires.

disconnection from the endotracheal tube (to avoid blow torch affect of continued flow through the burning tube). Residual fire and embers in the airway should be *extinguished* with normal saline. Mask ventilation should be initiated and once the patient is stabilized a thorough *evaluation* of the upper and lower airway must occur, and depending on the degree of injury reintubation or even tracheostomy may be indicated.

## POSTOPERATIVE CONCERNS

### Postoperative Croup/Stridor

Post intubation croup occurs in 1%–6% of pediatric patients and is more common in younger patients.[82] Pressure on the mucosa by the endotracheal tube at the level of the cricoid (the narrowest part of the pediatric airway) may cause mucosal irritation and edema. Laryngeal edema after surgery even in absence of intubation can manifest early in the postoperative period by inspiratory stridor. It may also manifest in patients who received a large quantity of fluids intraoperatively, maintained a strained lateral head position, or in patients who have a co-existing URI. The edema causing post-intubation croup usually peaks at four hours and subsides by 24 hours. Humidified oxygen, inhaled racemic epinephrine and intravenous steroids may improve symptoms. Because symptoms can recur up to two hours after treatment with racemic epinephrine, the child should be observed for at least two to three hours post-treatment for recurrence of symptoms. In extreme cases when oxygenation and ventilation cannot be maintained or if fatigue occurs reintubation may be indicated using an endotracheal tube that is up to one size smaller to prevent further injury.

### Apnea of Prematurity

Neonates and infants are prone to episodes of apnea presumably secondary to a "physiological" immaturity of respiratory control and the nervous system. Clinically significant apnea, defined as breathing pauses of >20 seconds or ten seconds, with bradycardia or oxygen desaturation occuring in greater than 50% of premature infants and is almost universal in infants who are less than 1000 grams at birth.[83,84] Preterm infants are shown to have an increased incidence of apnea after general anesthesia and this risk has been shown to increase regardless of the choice of agents.[85] The data from several studies examining risk of apnea in preterm infants was analyzed in 1995 by Cote and colleagues.[86] This analysis suggested that the likelihood of postoperative apnea was inversely proportional to both gestational age (GA) and post-conceptual age (PCA) so that with two infants who were now 55 weeks PCA — one born at 28 weeks and the other at 32 weeks GA, the infant born at 32 weeks would have a lower propensity toward postoperative apnea than the one born at 28 weeks GA. For infants with a gestational age of 35 weeks the risk of apnea was 5% until 48 weeks post-conceptual Furthermore, they determined that for non-anemic infants free of recovery room apnea, the probability of apnea was not less than 1% until 56 weeks post-conceptual age in patients born at 32 weeks gestational age or post-conceptual age of 54 in those born at 35 weeks.

While the presence of postoperative apnea is accepted there exists controversy amongst practitioners and a paucity of evidence in the literature as to what age range an ex-premature patient must be admitted for observation after anesthesia. Further controversy exists as to whether a term infant (defined as being born at 37 weeks PCA or later) is at risk for apnea and at what age outpatient surgery is acceptable. Because of this no formal guidelines exist and practitioner and institutional biases exist. Recommendations for postoperative monitoring range from 12 to 24 hours and include at minimum, pulse oximetry and heart rate. Some evidence exists that neonates and infants with anemia, history of apnea or other coexisting disease are at increased risk of apnea post-anesthesia and may require prolonged monitoring despite post-conceptual age.[83,86] Further consideration of the type of procedure (and resultant physiologic changes) and the postoperative narcotic requirements may also guide the need for prolonged monitoring. A sample guideline is shown in Table 5.

**Table 5. Recommendations for admission for infants undergoing general anesthesia and deep sedation**

| Age at birth | Age admission required |
|---|---|
| Full term (born 37 weeks PCA or greater) | <44 weeks PCA |
| Premature (<37 weeks PCA) | <52 weeks PCA* |

*Anemia, ongoing apnea or other comorbidities may require admission despite age.
Adapted from Ronald Reagan — UCLA admission guidelines.

## Postoperative Nausea and Vomiting

Postoperative nausea and vomiting can diminish patient satisfaction, delay discharge from the recovery room and potentially lead to dehydration. Since nausea is subjective, the incidence in young children is difficult to determine. Most studies therefore focus on incidence of vomiting in children. Infants have the lowest incidence with a peak incidence occurring in school age children.[87] The incidence depends on the type of anesthetic used, the gender and age of the patient, whether there is a history of motion sickness and the degree of hydration. Ophthalmologic procedures and otolaryngology procedures such as tonsillectomy and middle ear surgery are associated with a high incidence of vomiting. Nitrous oxide and narcotic use can increase the risk of vomiting. The use of a low dose infusion of propofol intraoperatively may provide an antiemetic effect.

In high risk patients multimodal prophylactic therapy is recommended. Medications used with some frequency include metoclopramide (0.1 mg/kg) which speeds up gastric emptying and has central antidopaminergic antiemetic effects. Droperidol (10–20 mcg/kg) while an effective antiemetic, is associated with sedation and extrapyramidal side effects that may be undesirable in patients undergoing airway surgery. A 2001 FDA black box warning about potential QT prolongation has also decreased its use as a first line therapy. While the risk of QT prolongation at the low antiemetic doses is not known, many practitioners have chosen to make droperidol a second line therapy when other modalities fail to control symptoms.[88,89] Because the 5-$HT_3$ antagonists have demonstrated efficacy in preventing vomiting, they are recommended as a first line therapy for postoperative vomiting in children. Ondansetron (0.1 mg/kg to max 4 mg) is the most commonly used antiemetic in this category. Its effectiveness in preventing nausea and vomiting has lead to its widespread use in chemotherapy patients. In a study of children undergoing outpatient tonsillectomy, the frequency of in-hospital emesis was 16% in patients given ondansetron and 30% in the droperidol group.[90] Another benefit of ondansetron is its oral dosing. Oral ondansetron disintegrating tablets are ideal for use in patients who do not have intravenous access. A study in pediatric patients undergoing outpatient tonsillectomy and adenoidectomy found that patients who received ondansetron ODT's had less at-home emesis in the first three postoperative days (14.5%) compared to those who received placebo (32%).[91] While this benefit was only seen in patients who did not require a rescue dose of antiemetic in the recovery room, the usefulness of oral dosing of this effective antiemetic are apparent. A single intraoperative dose of dexamethasone has been shown to decrease the incidence of PONV. A wide range of recommended doses (0.0625–1.0 mg/kg) has been suggested in the literature. A recent study[92] showed that the lowest dose was as effective in reducing PONV as the highest dose. Additionally, children receiving dexamethasone were more likely to advance to a soft/solid diet on post-tonsillectomy day 1 than those children receiving placebo.[93]

Finally, while no studies have been done in pediatric patients to substantiate the fact that adequate intraoperative hydration can help to prevent PONV, adult studies have shown that replacing deficit fluids during the intraoperative period decreased postoperative emesis and dizziness in adults.[94,95] Adequate intravenous hydration also allows oral intake of fluids to be safely delayed until the child asks for it as the practice of insisting upon oral intake prior to discharge is associated with vomiting and delays in discharge. Therefore, this is no longer a recommended practice.[96]

**Pain Management**

Recognition and treatment of postoperative pain in preverbal or developmentally delayed children remains a challenge. While older children (greater than three to four years) may be able to verbalize pain and use simple pain scales to quantify the severity, younger patients are unable to do so reliably so observational pain scales may be used. Furthermore, a parent's interpretation of the child's behavior can also provide valuable clues to the presence of pain. Physiologic indices such as tachycardia, tachypnea, elevated blood pressure and diaphoresis may also be signs of pain but other causes such as hypoxemia, hypercapnia, etc. must be considered and ruled out. Considerations in treatment of postoperative pain include the severity of the pain, the route available for delivery (presence of intravenous access), the potential complications from side effects (respiratory depression, over-sedation, bleeding), and finally, the setting in which it is treated (inpatient versus outpatient).[97]

Multimodal therapy is ideal in minimizing the potential side effects of each class of drugs. For head and neck procedures such as laryngoscopy and bronchoscopy the post-surgical pain may be minimal or of short duration so that the acetaminophen given as a suppository (30–40 mg/kg) during the procedure or orally in the recovery room (10–15 mg/kg) may be adequate. Note that a higher dose of rectal acetaminophen is needed to achieve the same serum levels as that given orally.[98] For more severe pain oral acetaminophen in combination with oxycodone (0.1–0.2 mg/kg) or codeine (0.5–1.0 mg/kg) can be used. Both of these combinations are often used to treat postoperative pain from adenotonsillectomy and can be repeated every four to six hours. Immediately postoperatively or for severe pain and more immediate effect, intravenous opioids such as fentanyl (0.5–1.0 mcg/kg) or longer acting morphine can be used taking care to monitor the patient closely for signs of respiratory depression or airway obstruction. Fentanyl can also be given multiple routes (nasal, intravenous, transmucosal, transdermal) so it is of benefit in patients without intravenous access such as patients undergoing myringotomy tube placement. Fentanyl 2.0 mcg/kg given nasally at the start of the procedure (with or without rectal acetaminophen) can provide adequate postoperative analgesia. Ketorolac a non-steroidal anti-inflammatory agent is a potent analgesic effective for postoperative pain, and is the only NSAID available in the United States that can be given intravenously as well as the typical oral route. However, caution is warranted in patients with renal insufficiency and because of its inhibition of platelet aggregation, it should be avoided after procedures with a high risk of bleeding.

Regardless of the class of drugs used, adequate pain management prior to discharge from the recovery room is the goal. If the patient is discharged home or to an unmonitored bed and narcotic analgesics are given the patient must be observed for respiratory depression, nausea and vomiting and other side effects before discharge. Finally, specific instructions should be given to the parents regarding potential side effects and when the next dose of pain medicine may be given. Strict adherence to dosing schedule should be stressed to avoid overdose of narcotics or acetaminophen causing potentially devastating complications such as respiratory depression or hepatic necrosis.

## REFERENCES

1. Morgan GE, Mikhail MS, Murray MJ. *Clinical Anesthesiology*, 4th Ed. New York: McGraw-Hill Companies, 2006.
2. Miller RD, ed. *Miller's Anesthesia*, 7th Ed. Florida: Churchill Livingstone, 2007.
3. Cohen MM, Cameron CB, Duncan PG. Pediatric anesthesia morbidity and mortality in the perioperative period. *Anesth Analg* 1990;70:160–167.
4. Jimenez N, Posner K, Cheney F, *et al.* An update on pediatric anesthesia liability: a closed claims analysis. *Anesth Analg* 2007;104:147–153.
5. Lee C, Mason L. Complications in paediatric anesthesia. *Curr Opin Anesthesiol* 2006;19:262–267.
6. Morray JP, Geiduschek JM, Caplan RA, *et al.* A comparison of pediatric and adult anesthesia closed malpractice claims. *Anesthesiology* 1993;78: 461–463.

7. Tiret L, Nivoche Y, Hatton JM, *et al.* Complications related to anaesthesia in infants and children. A prospective survey of 40240 anaesthetics. *Br J Anaesth* 1988;61:263–269.
8. Lema MJ. Using the ASA physical status classification may be risky business. *ASA Newslett* 2002 Sep;66(9).
9. Owens WD. American Society of Anesthesiologists physical status classification system is not a risk classification system. *Anesthesiology* 2001;94:378.
10. Bhananker S, Ramamoorthy C, Geiduschek JM, *et al.* Anesthesia-related cardiac arrests in children: update from pediatric perioperative cardiac arrest registry. *Anesth Analg* 2007;105:344–350.
11. Mellon RD, Simone AF, Rappaport BA. Use of anesthetic agents in neonates and young children. *Anesth Analg* 2007;104:509–520.
12. Soriano SG, Anand KJ. Anesthetics and brain toxicity. *Curr Opin Anesthesiol* 2005;18:293–297.
13. Tait AR, Malviya S. Anesthesia for the child with an upper respiratory tract infection: still a dilemma? *Anesth Analg* 2005;100:59–65.
14. Cohen MM, Cameron CB. Should you cancel the operation when a child has an upper respiratory tract infection? *Anesth Analg* 1991;72:282–288.
15. Parnis SJ, Barker DS, Van Der Walt JH. Clinical predictors of anaesthetic complications in children with respiratory tract infections. *Paediatr Anaesth* 2001;11:29–40.
16. Tait AR, Malviya S, Voepel-Lewis T, *et al.* Risk factors for perioperative adverse respiratory events in children with upper respiratory tract infections. *Anesthesiology* 2001;95:299–306.
17. Rolf N, Cote´ CJ. Frequency and severity of desaturation events during general anesthesia in children with and without upper respiratory infections. *J Clin Anesth* 1992;4:200–203.
18. Tait AR, Knight PR. The effects of general anesthesia on upper respiratory tract infections in children. *Anesthesiology* 1987;67:930–935.
19. Skolnick ET, Vomvolakis MA, Buck KA, Mannino SF, Sun LS. Exposure to environmental tobacco smoke and the risk of adverse events in children receiving general anesthesia. *Anesthesiology* 1998;88:1144–1153.
20. Warner TO, Warner WA, Barnes RD, *et al.* Peri-operative respiratory complications in patients with asthma. *Anesthesiology* 1996;85:460–467.

21. Schreiner MS, O'Hara I, Markakis DA, Politis GD. Do children who experience laryngospasm have an increased risk of upper respiratory tract infection? *Anesthesiology* 1996;85:475–480.
22. American Society of Anesthesiologists. Practice guidelines for preoperative fasting and the use of pharmacologic agents to reduce the risk of pulmonary aspiration: application to healthy patients undergoing elective procedures. *Anesthesiology* 1999;90:896–905.
23. Section on Pediatric Pulmonology, Subcommittee on Obstructive Sleep Apnea Syndrome, American Academy of Pediatrics. Clinical practice guideline: diagnosis and management of childhood obstructive sleep apnea syndrome. *Pediatrics* 2002;109:704–712.
24. Marcus CL, Greene MG, Carroll JL. Blood pressure in children with obstructive sleep apnea. *Am J Respir Crit Care Med* 1998;157: 1098–1103.
25. Graham RJ, Wachendorf MT, Burns JP, *et al.* Successful and safe delivery of anesthesia and perioperative care for children with complex special health care needs. *J Clin Anesth* 2009;21:165–172.
26. Meitzner MC, Skurnowicz JA. Anesthetic considerations for patients with Down syndrome. *AANA Journal* 2005;73:103–107.
27. Pueschel SM, Findley TW, Furia J, *et al.* Atlantoaxial instability in Down syndrome: roentgenographic, neurologic, and somatosensory evoked potential studies. *J Pediatr* 1987;110:515–521.
28. Kopel M, Creighton RE, Steward DJ. Anesthetic considerations in Down's syndrome: experience with 100 patients and a review of literature. *Can Anaesth Soc J* 1982 Nov;29(6):593–599.
29. Cunningham MJ, Ferrari LR, Kearse LA, *et al.* Intraoperative somatosensory evoked potential monitoring in achondroplasia. *Paediatr Anaesth* 1994;4:129–132.
30. Lake CL. *Pediatric Cardiac Anesthesia* 3rd Ed. Connecticut: Appleton and Lange, 1998.
31. Nishimura RA, Carabello BA, Faxon DP, *et al.* ACC/AHA 2008 guideline update on valvular heart disease: focused update on infective endocarditis. *Circulation* 2008;118:887–896.
32. Wilson W, Taubert KA, Gewitz M, *et al.* Prevention of infective endocarditis — Guidelines from the American Heart Association. *Circulation* 2007;106:1736–1754.

33. Olsson GL, Hallen B, Hambraeus-Jonzon K. Aspiration during anaesthesia: a computer-aided study of 185,358 anaesthetics. *Acta Anaesthesiol Scand* 1986;30:84–92
34. Splinter WM *et al.* Large volumes of apple juice preoperatively do not affect gastric pH and volume in children. *Can J Anaesth* 1990;37(1): 36–39.
35. Nicolson SC, Dorsey AT, Schreiner MS. Shortened preanesthetic fasting interval in pediatric cardiac surgical patients. *Anesth Analg* 1992;74:694–697.
36. Green CR, Pandit SK, Schork MA. Preoperative fasting time: is the traditional policy changing? Results of a national survey. *Anesth Analg* 1996;83:123–128.
37. Cote CJ. NPO after midnight for children — a reappraisal. *Anesthesiology* 1990;72:589–592.
38. Fortier MA, Chorney JM, Rny RY, *et al.* Children's desire for perioerative information. *Anesth Analg* 2009;109:1085–1090.
39. Kain A, Caramico I, Mayes I, *et al.* Preoperative preparation programs in children: a comparative study. *Anesth Analg* 1998;87:1249–1255.
40. Kain ZN, Caldwell-Andrews AA, Maranets I, *et al.* Preoperative anxiety and emergence delirium and postoperative maladaptive behaviors. *Anesth Analg* 2004;99:1648–1654.
41. Kain ZN, Mayes IC, O'Connor TZ, Cicchetti DV. Preoperative anxiety in children: predictors and outcomes. *Arch Pediatr Adolesc Med* 1996; 150:1238–1245.
42. McCann ME, Kain ZN. The management of preoperative anxiety in children: an update. *Anesth Analg* 2001;93:98–105
43. Synera package insert.
44. Viitanen H, Annila P, Viitanen M, *et al.* Premedication with midazolam delays recovery after ambulatory sevoflurane anesthesia in children. *Anesth Analg* 1999;89:75–79.
45. Hannallah RS, Rosales JK. Experience with parent's presence during anesthesia induction in children. *Can Anaesth Soc J* 1983;30: 286–289.
46. Kain Z, Mayes I, Wang S, *et al.* Parental presence and a sedative premedicant for children undergoing surgery: a hierarchical study. *Anesthesiology* 2000;92:939–946.

47. Chen L, Zhang S, Li S, *et al.* The risk factors for hypoxemia in children younger than 5 years old undergoing rigid bronchoscopy for foreign body removal. *Anesth Analg* 2009;109:1079–1084.
48. American Society of Anesthesiologists. *Standards for Basic Anesthetic Monitoring: 2005 Committee on Standards and Practice Parameters.* Park Ridge, Illinois: American Society of Anesthesiology, 2005.
49. Munson ES: Transfer of nitrous oxide into body air cavities. *Br J Anaesth* 1974:46:202–209.
50. Perrault L, Roussea P: Problem of gas diffusion into the middle ear during anaesthesia for tympanoplasty. *Can Anaesth Soc J* 1981;28:136–210.
51. Lerman J, Robinson S, Willis MM, *et al.* Anesthetic requirements for halothane in young children 0–1 month and 1–6 months of age. *Anesthesiology* 1983;59:421–424.
52. Kenna JG, Neuberger J, Mieli-Vergani G, *et al.* Halothane hepatitis in children. *Br Med J* 1987;294:1209–1211.
53. Holzman RS, van der Velde Me, Kaus SJ, *et al.* Sevoflurane depresses myocardial contractility less than halothane during induction of anesthesia in children. Anesthesiology 1996;85:1260–1267.
54. Welborn LG, Hannallah RS, Norden JM, *et al.* Comparison of emergence and recovery characteristics of sevoflurane, desflurane, and halothane in pediatric ambulatory patients. *Anesth Analg* 1996;83:917–920.
55. Zwass MS, Fisher DM, Welborn LG, *et al.* Induction and maintenance characteristics of anesthesia with desflurane and nitrous oxide in infants and children. *Anesthesiology* 1992;76:373–378.
56. Yaster M. The dose response of fentanyl in neonatal anesthesia. *Anesthesiology* 1987;66:136–139.
57. Burtin P, Jacqz-Aigrain E, Girard P, *et al.* Population pharmacokinetics of midazolam in neonates. *Clin Pharmacol Ther* 1994;56:615–625.
58. Cote CJ, Cohen IT, Suresh S, *et al.* A comparison of three doses of commercially prepared oral midazolam syrup in children. *Anesth Analg* 2002;94:37–43.
59. Buck ML. Dexmedetomidine for sedation in the pediatric intensive care setting. *Pediatr Pharm* 2006;12(1).
60. Jooste EH, Ohkawa S, Sun LS. Fiberoptic intubation with dexmedetomidine in two children with spinal cord impingements [letter]. *Anesth Analg* 2005;101:1238–1248.

61. Ibacache ME, Munoz HR, Brandes V, *et al.* Single-dose dexmedetomidine reduces agitation after sevoflurane anesthesia in children. *Anesth Analg* 2004;98:60–63.
62. Strazis KP, Fox AW. Malignant hyperthermia: a review of published cases. *Anesth Analg* 1993;77(2):297–304.
63. Klinger W, Rueffert H, Lehmann-Horn F, *et al.* Core myopathes and risk of makgnant hyperthermia. *Anesth Analg* 2009;109:1167–1173.
64. Davis PJ, Brandom, BW. The association of malignant hyperthermia and unusual disease: when you're hot you're hot or maybe not. *Anesth Analg* 2009;109:1001–1003.
65. Gurnaney H, Brown A, Litman RS. Malignant hyperthermia and muscular dystrophies. *Anesth Analg* 2009;109:1043–1048.
66. Brown KA, Laferriere A, Lakheeram I, *et al.* Recurrent hypoxemia in children is associated with increased analgesic sensitivity to opiates. *Anesthesiology* 2006;105:665–669.
67. Stauss, SG, Lynn AM, Bratton SL. Ventilatory response to $CO_2$ in children with obstructive sleep apnea from adenotonsillar hypertrophy. *Anesth Analg* 199;89:328–332.
68. Holzman RS, Mancuso TJ, Polaner DM, *A Practical Approach to Pediatric Anesthesia.* Philadelphia: Lippincott Williams & Wilkins, 2008: pp. 253–255.
69. Shah RK, Boberson DW, Jones DT. Epiglottitis in the *hemophilus influenzae* type B vaccine era: changing trends. *Laryngoscope* 2004;114:557–560.
70. Colman MF. Epiglottis in immunocompromised patients. *Head Neck Surg* 1986;8:466–468.
71. Yao FS, Malhotra V, Fontes ML, eds. *Anesthesiology Problem-Oriented Patient Management,* 6th Ed. Philadelphia: Lippincott Williams & Wilkins, 2008, pp. 1038–1048.
72. Wolf G. Danger from OR fires still a serious problem, ASA Panel reports risks. *APSF Newslett* 1999.
73. Practice Advisory for the Prevention and Management of Operating Room Fires: A Report by the American Society of Anesthesiologists Task Force on Operating Room Fires. *Anesthesiology* 2008;108:785–801.
74. Niskanen M, Purhonen S Koljonen A, *et al.* Fatal inhalation injury caused by airway fire during tracheostomy. *Acta Aneaesthesiol Scand* 2007;51:509–513.

75. Chee, WK, Benumof, JL Airway fire during tracheostomy: extubation may be contraindicated. *Anesthesiology*: 1998 Dec;89:1576–1578.
76. Lin I, Hwang C, Kao, Y, *et al.* Tracheostomal fire during an elective tracheostomy. *Chang Gung Med J* 2005 Mar;28(3):186–189.
77. Wheatley TJ, Maddern GJ. Airway fire during formation of tracheostomy. *ANZ J Surg* 2002;72:157–158.
78. Varcoe RL, MacGowan KM, Cass AJ. Airway fire during tracheostomy. *ANZ J Surg* 2004;74:507–508.
79. Sesterhenn AM, Dunne AA, Baulke D, *et al.* Value of endotracheal tube safety in laryngeal laser surgery. *Lasers Surg Med* 2003;32:384–390.
80. Rogers ML, Nickalls RWD, Brackenbury ET, *et al.* Airway fire during tracheostomy: prevention strategies for surgeons and anaesthetists. *Ann R Coll Surg Engl* 2001;83:376–380.
81. Barker SJ, Polson JS. Fire in the operating room: a case report and laboratory study. *Anesth Analg* 2001;93:960–965.
82. Hall, SC. Pediatric postanesthesia recovery care. *J Clin Anesth* 1995; 7:600–605.
83. Abu-Shaweesh JM, Martin RJ. Neonatal apnea: what's new? *Pediatric Pulmonol* 2008; 43:937–944.
84. Finer NN, Higgins R, Kattwinkel J, *et al.* Summary proceedings from the apnea-of-prematurity group. *Pediatrics* 2006;117:S47–S51.
85. Krane E, Haberkern C, Jacobson L. Postoperative apnea, bradycardia and oxygen desaturation in formerly premature infants: prospective comparison of spinal and general anesthesia. *Anesth Analg* 1995;80:7–13.
86. Cote CJ, Zaslavsky A, Downes JJ, *et al.* Postoperative apnea in former preterm infants after inguinal herniorrhaphy. *Anesthesiology* 1995;82: 809–821.
87. Rose JB, Watcha MF. Postoperative nausea and vomiting in paediatric patients. *Br J Anaesth* 1998;83:104–117.
88. Gan TJ. "Black box" warning on droperidol: a report of the FDA convened expert panel. Letter to the editor. *Anesth Analg* 2004;98(6):1809.
89. Rappaport BA. Letter to the editor: FDA response to droperidol black box warning editorials. *Anesth Analg* 2008;106(5):1585.
90. Splinter WM, Rhine EJ, Roberts DW, *et al.* Ondansetron is a better prophylactic antiemetic than droperidol for tonsillectomy in children. *Can J Anaesth* 1995;42:848–851.

91. Davis PJ, Fertal KM, Boretsky KR. The effects of oral ondansetron disintegrating tablets for prevention of at-home emesis in pediatric patients after ear-nose-throat surgery. *Anesth Analg* 2008;106:1117–1121.
92. Kim MS, Cote CJ, Cristoloveanu C, *et al.* There is no dose-escalation response to dexamethasone (0.0625–1.0 mg/kg) in pediatric tonsillectomy or adenotonsillectomy patients for preventing vomiting, reducing pain, shortening time to first liquid intake, or the incidence of voice change. *Anesth Analg* 2007;104(5):1052–1058.
93. Steward DL, Welge JA, Myer CM. Steroids for improving recovery following tonsillectomy in children. *Cochrane Database Syst Rev* 2003; 1:CD003997.
94. Yogendran S, Asokumar B, Cheng DC, *et al.* A prospective randomized double-blinded study of the effect of intravenous fluid therapy on adverse outcomes on outpatient surgery. *Anesth Analg* 1995;80:682–686.
95. Maharaj CH, Kallam SR, Malik A, *et al.* Preoperative intravenous fluid therapy decreases postoperative nausea and pain in high risk patients. *Anesth Analg* 2005;11:675–682.
96. Cohen MM, Cameron CB, Duncan PG. Pediatric anesthesia morbidity and mortality in the perioperative period. *Anseth Analg* 1990;70:160–167.
97. Burd RS, Mellender SJ, Tobias JD. Neonatal and childhood perioperative considerations. *Surg Clin N Am* 2006;86:227–247.
98. Birmingham PK, Tobin MJ, Henthorn TK, *et al.* Twenty-four hour pharmacokinetics of rectal acetaminophen in children. *Anesthesiology* 1997; 87:244–248.
99. Cote CJ. NPO guidelines: children and adults. In: McGoldrick KE, ed. *Ambulatory Anesthesiology: A Problem-Oriented Approach.* Baltimore: Williams & Wilkins, 1995, pp. 20–32.

20

# Guidelines in Pediatric Otolaryngology

*Craig S. Derkay, Amy S. Ketcham*
*and Thomas S. Higgins*

## INTRODUCTION

Guidelines serve an important role in medicine today. They facilitate evidence-based decisions in clinical practice and influence public policy. The creation of quality guidelines is a multidisciplinary task that involves a rigorous systematic process of review. The American Academy of Otolaryngology–Head and Neck Surgery (AAO–HNS) has recommended guidelines be *systematic, transparent,* and *evidence-based.*[1]

The purpose of guidelines is to assist, but not supplant, professional clinical judgment. They should not be considered in reimbursement policies, performance measures, or legal precedents.[1] The Conference on Guideline Standardization (COGS) identified 18 characteristics for quality standards on guidelines required for inclusion in the National Guidelines Clearinghouse (NGC) database. These standards require detailed description of the guidelines' data acquisition, style of reporting, and rationale for recommendations. The group members are identified and any conflicts of interest, including funding source/sponsor, should be published. The guidelines document is also expected to provide definitions of terms, potential benefits and harms associated with the guidelines,

**Table 1. Evidence quality for grades of evidence.**[1]

| Grade | Evidence quality |
|---|---|
| A | Well-designed randomized controlled trials or diagnostic studies performed on a population similar to the guideline's target population. |
| B | Randomized controlled trials or diagnostic studies with minor limitations; overwhelmingly consistent evidence from observational studies. |
| C | Observational studies (case control and cohort design). |
| D | Expert opinion, case reports, reasoning from first principles (bench research or animal studies). |
| X | Exceptional situations where validating studies cannot be performed and there is a clear preponderance of benefit over harm. |

as well as algorithms that graphically describe stages of decision making. The guideline content is expected to be produced under the auspices of medical specialty groups and be a corroborating document based on results of a systematic literature search with review of existing scientific evidence published in peer-reviewed journals.[2]

Guidelines include evidence-based statements that are characterized in one of four ways based on the reliability of the current evidence: (1) Strong recommendation, (2) Recommendation, (3) Option, or (4) No recommendation. These statements are based on the quality of studies evaluated. Table 1 provides a summary of the grading system used by the (AAO–HNS).

Guidelines related to pediatric otolaryngology have been collaboratively compiled through the efforts of the AAO–HNS, the American Society for Pediatric Otolaryngologists (ASPO), the American Academy of Pediatrics (AAP), and the American Academy of Family Physicians (AAFP). The remainder of this chapter will summarize the currently available guidelines.

## ACUTE OTITIS MEDIA (AOM)[3]

As the most common infection requiring antibiotics in children ages two months to 12 years, acute otitis media (AOM) is a logical target for practice guidelines. Appropriate initial treatment of AOM is key to preventing complications of AOM such as hearing loss, mastoiditis, facial nerve paresis, petrous apicitis, subdural abscess, meningitis, and Bezold's abscess. On the other hand, judicious use of antibiotics is crucial to curbing the trend of increasing antibiotic resistance among otitis media-causing bacteria. In order to produce a set of guidelines on uncomplicated AOM geared toward the primary care practitioner, the Subcommittee on Management of Acute Otitis Media was formed. Pediatricians, otolaryngologists, epidemiologists, infectious disease specialists, and medical informatics specialists from the AAP, AAFP, Agency for Healthcare Research and Quality, and the Southern California Evidence-Based Practice Center partnered together to form this subcommittee. They reviewed 124 papers and published the AOM guidelines listed in Table 2 in 2004.

A diagnosis of AOM can be confounded with otitis media with effusion (OME) and viral infections unless a clear history is correlated with an AOM-consistent physical examination of the tympanic membrane. The differentiation between AOM and OME is key to preventing superfluous antibiotic administration. Tympanometry, audiometry and acoustic reflectometry can be useful if the history and physical do not solidify a child's diagnosis. Table 3 summarizes the three requirements for a diagnosis of AOM.

Appropriate treatment of AOM includes pain control and either antibiotics or observation. Table 4 further explains the role of watchful waiting vs. treatment with antibiotics.

## OTITIS MEDIA WITH EFFUSION (OME)[4]

OME is nearly universally experienced at some point in childhood. It often resolves spontaneously, and rarely do antibiotics, antihistamines, decongestants, homeopathic medications or chiropractic manipulations treat the condition or shorten its duration. As a result, it is necessary to differentiate this condition from AOM in order to prevent side effects from unneeded medications and maintain cost-effective care. If OME does not resolve on its own, it may cause impairment of speech development, hearing, and learning.

**Table 2. Guidelines for AOM.**[3]

**Recommendation 1:**
To diagnose AOM, the clinician should confirm a history of acute onset, identify signs of middle-ear effusion (MEE), and evaluate for the presence of signs and symptoms of middle-ear inflammation. *(This recommendation is based on observational studies and a preponderance of benefit over risk.)*

**Recommendation 2:**
The management of AOM should include an assessment of pain. If pain is present, the clinician should recommend treatment to reduce pain. *(This is a strong recommendation based on randomized clinical trials with limitations and a preponderance of benefit over risk.)*

**Recommendation 3a:**
Observation without use of antibacterial agents in a child with uncomplicated AOM is an option for selected children based on diagnostic certainty, age, illness severity, and assurance of follow-up. *(This option is based on randomized controlled trials with limitations and a relative balance of benefit and risk.)*

**Recommendation 3b:**
If a decision is made to treat with an antibacterial agent, the clinician should prescribe amoxicillin for most children. *(This recommendation is based on randomized clinical trials with limitations and a preponderance of benefit over risk.)*

When amoxicillin is used, the dose should be 80 to 90 mg/kg per day. *(This option is based on extrapolation from microbiologic studies and expert opinion, with a preponderance of benefit over risk.)*

**Recommendation 4:**
If the patient fails to respond to the initial management option within 48–72 hours, the clinician must reassess the patient to confirm AOM and exclude other causes of illness. If AOM is confirmed in the patient initially managed with observation, the clinician should begin antibacterial therapy. If the patient was initially managed with an antibacterial agent, the clinician should change the antibacterial agent. *(This recommendation is based on observational studies and a preponderance of benefit over risk.)*

**Recommendation 5:**
Clinicians should encourage the prevention of AOM through reduction of risk factors. *(This recommendation is based on strong observational studies and a preponderance of benefits over risks.)*

**Recommendation 6:**
No recommendations for complementary and alternative medicine (CAM) for treatment of AOM are made based on limited and controversial data.

**Table 3. Diagnostic requirements of AOM.**[3]

1. Recent, usually abrupt, onset of signs and symptoms of middle-ear inflammation and middle ear effusion (MEE).
2. The presence of MEE that is indicated by any of the following:
   a. bulging of the tympanic membrane,
   b. limited or absent mobility of the tympanic membrane,
   c. air-fluid level behind the tympanic membrane, or
   d. otorrhea.
3. Signs or symptoms of middle-ear inflammation as indicated by either
   a. distinct erythema of the tympanic membrane, or
   b. distinct otalgia (discomfort clearly referable to the ear[s] that results in interference with or precludes normal activity or sleep).

**Table 4. AOM treatment algorithm**[3]

| Age | Certain diagnosis | Uncertain diagnosis |
|---|---|---|
| ≤6 months | Antibacterial therapy | Antibacterial therapy |
| 6 months–2 years | Antibacterial therapy | Antibacterial therapy if severe illness; observation if non-severe illness* |
| ≥2 years | Antibacterial therapy if severe illness; observation if non-severe illness* | Observation |

* Observation is an appropriate option only when follow-up can be ensured with the resulting capability of starting antibiotics if symptoms persist or worsen. Non-severe illness is defined as mild otalgia and fever of less than 39°C in the past 24 hours. Severe illness is defined as moderate to severe otalgia and fever of 39°C or above. A certain diagnosis of AOM meets all three criteria: (1) rapid onset, (2) signs of MEE, and (3) signs and symptoms of middle-ear inflammation.

To address the diagnosis and management of this common condition, the Agency for Healthcare Policy and Research published a clinical guideline for OME for children in 1994. As the importance of practice guidelines became more accepted, a subcommittee on OME created by the AAFP, the AAO–HNS, and the AAP updated the OME guidelines. The subcommittee was composed of otolaryngologists, pediatricians, family practitioners, infectious disease specialists, epidemiologists, audiologists, otologists, speech and language pathologists, and nurse practitioners. From 2003 to 2004 they reviewed 970 selected articles. The new guidelines clarified their target population as two month to 12 year old children. They also expanded the earlier guidelines to include patients with congenital anomalies or other conditions that predispose to OME. After review by the Yale Center for Medical Informatics Guidelines Review Group, the revised guidelines were published in the May 2004 edition of *Pediatrics*. They were subsequently reprinted in the various sponsor organizations' publications. Table 5 summarizes the new guidelines. The subcommittee will review these guidelines every five years with a plan to address numerous areas that currently lack quality research.

**Table 5. Guidelines for OME.**[4]

**Recommendation 1a: pneumatic otoscopy**
Clinicians should use pneumatic otoscopy as the primary diagnostic method for OME. OME should be distinguished from AOM. *(Strong recommendation based on systematic review of cohort studies and preponderance of benefit over harm.)*

**Recommendation 1b: tympanometry**
Tympanometry can be used to confirm the diagnosis of OME. *(Option based on cohort studies and a balance of benefit and harm.)*

**Recommendation 1c: screening**
Population-based screening programs for OME are not recommended in healthy, asymptomatic children. *(Recommendation based on randomized, controlled trials and cohort studies with a preponderance of harm over benefit.)*

**Recommendation 2: documentation**
Clinicians should document the laterality, duration of effusion, and presence and severity of associated symptoms at each assessment of the child with OME. *(Recommendation based on observational studies and strong preponderance of benefit over harm.)*

**Recommendation 3: child at risk**
Clinicians should distinguish the child with OME who is at risk for speech, language, or learning problems from other children with OME, and should more promptly evaluate hearing, speech, language, and need for intervention. *(Recommendation based on case series, preponderance of benefit over harm, and ethical limitations in studying children with OME who are at risk.)*

(*Continued*)

**Table 5. (*Continued*)**

**Recommendation 4: watchful waiting**
Clinicians should manage the child with OME who is not at risk with watchful waiting for three months from the date of effusion onset (if known) or from the date of diagnosis (if onset is unknown). *(Recommendation based on systematic review of cohort studies and preponderance of benefit over harm.)*

**Recommendation 5: medication**
Antihistamines and decongestants are ineffective for OME and are not recommended for treatment. Antimicrobials and corticosteroids do not have long-term efficacy and are not recommended for routine management. *(Recommendation based on systematic review of randomized, controlled trials and preponderance of harm over benefit.)*

**Recommendation 6: hearing and language**
Hearing testing is recommended when OME persists for three months or longer, or at any time that language delay, learning problems, or a significant hearing loss is suspected in a child with OME. Language testing should be conducted for children with hearing loss. *(Recommendation based on cohort studies and preponderance of benefit over risk.)*

**Recommendation 7: surveillance**
Children with persistent OME who are not at risk should be re-examined at three- to six-month intervals until the effusion is no longer present, significant hearing loss is identified, or structural abnormalities of the eardrum or middle ear are suspected. *(Recommendation based on randomized, controlled trials and observational studies with a preponderance of benefit over harm.)*

**Recommendation 8: referral**
When children with OME are referred by primary care clinicians for evaluation by an otolaryngologist, audiologist, or speech-language pathologist, the referring clinician should document the effusion duration and specific reason for referral (evaluation, surgery), and provide additional relevant information such as history of AOM and developmental status of the child. *(Option based on panel consensus and a preponderance of benefit over harm.)*

**Recommendation 9: surgery**
When a child becomes a surgical candidate, tympanostomy tube insertion is the preferred initial procedure; adenoidectomy should not be performed unless a distinct indication exists (nasal obstruction, chronic adenoiditis). Repeat surgery consists of adenoidectomy plus myringotomy, with or without tube insertion. Tonsillectomy alone or myringotomy alone should not be used to treat OME. *(Recommendation based on randomized, controlled trials with a preponderance of benefit over harm.)*

(*Continued*)

**Table 5. (*Continued*)**

| |
|---|
| **Recommendation 10: complementary and alternative medications (CAM)**<br>No recommendation is made regarding CAM as a treatment for OME. *(No recommendation based on lack of scientific evidence documenting efficacy and an uncertain balance of harm and benefit.)* |
| **Recommendation 11: allergy management**<br>No recommendation is made regarding allergy management as a treatment for OME. *(No recommendation based on insufficient evidence of therapeutic efficacy or a causal relationship between allergy and OME.)* |

## OTITIS EXTERNA[5]

Acute otitis externa (AOE) is a common otolaryngologic infection defined as "diffuse inflammation of the external ear canal, which may also involve the pinna or tympanic membrane."[5] It is characterized by onset in less than 48 hours. The most common causative pathogens are *Pseudomonas aeruginosa* and *Staphylococcus aureus*, but multiple organisms are often involved. Table 6 lists the key elements of a diagnosis of AOE.

AOE is quite common, and primary care practitioners and urgent care/emergency room physicians are often the first to see patients with this disease. In addition, the appropriate use of oral antibiotics, topical antibiotics, and pain medications in this disease is often confused. Topical medications are the most effective treatment of AOE, and oral antibiotics add very little. However, 40% of

**Table 6. Elements of the diagnosis of diffuse AOE.**[5]

1. Rapid onset (generally within 48 hours) in the past three weeks, AND
2. Symptoms of ear canal inflammation that include:
   a. otalgia (often severe), itching, or fullness,
   b. WITH OR WITHOUT hearing loss or jaw pain, AND
3. Signs of ear canal inflammation that include:
   a. tenderness of the tragus, pinna, or both,
   b. OR diffuse ear canal edema, erythema, or both,
   c. WITH OR WITHOUT otorrhea, regional lymphadenitis, tympanic membrane erythema, or cellulitis of the pinna and adjacent skin.

**Table 7. Common topical otic preparations approved by the FDA for treating diffuse AOE.**[5]

| Active drug(s) | Trade name |
|---|---|
| Acetic acid, aluminum acetate | Otic Domeboro |
| Acetic acid, hydrocortisone | VoSol HC |
| Ciprofloxacin, hydrocortisone | Cipro HC |
| Ciprofloxacin, dexamethasone | Ciprodex |
| Neomycin, polymyxin B, hydrocortisone | Cortisporin Otic |
| Ofloxacin | Floxin Otic |

patients with AOE are still given oral antibiotics and exposed to more risk than benefit.[5] Table 7 lists the approved ototopical medications for AOE as adapted from the AAO–HNSF guidelines.

The American Academy of Otolaryngology Foundation (AAO–HNSF) formed a committee to review the literature regarding AOE and to create a guideline for the treatment of AOE in children aged two and above. This committee included head and neck surgeons, pediatric otolaryngologists, family practitioners, infectious disease specialists, emergency medicine physicians, and medical information specialists. Two-hundred and forty articles were selected for review from a MEDLINE search. In addition, 20 articles were chosen for use in a meta-analysis comparing the various topical treatments for AOE. Published data through September 2005 were used to create the AOE guidelines. These guidelines were then analyzed by the Yale Center for Medical Informatics. The final version was published in April 2006 and scheduled for review every five years. Interestingly, this guideline for AOE was the first independent guideline that the AAO–HNSF spearheaded. The guidelines are listed in Table 8.

## TONSILLECTOMY[6]

As the most common major surgical procedure performed on children, tonsillectomy is a natural topic for evidence-based guidelines. Accordingly, the first comprehensive guideline was released in January 2011 as composed by a team of anesthesiologists, sleep medicine physicians, nurse practitioners, family medicine physicians,

**Table 8. Guidelines for AOE.**[5]

**Recommendation 1a: differential diagnosis**
Clinicians should distinguish diffuse AOE from other causes of otalgia, otorrhea, and inflammation of the external ear canal. *(Recommendation based on observational studies with a preponderance of benefit over risk.)*

**Recommendation 1b: modifying factors**
Clinicians should assess the patient with diffuse AOE for factors that modify management (non-intact tympanic membrane, tympanostomy tube, diabetes, immunocompromised state, prior radiotherapy). *(Recommendation based on observational studies with a preponderance of benefit over risk.)*

**Recommendation 2: pain management**
The management of diffuse AOE should include an assessment of pain. The clinician should recommend analgesic treatment based on the severity of pain. *(Strong recommendation based on well-designed randomized trials with a preponderance of benefit over harm.)*

**Recommendation 3: initial therapy**
Clinicians should use topical preparations for initial therapy of diffuse, uncomplicated AOE. Systemic antimicrobial therapy should not be used unless there is extension outside the ear canal or the presence of specific host factors that would indicate a need for systemic therapy. *(Recommendation based on randomized controlled trials with minor limitations and a preponderance of benefit over harm.)*

**Recommendation 4: topical therapy**
The choice of topical antimicrobial for initial therapy of diffuse AOE should be based upon efficacy, low incidence of adverse events, likelihood of adherence to therapy, and cost. *(Recommendation based on randomized trials with some heterogeneity and a preponderance of benefit over harm.)*

**Recommendation 5: drug delivery**
Clinicians should inform patients how to administer topical drops. When the ear canal is obstructed, delivery of topical preparations should be enhanced by aural toilet, placement of a wick, or both. *(Recommendation based on observational studies with a preponderance of benefit over harm.)*

**Recommendation 6: non-intact tympanic membrane**
When the patient has a tympanostomy tube or known perforation of the tympanic membrane, the clinician should prescribe a non-ototoxic topical preparation. *(Recommendation based on reasoning from first principles and on exceptional circumstances where validating studies cannot be performed and there is clear preponderance of benefit over harm.)*

**Recommendation 7: outcome assessment**
If the patient fails to respond to the initial therapeutic option within 48–72 hours, the clinician should re-assess the patient to confirm the diagnosis of diffuse AOE and to exclude other causes of illness. *(Recommendation based on observational studies and a preponderance of benefit over harm.)*

otolaryngologists, infectious disease physicians, pediatricians, and consumers. The guideline was created for patients one to 18 years old with diagnoses of (1) recurrent throat infection (pharyngitis and/or tonsillitis) or (2) sleep disordered breathing (SDB; abnormal breathing and/or ventilation during sleep). The overall goals were to identify which patients would benefit from tonsillectomy and to promote quality improvement. *A priori* criteria were used to gather previous consensus and evidence-based guidelines less than ten years old, systemic reviews less than 15 years old, and randomized controlled trials published through April 2010. The guideline is not intended to address patients with diabetes mellitus, coagulation disorders, sickle cell disease, cardiac disease, or craniofacial anomalies. Table 9 lists the final recommendations.

**Table 9. Guidelines for Tonsillectomy.**[6]

| |
|---|
| **Recommendation 1: watchful waiting for recurrent throat infection**<br>Clinicians should recommend watchful waiting for recurrent throat infection if there have been fewer than 7 episodes in the past year, 5 episodes per year in the past 2 years, or 3 episodes per year in the past 3 years. *(Recommendation based on randomized trials with limitations and observational studies with a preponderance of benefit over harm.)* |
| **Recommendation 2: recurrent throat infection with documentation**<br>Clinicians may recommend tonsillectomy for recurrent throat infection with a frequency of at least 7 episodes the past year, 5 episodes per year for 2 years, or 3 episodes per year for 3 years with documentation in the medical record for each episode of sore throat and one or more of the following: T > 38.3°C, cervical adenopathy, tonsillar exudate, or positive test for group A beta-hemolytic streptococcus. *(Option based on systematic review, randomized controlled trials with minor limitations, as well as observational studies, with an uncertain relationship of benefit to harm.)* |
| **Recommendation 3: tonsillectomy for recurrent infection with modifying factors**<br>Clinicians should assess the child with recurrent throat infection who does not meet criteria for tonsillectomy (in statement 2) for modifying factors that include febrile seizures, multiple antibiotic allergy/intolerance, PFAPA, or history of peritonsillar abscess. *(Recommendation based on randomized trials and observational studies with a preponderance of benefit over harm.)* |

(*Continued*)

**Table 9. (*Continued*)**

**Recommendation 4: tonsillectomy for sleep-disordered breathing**
Clinicians should ask caregivers of children with sleep disordered breathing and tonsil hypertrophy about co-morbid conditions that might improve after tonsillectomy, including growth retardation, poor school performance, enuresis, and behavioral problems. *(Recommendation based on observational, before-and-after, studies with a preponderance of benefit over harm.)*

**Recommendation 5: tonsillectomy and polysomnography**
Clinicians should counsel caregivers about tonsillectomy as a means to improve health in children with sleep disordered breathing, abnormal polysomnography, and tonsil hypertrophy. *(Recommendation based on observational, before-and-after studies with a preponderance of benefit over harm.)*

**Recommendation 6: outcome assessment for sleep-disordered breathing (SDB)**
Clinicians should counsel caregivers and explain that SDB may persist or recur after tonsillectomy and may require further management. *(Recommendation based on observational studies, case-control and cohort design, with a preponderance of benefit over harm.)*

**Recommendation 7: intraoperative steroids**
Clinicians should administer a single intraoperative dose of intravenous dexamethasone to children undergoing tonsillectomy. *(Strong recommendation based on randomized controlled trials and systematic reviews of randomized controlled trials with a preponderance of benefit over harm.)*

**Recommendation 8: perioperative antibiotics**
Clinicians should not routinely administer or prescribe perioperative antibiotics to children undergoing tonsillectomy. *(Strong recommendation against based on randomized controlled trials and systematic reviews with a preponderance of benefit over harm.)*

**Recommendation 9: postoperative pain control**
The clinician should advocate for pain management after tonsillectomy and educate caregivers about the importance of managing and reassessing pain. *(Recommendation based on randomized controlled trials with limitations and observational studies with a preponderance of benefit over harm.)*

**Recommendation 10: post-tonsillectomy hemorrhage**
Clinicians who perform tonsillectomy should determine their rate of primary and secondary post-tonsillectomy hemorrhage at least annually. *(Recommendation based on observational studies with a preponderance of benefit over harm.)*

Several things should be taken into account when considering tonsillectomy for recurrent throat infections: (1) the overall number of infections, (2) the impact of those infections on a child's health, and (3) the child's quality of life pre- and post-tonsillectomy. Bearing these things in mind, clinicians should practice watchful waiting for at least one year prior to tonsillectomy. Many patients' symptoms will resolve over the course of one year without surgical treatment. Yet if strict criteria are met by accurately documented symptoms over the course of that year, tonsillectomy may be beneficial, reducing the incidence of sore throat by 43%. It takes 11 tonsillectomies to prevent 1 episode of sore throat per month. Patients with modifying factors such as significant obstructive sleep disorders, severe or debilitating symptoms, peritonsillar abscess, PFAPA, halitosis, febrile seizures, or tonsillar asymmetry concerning for underlying tumor or lymphoma may also benefit from tonsillectomy even without meeting strict infectious criteria.

Sleep disordered breathing (SDB) ranges from primary snoring to true obstructive sleep apnea syndrome. A combination of history, physical examination, videotape, audiotape, pulse oximetry, and/or polysomnography (PSG) is used to diagnose SDB. Physical exam may show adeno-tonsillar hypertrophy, craniofacial dysmorphology, or altered neuromuscular tone. Often there will be a combination of several of these elements; thus, it is not only tonsil and adenoid size alone that determines SDB. There are no evidence-based criteria for using PSG to determine need for tonsillectomy. Even so, an apnea-hypopnea index (AHI) over 1 is considered abnormal in a child, and an AHI of > 5 is generally considered severe enough to consider an adeno-tonsillectomy.

Tonsillectomy has been shown to be beneficial for those meeting surgical criteria. Quality of life scores have improved after tonsillectomy in both patients with throat infections and patients with SDB.[7] School performance and overall behavior have improved in SDB patients.[8] Failure to thrive has been reversed in some; enuresis has been halted in others. Tonsillectomy equilibrates with watchful waiting at 2 years postoperatively. And despite other benefits, residual SDB after tonsillectomy may still cause problems for the patient, especially in children with other co-morbidities such as obesity. Thus, if a caregiver reports persistent symptoms postoperatively, even if somewhat improved, the patient should be evaluated further.

Risks associated with tonsillectomy must also be taken into account. The theoretical risk of decreased immunological health after removing these lymphoid organs has never been shown. However, administering anesthesia for surgery does risk allergic or pulmonary complications. Local trauma may occur during surgery. Patients will also face postoperative pain and a risk of postoperative hemorrhage, dehydration, and scarring. Death occurs in up to 1:17,000 tonsillectomies. Patients at greatest risk of complications following tonsillectomy are those with Trisomy 21, craniofacial disorders, clotting disorders, heart disease, or cerebral palsy. They are accordingly excluded from the targeted audience for the tonsillectomy guideline as there are clearly more factors to consider in their care. For accurate preoperative counseling and overall quality control, individual surgeons should consider performing periodic self-assessment of significant complications, especially post-tonsillectomy hemorrhage.

The tonsillectomy guideline also includes recommendations for best peri-operative practices. First, one dose of intraoperative IV dexamethasone has been shown to decrease postoperative nausea and vomiting. This is an important intervention since 70% of patients undergoing tonsillectomy will have postoperative nausea and vomiting without treatment. Preventing this complication may prevent pain, dehydration, and the resultant increase in likelihood of postoperative hemorrhage. Contrary to a few isolated studies, there is not sufficient evidence to indicate that the rate of hemorrhage is higher with dexamethasone given at the standard 0.5 mg/ kg/dose. Second, peri-operative antibiotics have not been shown to confer a significant enough postoperative benefit to outweigh their potential risk, and as a result, they are not recommended. This is perhaps the most controversial aspect of the guideline as the vast majority of practicing otolaryngologists currently utilize antibiotics in the peri-operative period. Third, the literature concerning intra-operative local anesthetic injection does not show a statistically significant decrease in postoperative pain, and thus is not recommended. However, adequate postoperative pain medication is needed. Tylenol with codeine has questionable adequacy. Scheduled doses of Tylenol with Hydrocodone have been shown to be more effective than PRN dosing. Non-steroidal anti-inflammatory drugs (NSAIDs), other than ketorolac, are considered to be safe to give after tonsillectomy and do not increase risk of post-operative hemorrhage, contrary to prior early literature reports.

Prior to this guideline, tonsillectomy rates varied widely internationally due to a lack of consensus on timing and indications. The 2011 guideline is hoped to bring about a more uniform quality of care for these patients. It also highlights areas needing better research. Two such areas are (1) effect of tonsillectomy techniques (e.g. intracapsullar tonsillectomy, which is excluded from the current guideline due to lack of evidence), and (2) PSG indications and interpretation in children (guideline currently being formulated). As is appropriate for all evidence-based guidelines, the tonsillectomy guideline will be reviewed and revised in five years.

## OBSTRUCTIVE SLEEP APNEA SYNDROME[9]

Obstructive sleep apnea syndrome (OSAS) is a common disorder of childhood (2% prevalence) that is most commonly caused by adenotonsillar hypertrophy and obesity. The diagnosis of this disorder has evolved with the understanding that OSAS, as opposed to primary snoring (PS), is based on both a patient's neuromuscular tone and physical characteristics; it is not clinched by physical examination alone. The polysomnogram (PSG) has become the gold standard for diagnosing OSA; however, the number of pediatric sleep centers equipped and staffed to test children, and the cost of performing and interpreting these studies, limits this test's universal usefulness.

The effects of untreated OSAS are significantly detrimental and include neurocognitive deficits, behavior disorders, learning disorders, enuresis, daytime somnolence, and can lead to cor pulmonale. Adenotonsillectomy has been shown to be the most effective treatment of OSAS in children. However, surgical treatment should not be undertaken cavalierly because children with

**Table 10. Risk factors for postoperative respiratory complications in children with OSAS undergoing adenotonsillectomy.[9]**

| |
|---|
| Age less than three years |
| Severe OSAS on PSG |
| Cardiac complications of OSAS |
| Failure to thrive |
| Obesity |
| Prematurity |
| Recent respiratory infection |
| Craniofacial anomalies |
| Neuromuscular disorders |

more severe OSAS also are at-risk for increased postoperative and perioperative pulmonary complications. PSG can improve clinical decision-making with respect to choosing treatment in addition to identifying the most appropriate venue for surgery and the most ideal form of postoperative monitoring (see Table 10).

Given the prevalence and impact of OSAS, the AAP Section on Pediatric Pulmonology formed a subcommittee to establish guidelines for the management of OSA in children. The subcommittee, which consisted of pediatricians, pulmonologists, otolaryngologists, and epidemiologists, produced a set of guidelines geared toward primary practitioners. These were based on a review of 278 selected evidence-based papers and were published in 2002 (Table 11).

Already, strict adherence to the Conference on Guideline Standardization would require that this guideline be updated. However the difficulty of performing randomized controlled trials in children remains an impediment to research in this field, as in others. When a treatment has been shown to effectively reverse attention disorders and improve a child's overall health and wellbeing, it is difficult to ethically justify intentionally withholding that treatment. The OSAS literature is constantly evolving, but its quality has not reached the point of commanding a solid revised guideline. Further research differentiating between primary snoring and OSAS is still needed. A good summary of the areas of OSAS needing further research was given by the American Thoracic Society and is listed in Table 12.

**Table 11. Guidelines for OSAS.**[9]

**Recommendation 1:**
All children should be screened for snoring. As part of routine health care maintenance for all children, pediatricians should ask whether the patient snores. An affirmative answer should be followed by a more detailed evaluation. *(Evidence for this recommendation is good, and the strength of the recommendation is strong.)*

**Recommendation 2:**
Complex, high-risk patients should be referred to a specialist. *(Evidence is good that these children are at increased surgical risk and require more complex management; the strength of the recommendation is strong.)*

**Recommendation 3:**
Patients with cardiorespiratory failure cannot await elective evaluation. It is expected that these patients will be in an intensive care setting and will be treated by a specialist; thus, these patients are not covered in this practice guideline.

**Recommendation 4:**
Thorough diagnostic evaluation should be performed. History and physical examination have been shown to be poor at discriminating between PS and OSAS. *(Evidence is strong.)*

Polysomnography is the only method that quantifies ventilator and sleep abnormalities and is recommended as the diagnostic test of choice. Other diagnostic techniques, such as videotaping, nocturnal pulse oximetry, and daytime nap studies, may be useful in discriminating between PS and OSAS if results of polysomnography are positive. However, they do not assess the severity of OSAS, which is useful for determining treatment and follow-up. In any case, because of their high rate of false-negative results, polysomnography should be performed in the event of negative results of the other diagnostic techniques. Additional study of audiotaping is necessary. *(Evidence for and strength of the recommendation are strong.)*

**Recommendation 5:**
Adenotonsillectomy is the first line of treatment for most children. CPAP is an option for those who are not candidates for surgery or do not respond to surgery. *(Evidence for and strength of the recommendation are strong.)*

**Recommendation 6:**
High-risk patients should be monitored as inpatients postoperatively. *(Evidence that these patients are at high risk of postoperative complications is strong. Strength of the recommendation is strong.)*

(*Continued*)

**Table 11. (*Continued*)**

**Recommendation 7:**
Patients should be re-evaluated postoperatively to determine whether additional treatment is required. All patients should undergo clinical reevaluation. High-risk patients should undergo objective testing. *(Evidence is good, and strength of the recommendation is strong.)*

**Table 12. Areas of future research in OSAS.**[9]

| |
|---|
| Accurate prevalence data. |
| Identification of risk factors of complications resulting from OSAS, including the relationship of OSAS severity to specific outcomes. |
| Development and evaluation of low-cost, high-sensitivity, and high-specificity screening methods for OSAS. |
| Delineation of the natural history of treated and untreated PS and OSAS. |
| Assessment of long-term efficacy of adenotonsillectomy, CPAP, and other OSAS treatments. |

## SINUSITIS[10,11]

Acute sinusitis is one of the most common complications of viral upper respiratory infections (URIs) and a frequent indication for antimicrobial therapy. Six to eight yearly URIs are typical for children; "5%–13% of these infections may be complicated by a secondary bacterial infection of the paranasal sinuses."[10]

The AAP guidelines for the diagnosis and treatment of sinusitis in children and the AAO–HNS guidelines for adult sinusitis are summarized in Tables 13 and 14. The AAP guidelines were created by a subcommittee of pediatricians with expertise in infectious disease, allergy, epidemiology, family practice, and pediatric practice, as well as an otolaryngologist and a radiologist. The guideline was reviewed by several groups, including members of the American College of Emergency Physicians, the AAO–HNS, the American Academy of Asthma, Allergy and Immunology, as well as sections of the AAP Pediatrics. The guideline focused on the diagnosis, evaluation, and treatment of children, ages one to 21 years, with uncomplicated

**Table 13. Guidelines for pediatric sinusitis.**[10]

**Recommendation 1:**
The diagnosis of acute bacterial sinusitis is based on clinical criteria in children who present with upper respiratory symptoms that are either persistent or severe. *(Strong recommendation based on limited scientific evidence and strong consensus of the panel.)*

**Recommendation 2a:**
Imaging studies are not necessary to confirm a diagnosis of clinical sinusitis in children less than six years of age. *(Strong recommendation based on limited scientific evidence and strong consensus of the panel.)*

**Recommendation 2b:**
CT scans of the paranasal sinuses should be reserved for patients in whom surgery is being considered as a management strategy. *(Strong recommendation based on good evidence and strong panel consensus.)*

**Recommendation 3:**
Antibiotics are recommended for the management of acute bacterial sinusitis to achieve a more rapid clinical cure. *(Strong recommendation based on good evidence and strong panel consensus.)*
Adjuvant therapies:
No recommendations are made based on controversial and limited data.
Antibiotic prophylaxis:
No recommendations are made based on limited and controversial data.

**Recommendation 4:**
Children with complications or suspected complications of acute bacterial sinusitis should be treated promptly and aggressively. This should include referral to an otolaryngologist usually with the consultation of an infectious disease specialist, ophthalmologist, and neurosurgeon. *(Strong recommendation based on strong consensus of the panel.)*

acute, subacute, and recurrent acute bacterial sinusitis. It excludes neonates and children younger than one year of age, as well as children with anatomic abnormalities of the paranasal sinuses, immunodeficiencies, cystic fibrosis, or immotile cilia syndrome. It also does not include chronic sinusitis. The literature search found 21 qualifying studies, including five randomized controlled trials and eight case series on antimicrobial therapy, three controlled randomized trials on ancillary treatments, and eight studies with information on diagnostic tests.

**Table 14. Guidelines for adult sinusitis.**[11]

**Recommendation 1a: diagnosis of acute rhinosinusitis:**

Clinicians should distinguish presumed acute bacterial rhinosinusitis (ABRS) from acute rhinosinusitis caused by viral upper respiratory infections and non-infectious conditions.

A clinician should diagnose ABRS when:

(a) symptoms or signs of acute rhinosinusitis are present ten days or more beyond the onset of upper respiratory symptoms, or
(b) symptoms or signs of acute rhinosinusitis worsen within ten days after an initial improvement (double worsening).

*(Strong recommendation based on diagnostic studies with minor limitations and a preponderance of benefit over harm.)*

**Recommendation 1b: radiographic imaging and acute rhinosinusitis:**

Clinicians should not obtain radiographic imaging for patients who meet diagnostic criteria for acute rhinosinusitis, unless a complication or alternative diagnosis is suspected. *(Recommendation against based on diagnostic studies with minor limitations and a preponderance of benefit over harm).*

**Recommendation 2: symptomatic relief of viral rhinosinusitis (VRS):**

Clinicians may prescribe symptomatic relief in managing VRS. *(Option based on randomized trials with limitations and cohort studies with an unclear balance of benefit and harm that varies by patient.)*

**Recommendation 3a: pain assessment of acute bacterial rhinosinusitis (ABRS):**

The management of ABRS should include an assessment of pain. The clinician should recommend analgesic treatment based on the severity of pain. *(Strong recommendation based on randomized controlled trials of general pain relief in non-ABRS populations with a preponderance of benefit over harm.)*

**Recommendation 3b: symptomatic relief of acute bacterial rhinosinusitis (ABRS):**

Clinicians may prescribe symptomatic relief in managing ABRS. *(Option based on randomized trials with heterogeneous populations, diagnostic criteria, and outcome measures with a balance of benefit and harm.)*

**Recommendation 5: choice of antibiotic for acute bacterial rhinosinusitis (ABRS):**

If a decision is made to treat ABRS with an antibiotic agent, the clinician should prescribe amoxicillin as first line therapy for most adults. *(Recommendation based on randomized controlled trials with heterogeneity and non-inferiority design with a preponderance of benefit over harm.)*

(*Continued*)

**Table 14. (*Continued*)**

**Recommendation 6: treatment failure for acute bacterial rhinosinusitis (ABRS):**

If the patient worsens or fails to improve with the initial management option by seven days after diagnosis, the clinician should re-assess the patient to confirm ABRS, exclude other causes of illness, and detect complications. If ABRS is confirmed in the patient initially managed with observation, the clinician should begin antibiotic therapy. If the patient was initially managed with an antibiotic, the clinician should change the antibiotic. *(Recommendation based on randomized controlled trials with limitations supporting a cut point of seven days for lack of improvement and expert opinion and first principles for changing therapy with a preponderance of benefit over harm.)*

**Recommendation 7a: diagnosis of chronic rhinosinusitis or recurrent acute rhinosinusitis:**

Clinicians should distinguish chronic rhinosinusitis and recurrent acute rhinosinusitis from isolated episodes of acute bacterial rhinosinusitis and other causes of sinonasal symptoms. *(Recommendation based on cohort and observational studies with a preponderance of benefit over harm.)*

**Recommendation 7b: modifying factors:**

Clinicians should assess the patient with chronic rhinosinusitis or recurrent acute rhinosinusitis for factors that modify management, such as allergic rhinitis, cystic fibrosis, immunocompromised state, ciliary dyskinesia, and anatomic variation. (*Recommendation based on observational studies with a preponderance of benefit over harm.*)

**Recommendation 8a: diagnostic testing:**

The clinician should corroborate a diagnosis and/or investigate for underlying causes of chronic rhinosinusitis and recurrent acute rhinosinusitis. (*Recommendation based on observational studies with a preponderance of benefit over harm.*)

**Recommendation 8b: nasal endoscopy:**

The clinician may obtain nasal endoscopy in diagnosing or evaluating a patient with chronic rhinosinusitis or recurrent acute rhinosinusitis. *(Option based on expert opinion and a preponderance of benefit over harm.)*

(*Continued*)

**Table 14. (*Continued*)**

| |
|---|
| **Recommendation 8c: radiographic imaging:** |
| The clinician should obtain computed tomography (CT) of the paranasal sinuses in diagnosing or evaluating a patient with chronic rhinosinusitis or recurrent acute rhinosinusitis. *(Recommendation based on diagnostic and observational studies and a preponderance of benefit over harm.)* |
| **Recommendation 8d: testing for allergy and immune function:** |
| The clinician may obtain testing for allergy and immune function in evaluating a patient with chronic rhinosinusitis or recurrent acute rhinosinusitis. *(Option based on observational studies with an unclear balance of benefit vs. harm.)* |
| **Recommendation 9: prevention:** |
| Clinicians should educate/counsel patients with chronic rhinosinusitis or recurrent acute rhinosinusitis regarding control measures. *(Recommendation based on randomized controlled trials and epidemiologic studies with limitations and a preponderance of benefit over harm.)* |

The AAO–HNS guideline focuses on sinusitis in individuals older than 12 years of age, so not all the information can be extrapolated to the pediatric population. It does discuss chronic sinusitis and recurrent acute rhinosinusitis, which are not discussed in the AAP guidelines.

Accurate diagnosis, especially distinguishing viral URIs from acute bacterial sinusitis, is addressed in both guidelines. A viral URI is generally defined as acute rhinosinusitis symptoms lasting less than ten to 14 days and not worsening. The AAP guidelines also include severe symptoms, such as a temperature of at least 102°F (39°C) and purulent nasal discharge for at least three to four consecutive days in an ill-appearing child, as criteria to diagnose acute bacterial sinusitis (Table 15).

Both the AAP and AAO–HNS recommend amoxicillin as the first-line antibiotic for acute bacterial sinusitis. It is recommended in either the usual dose of 45 mg/kg/d in two divided doses or the high dose of 90 mg/kg/d in two divided doses. Choices for patients with amoxicillin allergies are summarized in Table 16.

**Table 15. Definitions related to acute bacterial sinusitis.**[11]

| Term | Definition |
|---|---|
| Acute rhinosinusitis | Up to four weeks of purulent nasal drainage (anterior, posterior, or both) accompanied by nasal obstruction, facial pain-pressure-fullness, or both:<br>• Purulent nasal discharge is cloudy or colored, in contrast to the clear secretions that typically accompany viral upper respiratory infection, and may be reported by the patient or observed on physical examination.<br>• Nasal obstruction may be reported by the patient as nasal obstruction, congestion, blockage, or stuffiness, or may be diagnosed by physical examination.<br>• Facial pain-pressure-fullness may involve the anterior face, periorbital region, or manifest with headache that is localized or diffuse. |
| Viral rhinosinusitis (VRS) | Acute rhinosinusitis that is caused by, or is presumed to be caused by, viral infection. A clinician should diagnose VRS when symptoms or signs of acute rhinosinusitis are present less than ten days and the symptoms are not worsening. |
| Acute bacterial rhinosinusitis (ABRS) | Acute rhinosinusitis that is caused by, or is presumed to be caused by, bacterial infection. A clinician should diagnose ABRS when:<br>a. symptoms or signs of acute rhinosinusitis are present ten days or more beyond the onset of upper respiratory symptoms, *or*<br>b. symptoms or signs of acute rhinosinusitis worsen within ten days after an initial improvement (double worsening). |

In general, imaging studies are not recommended in acute sinusitis. The AAP recommends reserving imaging studies for patients who are being considered for surgery. The AAO–HNS recommends a CT scan of the sinuses in patients with chronic sinusitis or recurrent acute sinusitis (Table 17).

**Table 16. AAP antibiotic recommendations for pediatric acute bacterial sinusitis.**[10]

| Situation | Antibiotic choice |
|---|---|
| No allergy | Amoxicillin (usual dose: 45 mg/kg/d in 2 divided doses, high dose: 90 mg/kg/d in 2 divided doses). |
| Mild penicillin allergy (non-type 1 hypersensitivity reaction) | Cefdinir (14 mg/kg/d in 2 divided doses).<br>Cefurozime (30 mg/kg/d in 2 divided doses).<br>Cefpodoxime (10 mg/kg/d once daily). |
| Severe penicillin allergy | Clarithromycin (15 mg/kg/d in 2 divided doses).<br>Azithromycin (10 mg/kg/d on day 1, then 5 mg/kd/d for 4 days once daily). |
| Penicillin allergy with penicillin-resistant *S. pneumoniae* | Clindamycin (30–40 mg/kg/d in 3 divided doses). |

**Table 17. Definitions of chronic and recurrent rhinosinusitis.**[11]

**Chronic rhinosinusitis (CRS)**

Twelve weeks or longer of two or more of the following signs and symptoms:

- mucopurulent drainage (anterior, posterior, or both),
- nasal obstruction (congestion),
- facial pain-pressure-fullness, or
- decreased sense of smell.

AND inflammation is documented by one or more of the following findings:

- purulent (not clear) mucus or edema in the middle meatus or ethmoid region,
- polyps in nasal cavity or the middle meatus, and/or
- radiographic imaging showing inflammation of the paranasal sinuses.

**Recurrent acute sinusitis**

Four or more episodes per year of ABRS without signs or symptoms of rhinosinusitis between episodes:

- each episode of ABRS should meet diagnostic criteria in Table 15.

Unfortunately, neither of the guidelines makes detailed recommendations for surgical management of sinonasal disease, including adenoidectomy as first line surgical management of sinonasal disease in children.

## HOARSENESS[12]

Hoarseness has a lifetime prevalence of 30%. The prevalence rates have varied from 3.9%–23.4% among children, with the most affected ages being eight to 14 years.[12] Hoarseness can greatly affect a child's quality of life, especially in crowded areas, such as schools or the playground, where lack of voice projection may limit their ability to communicate effectively.

Hoarseness is a symptom, not a diagnosis. A thorough history is the first step to identifying the etiology. Medications should be reviewed, as they can cause a change in voice by several different mechanisms. Table 18 lists several classes of medications that may cause hoarseness in the adult population; some have application in children and adolescents as well.

Recent surgical procedures, especially those surgeries placing the recurrent laryngeal nerve at risk such as patent ductus arteriosus (PDA) repair and thyroid surgery, should be reviewed. Infants usually present with an abnormal cry, and etiologies such as birth

**Table 18. Medications that may cause hoarseness.**[12]

| Medication | Mechanism of impact on voice |
|---|---|
| Coumadin, thrombolytics, phosphodiesterase-5 inhibitors | Vocal fold hematoma |
| Biphosphonates | " |
| Angiotensin-converting enzyme inhibitors | " |
| Antihistamines, diuretics, anticholinergics | Chemical laryngitis |
| Danocrine, testosterone | Cough |
| Antipsychotics, atypical antipsychotics | Drying effect on mucosa |
| Inhaled steroids | " |
| | Sex hormone production/ utilization alteration |
| | Laryngeal dystonia |
| | Dose-dependent mucosal irritation, fungal laryngitis |

trauma or intracranial pathology (Arnold-Chiari malformation or neuromuscular conditions) should be considered. School-aged and younger children may have vocal fold nodules from improper vocal hygeine ("screamer nodes") while infants may develop these from excessive crying due to colic or reflux. Craniofacial anomalies may also affect the voice through the development of compensatory vocal mechanisms.

Neonates with hoarseness should undergo laryngoscopy to identify vocal fold paralysis, laryngeal webs, or other congenital anomalies that might affect their ability to swallow or breathe. Hoarseness in children is generally caused by benign lesions of the larynx, such as vocal fold polyps, nodules, or cysts. Clinicians should, however, have a high suspicion for laryngeal papillomatosis as well. When dysphonia is progressive, especially if there are any signs of airway obstruction or stridor, then referral to an otolaryngologist should be initiated and an exam of the larynx is warranted. Other symptoms besides voice change to be considered include stridor, airway obstruction, or dysphagia, all of which can be signs of serious underlying problems such as Chiari malformations, hydrocephalus, skull base tumors, or a compressing neck or mediastinal mass. Vocal fold paralysis should be considered in children with neck masses, congenital heart disease, or previous cardiothoracic, esophageal, or neck surgery. Reflux medications can be considered for presumptive treatment in lieu of performance of EGD or imaging studies in children with hoarseness whose flexible laryngoscopy shows signs of inflammation and whose history suggests symptoms of reflux. Although routine use of corticosteroids is not recommended, children with recurrent croup, concomitant airway compromise, or autoimmune disorders may improve with corticosteroids. Antibiotics are warranted in children who have signs of infection. The AAO–HNS guidelines for hoarseness that can be applied to children are summarized in Table 19.

**Table 19. Guidelines for hoarseness.**[12]

**Recommendation 1: diagnosis**
Clinicians should diagnose hoarseness (dysphonia) in a patient with altered voice quality, pitch, loudness, or vocal effort that impairs communication or reduces voice-related QOL. *(Recommendation based on observational studies with a preponderance of benefit over harm.)*

**Recommendation 2: modifying factors**
Clinicians should assess the patient with hoarseness by history and/or physical examination for factors that modify management such as one or more of the following: recent surgical procedures involving the neck or affecting the recurrent laryngeal nerve, recent endotracheal intubation, radiation treatment to the neck, a history of tobacco abuse, and occupation as a singer or vocal performer. *(Recommendation based on observational studies with a preponderance of benefit over harm.)*

**Recommendation 3a: laryngoscopy and hoarseness**
Clinicians may perform laryngoscopy, or may refer the patient to a clinician who can visualize the larynx, at any time in a patient with hoarseness. *(Option based on observational studies, expert opinion, and a balance of benefit and harm.)*

**Recommendation 3b: indications for laryngoscopy**
Clinicians should visualize the patient's larynx or refer the patient to a clinician who can visualize the larynx if hoarseness fails to resolve by a maximum of three months after onset, or at any time if a serious underlying cause is suspected. *(Recommendation based on observational studies, expert opinion, and a preponderance of benefit over harm.)*

**Recommendation 4: imaging**
Clinicians should not obtain computed tomography (CT) or magnetic resonance imaging (MRI) of the patient with a primary complaint of hoarseness prior to visualizing the larynx. *(Recommendation against imaging based on observational studies of harm, absence of evidence concerning benefit, and a preponderance of harm over benefit.)*

**Recommendation 5a: anti-reflux medication and hoarseness**
Clinicians should not prescribe anti-reflux medications for patients with hoarseness without signs or symptoms of gastroesophageal reflux disease (GERD). *(Recommendation against prescribing based on randomized trials with limitations and observational studies with a preponderance of harm over benefit.)*

(*Continued*)

**Table 19. (*Continued*)**

**Recommendation 5b: anti-reflux medication and chronic laryngitis**
Clinicians may prescribe anti-reflux medication for patients with hoarseness and signs of chronic laryngitis. *(Option based on observational studies with limitations and a relative balance of benefit and harm.)*

**Recommendation 6: corticosteroid therapy**
Clinicians should not routinely prescribe oral corticosteroids to treat hoarseness. *(Recommendation against prescribing based on randomized trials showing adverse events and absence of clinical trials demonstrating benefits with a preponderance of harm over benefit for steroid use.)*

**Recommendation 7: antimicrobial therapy**
Clinicians should not routinely prescribe antibiotics to treat hoarseness. *(Strong recommendation against prescribing based on systematic reviews and randomized trials showing ineffectiveness of antibiotic therapy and a preponderance of harm over benefit.)*

**Recommendation 8a: laryngoscopy prior to voice therapy**
Clinicians should visualize the larynx before prescribing voice therapy and both document and communicate the results to the speech-language pathologist. *(Recommendation based on observational studies showing benefit and a preponderance of benefit over harm.)*

**Recommendation 8b: advocating for voice therapy**
Clinicians should advocate voice therapy for patients diagnosed with hoarseness (dysphonia) that reduces voice-related QOL. *(Strong recommendation based on systematic reviews and randomized trials with a preponderance of benefit over harm.)*

**Recommendation 9: surgery**
Clinicians should advocate for surgery as a therapeutic option in patients with hoarseness with suspected:

1) laryngeal malignancy,
2) benign laryngeal soft tissue lesions, or
3) glottic insufficiency.

*(Recommendation based on observational studies demonstrating a benefit of surgery in these conditions and a preponderance of benefit over harm.)*

**Recommendation 10: prevention**
Clinicians may educate and counsel patients with hoarseness about control and preventive measures. *(Option based on observational studies and small randomized trials of poor quality.)*

(*Continued*)

## SUMMARY

Guidelines are dynamic documents. As such, they are modified periodically to reflect new evidence-based findings. Future guidelines that may be beneficial for pediatric otolaryngologists could include such conditions as reflux, allergy, ankyloglossia, and bilateral simultaneous cochlear implantations.

The preparation of guidelines is exhaustive, time-consuming, and requires funding. Several considerations must be made when choosing the clinical topics for future guidelines. The condition must be common enough that (1) adequate research has been performed to provide evidence-based recommendations and (2) a sufficient number of clinicians would benefit from the guidelines to justify the effort. Although double-blinded, placebo-controlled randomized controlled trials are the standard for clinical therapy efficacy and effectiveness, they can be difficult to perform in both the pediatric and surgical specialties. Many medications routinely used in pediatrics are used "off-label" because of the risks involved in doing randomized controlled trials in the pediatric population. Thus, many guidelines are based on management of adults. These guidelines cannot simply be extrapolated to children, and in order to establish pediatric evidence-based guidelines, adequate studies need to be performed.

## REFERENCES


1. Rosenfeld RM, Shiffman RN. Clinical practice guidelines: a manual for developing evidence-based guidelines to facilitate performance measurement and quality improvement. *Otolaryngol Head Neck Surg* 2006 Oct;135(4 Suppl):S1–28.
2. www.guideline.gov.
3. Lieberthal AS, *et al.* Diagnosis and management of acute otitis media: subcommittee on management of acute otitis media. *Pediatrics* 2004;113:1451–1465.
4. Rosenfeld RM, *et al.* Otitis media with effusion: subcommittee on otitis media with effusion. *Pediatrics* 2004;113:1412–1429.

5. Rosenfeld RM, *et al.* Clinical practice guideline: acute otitis externa. *Otolaryngol Head Neck Surg* 2006;134:S4–S23.
6. Baugh RF, *et al.* Clinical practice guideline: tonsillectomy in children. *Otolaryngol Head Neck Surg* 2011;144(IS):S1–S30.
7. DeSerres LM, Derkay C, *et al.* Impact of adenotonsillectomy on quality of life in children with obstructive sleep disorders. *Arch Otolarygol Head Neck Surg* 2002;128(5):489–496.
8. Mitchell RB, Kelly J. Child behavior after adenotonsillectomy for obstructive sleep apnea syndrome. *Laryngoscope* 2005;115:2051–2055.
9. Marcus CL, *et al.* Clinical practice guidelined: diagnosis and management of childhood obstructive sleep apnea syndrome. Section on pediatric pulmonology and subcommittee on obstructive sleep apnea syndrome. *Pediatrics* 2002;109:704–712.
10. Wald ER, *et al.* Clinical practice guideline: management of sinusitis: subcommittee on management of sinusitis and committee on quality improvement. *Pediatrics* 2001;108(3):798–808.
11. Rosenfeld RM, *et al.* Clinical practice guideline: adult sinusitis. *Otolaryngol Head Neck Surg* 2007;137:S1–S31.
12. Schwartz SR, *et al.* Clinical practice guideline: hoarseness (dysphonia). *Otolaryngol Head Neck Surg* 2009;141:S1–S31.

21

# Medical Error in Pediatric Otolaryngology

*Douglas Sidell and Nina L. Shapiro*

## INTRODUCTION

A significant body of evidence has amassed over the past decade reflecting a universal effort by the healthcare system to improve the quality of medical care, enhance patient safety and decrease the incidence of medical error.

Commonly defined as the failure of planned action to be completed as intended, or the use of an incorrect plan to achieve an aim, medical error has been highlighted as a significant source of morbidity and mortality.[1,2]

Historically, unexpected outcomes resulting from medical errors have been temporized or managed on an individual basis. This form of "damage control" (rather than problem solving at the root-cause level) has been criticized for perpetuating the problem of error in the medical system.[3] Now, in an era where medical errors are understandably becoming less acceptable, there is a push for the prevention of error, the recognition and reporting of error, and the development of systems and technology to avoid error in the future.

In both the pediatric and adult patient population, these regulatory mechanisms are born from the analysis of medical errors and the specific settings in which they take place. Examples in the operative and perioperative environment include structured patient checklists, repetitive nursing evaluation of patient identification, and preoperative surgical site marking. The inpatient ward has likewise adopted charting checks, patient identification checks, and paperwork regulations. In addition, computer systems have been implemented at many institutions to reduce human error before it reaches the patient. In a similar effort to reduce medical error, departmental meetings such as the Morbidity and Mortality conference are held as a form of monthly internal audit of adverse events. At these meetings, medical errors and adverse events (injury resulting directly from medical or surgical management rather than the underlying disease)[4] are discussed in an interdisciplinary setting with the goal of recognizing medical error, thereby reducing future errors of a similar nature.

Despite the regulatory and preventative mechanisms used in the healthcare industry and the body of research aimed at their reduction, medical errors and adverse outcomes continue to occur. The detection and reporting of error are recognized as key steps in overall reduction of medical error. Only after an error is recognized and reported can it be fully understood and, hopefully, avoided. Unfortunately, medical error is an underreported phenomenon. Efforts have been made to analyze behavior patterns which influence the reporting of medical error, as well as the potential barriers which deter physicians from recognizing, reporting or disclosing errors.

Malpractice litigation is a frequently cited barrier to the disclosure of medical error, and is becoming a more common topic of interest in the medical and surgical literature. The fields of surgery and anesthesia account for nearly 75% of adverse events in the healthcare system based on numbers of legal claims. Malpractice litigation is therefore a necessary component of any discussion of medical error, and an understandable driving force for change.[5]

With an emphasis on the pediatric surgical patient, this section aims to (1) discuss the various forms of medical error and adverse events in the healthcare system, (2) discuss some of the current mechanisms in place to detect, reduce, and/or prevent medical error, and (3) to provide a brief, yet up-to-date discussion of malpractice litigation associated with the surgical patient.

## REPORTING MEDICAL ERROR

The vast majority of literature discussing the incidence and prevalence of medical error and adverse events involves self-reporting mechanisms. It is therefore negatively influenced by recall bias and reporting error. With this in mind, several studies exist which objectively evaluate the prevalence of medical error in the pediatric surgical patient. When considering a "zero defect" or "zero tolerance" system of error evaluation, in which all errors are investigated (ranging from small charting errors to large errors resulting in major adverse events), a significant percentage of patient care is noted to be subject to medical error.[1,6]

In a 2009 study involving the review of pediatric otolaryngology patients at Children's National Medical Center in Washington DC, the rate of errors using this "zero-defect paradigm" was greater than 6000 errors per 1000 admission days. Nearly 92 errors resulted in moderate adverse events requiring prolonged hospitalization or intervention, but were without permanent patient harm.[1] Other studies have similar rates of error, suggesting the frequency of moderate adverse events at large tertiary care medical centers to range from 80 to 90 events per 1000 admission days.[7,8]

Considering the high incidence of medical error in the pediatric setting, it may be comforting to know that the bulk of medical error identified in closely scrutinized chart audits does not directly affect the patient. As outlined in a 2003 prospective analysis at the Hospital for Sick Children in Toronto, Canada, the vast majority of medical error reported (>50% of admissions), does not result in direct patient harm.[8] Although this may at first seem reassuring, these small errors may suggest a larger problem in the system, as the accumulation of multiple small errors likely contributes to more significant adverse events.[1]

Understanding that a significant percentage of patient care is associated with medical error when thoroughly investigated, it is evident that errors are underreported.[9] The pediatric patient environment is a common location for medical error and an especially challenging arena when considering error reporting. As a result, efforts have been made to better understand the reasons for under-reporting of medical errors, specifically in the pediatric population.

Garbutt *et al.* attempt to illuminate specific barriers to reporting error in a 2007 survey-based study. In their report, it was revealed that, while the majority of pediatrician respondents endorsed disclosure of serious error to families, few endorsed disclosure of "near miss" events (in which no harm is done to the patient). The specific barriers to reporting error investigated in this report were similar to other studies, and include insufficient time to report error and fear of punishment such as malpractice litigation.[9]

Specific to the pediatric patient, the inclusion of parents as a third party adds a challenging element to the disclosure of medical error in this patient population. The difficulties associated with the disclosure of medical error to families of pediatric patients in the abovementioned study included the notion that the patient's family (1) would not understand the error, (2) were unaware of the error, or (3) would not want to know about the error. Interestingly, although commonly cited as a barrier to reporting medical error, the fear of malpractice litigation was not concluded to be a contributing factor in this study. On the contrary, three of four physicians thought that disclosure would actually decrease the likelihood of malpractice litigation.[9–12]

In a 2008 analysis, Loren *et al.* sought to further elucidate the conceptions held by physicians as well as patients and families with regard to disclosure of medical errors. Specifically, this study emphasized the disparity between inconsistent physician disclosure and the common desire for patients and families to be thoroughly informed of all adverse events. Attributed in part to the pediatric environment being a complicated setting in which to deliver bad news, this study discusses parental knowledge of the error as a large influence on the presence or absence of disclosure. If patients and their families were unaware of the events, they were less likely to receive complete disclosure. As pointed out by Loren *et al.*, this is in conflict with the Joint Commission on Accreditation of Healthcare Organizations (JCAHO) standards, which support the creation of error reporting systems, and can understandably become an ethical dilemma.[13]

The issues surrounding the reporting or disclosing of medical errors have resulted in the establishment of training strategies at several institutions in efforts to encourage appropriate reporting protocols and behavior. This ranges from hospital-based teaching to the classroom environment, where medical schools are incorporating disclosure of medical error into the standard curriculum thereby eliminating uncertainty among young physicians. Over time, it is hoped that this will contribute to an overall reduction in the prevalence of adverse events in the pediatric patient population.

## PREVENTATIVE MEASURES

Knowing that medical errors do occur, that they are a significant source of morbidity and mortality, and are an underreported phenomenon, the question becomes, "how can they be prevented effectively?" Institutions across the nation have adopted several mechanisms to approach this question systematically:

### Pharmaceutical Error

Medication dosing and prescribing errors are of the most frequently implicated errors in the pediatric patient population.[14] Because medication administration is a common occurrence with frequent room for error, adverse events must be recognized and diverted prior to negatively affecting the patient. One of the greatest improvements in risk reduction involves the adoption of zero-tolerance policies in the pharmaceutical department.[6,15] Suggested as a "first step" for any pediatric surgical service, the zero tolerance policy for medication administration is said to result in positive changes in behavior, which thereby reduce potential adverse events resulting from the accumulation of several small medical errors. Other effective preventative measures include redundancy and "double-check" methods used by the pharmacist. As a result, the majority of errors (>75% in one report) are identified before reaching the patient.[6] In a similar fashion, the use of mg/kg dosing information in all pediatric orders, also checked by the pharmacist, helps to reduce dosing errors on the pediatric wards. Likewise, dosing charts, readily available on the wards, distributed to residents, at the bedside, and on anesthesia carts, have also helped to decrease the incidence of dosing error.

At the expense of extensive training and a hospital-wide culture change, the adoption of computerized order entry systems at some institutions has also contributed to a significant improvement in the incidence of medication errors. The addition of a pharmacist to the surgical team during rounds, or individual pharmacist ward-rounds (where the pharmacist rounds independently on the patients) has also been shown to significantly reduce adverse events. Finally, to review and alert the team to common errors, interval pharmacy meetings or the incorporation of a pharmacist in the morbidity and mortality meetings of a surgical service is highly effective.[16]

## Charting Error

Charting errors do not always directly affect patient care, however as described by Shah *et al.*, their collective presence likely contributes to more noteworthy adverse events. Ranging from record keeping errors (such as failure to document a procedure or absence of physician signature) to illegible or incorrect patient orders, these errors may go unnoticed or result directly in patient harm. As a result, charting checks or order-review services have been developed at several institutions, and when implemented, effectively reduce error. For example, at a Los Angeles County tertiary care hospital, a medical record review service evaluates patient charts on a daily basis for signatures and note legibility. Similarly, at Children's Hospital Boston, a review committee performs chart reviews on a quarterly basis, and generates reports for all physicians in the pediatric otolaryngology department.[1] This reduction of charting errors, while individually small, together helps to eliminate the occurrence of more significant adverse events.

## Communication Error in the Operating Room

The operating room is a unique environment which demands communication between individuals from several disciplines, including anesthesiologists, technicians, nurses, and surgeons. Hindrances to effective communication include: differences in job responsibility, training, and specific goals associated with each individual and their duties. Communication error is therefore an undeniable influence on medical error in the operating room. Contributing to the 47–50% rate of error associated with the surgical patient, communication errors are the number one reason for wrong-site surgery and sentinel events in the United States.[17,18]

In a single-center, survey-based study, Catchpole *et al.* analyzed communication skills and their influence on "technical outcomes" in the operating room. This study exemplifies a feasible analysis of team interactions and dynamics in the operating room, and demonstrates that, with proper evaluation, interventions aimed at improving this communication process can be well designed and calculated. As previous studies have shown, this study suggests that multiple small errors, although indirectly related to surgical techniques or the operative field, have a cumulative negative effect on patient outcomes and operating room time.[17,19] The reduction of communication error is therefore a critical component in the reduction of adverse events associated with the surgical patient.

One technique used at many medical centers to reduce perioperative morbidity and mortality involves the use of operating room checklists or briefings to assist the coordination of patient care. Included in this technique is the preoperative "time-out," whereby critical information such as patient identification, surgical site, instrument availability, and patient positioning are all reviewed by the OR team. Lingard *et al.* evaluated the effectiveness of checklists in a large multicenter prospective analysis in which nurses, surgeons and technicians use a standard checklist and preprocedure meeting. A greater than three-fold increase in communication failures in the operating room was reported when the preoperative briefing and checklist were not used.[20] Likewise, a study seeking to evaluate preoperative checklists and briefings at the Hospital for Sick Children in Toronto, Canada, demonstrated a measurable reduction in wrong-site surgeries with the institution of surgical time-outs. In addition, this study demonstrates a significant improvement in the perception of openness and communication by nurses in the operating room, who reported less "difficulty in discussing errors" after the institution of time-outs.[21] On a larger scale, when the use of a safe-surgery checklist was applied across eight major hospitals in eight diverse countries, Haynes *et al.* demonstrate a reduction in both the rate of death and the rate of inpatient complications. This study reflects the applicability of checklists across multiple diverse patient populations, and further emphasizes their feasibility.[22]

Checklists have been criticized as being time consuming and tedious, however it is being discovered that reductions in the rate of medical error may be directly associated with their use. Therefore, checklists arguably reflect a change in culture which is necessary to provide a safer environment for the surgical patient. With this concept in mind, several independent companies have been developed which provide systems-based services to hospitals in an attempt to reduce medical error. Knowing that human error will never be eliminated entirely, the concept of "systems science" is utilized to provide an algorithm-like system of redundancy to complex hospital processes. Similar to the airline industry, systems science is applied to the surgical and ICU settings as a means to enhance communication and to provide structured, goal-driven responsibilities for all individuals involved. In these systems, deviation from protocols designed to reduce errors is rarely tolerated, and all personnel involved, regardless of duty, are empowered without penalty to interject on behalf of the patient when concern for safety arises.[23]

## PHYSICIAN EDUCATION

The Chinese political figure and philosopher Confucius said, "Tell me and I will forget. Show me, and I may remember. Involve me and I will understand." As described by Kolb in 1984, this statement embodies the concept of the transition from a teacher-led learner to a learner-directed experience, and exemplifies the importance of continued education in the healthcare arena.[24,25] It is not surprising that a key concept in the reduction of medical error and the improvement of healthcare quality is the ongoing process of medical education and self-directed learning.

### The Practicing Physician

With the increasing awareness and decreased acceptance of medical errors in the healthcare system, physicians are being trained to recognize and reduce error. The American College of Surgeons (ACS) has developed communication-strengthening programs, recognizing that "communication is essential for modern surgeons."[26] Various seminars and computer-based courses are available for practicing physicians. In addition, practicing physicians are encouraged to continue self-directed learning by identifying their own deficiencies to work toward their improvement. Of course, a general desire for competence in an ever-changing environment is required for self-directed learning, and should be considered a fundamental requirement for all practicing physicians.[24]

### The Resident Physician

At the resident level, the Accreditation Council for Graduate Medical Education (ACGME) has added communication skills as a core-competency, and thereby developed requirements for residents to be "able to demonstrate interpersonal and communication skills that result in effective information exchange and teaming with patient, their patients' families, and professional associates."[27] Recently, "resident portfolios" have been suggested as a means to address the ACGME practice based learning and improvement competency. These portfolios are a tool through which residents may analyze cases in the context of errors and the events surrounding those errors, as a form of self-reflection.[24,28,29]

### The Medical Student

Medical schools nationwide have begun to incorporate the awareness of medical error, the mechanisms for disclosure or reporting error, and the delivery of bad news into their curriculums.[28] In addition, practice-based and self-directed learning methods are being introduced at the medical school level, fostering an ingrained method of learning for future physicians.

### The Morbidity and Mortality Audit

One of the most important mechanisms employed to reduce medical error is the Morbidity and Mortality (M&M) conference. A fundamental element of resident education and a cornerstone of surgical culture, the M&M audit is a means of reviewing both preventable and unpreventable adverse events. It functions to allow physicians to better understand the nature of the event and the circumstances which may have contributed to its occurrence.

Often held at a monthly or quarterly interval, the M&M conference is designed to reduce future error and has been the foundation of several well-defined protocols and guidelines developed to protect the surgical patient. Examples include medication dosing protocols, presurgical antibiotic prophylaxis protocols or surgery-specific technical advances.[3]

## INFORMED CONSENT AND MALPRACTICE LITIGATION

The potential for medical error or the occurrence of adverse events emphasizes the importance of appropriate informed consent practices during evaluation of the surgical patient. A discussion of risks, benefits and alternatives is a suggested component of all forms of treatment, and this is not with the exception of pediatric patients. Contrary to any misconceptions, informed consent is equally necessary in this patient population. In fact, studies have demonstrated that children actually want to be informed about their healthcare. In addition, the active participation of parents has been shown to improve overall patient satisfaction.[30–32]

Surgeons are in a unique position to inform their patients about the possibility of not only adverse events and surgical risk, but also of medical error. This physician-patient discussion will facilitate the disclosure of adverse events when they do occur, and it may encourage the reporting of error. This is not a suggestion that medical error should be accepted as an irreparable component of the medical system. In fact, the opposite is true. Medical errors should be understood as a dynamic segment of healthcare, which to be repaired, require constant recognition, reporting and, when possible, remedy.

As previously mentioned, the risk of malpractice litigation exists as a potential barrier to the reporting of error. Therefore, suboptimal patient-physician communication or inadequate consent preoperatively will likewise contribute to the difficulty associated with the disclosure of error when it does occur. In contrast, the adequately informed patient and parent who are active participants in the decision making process may be more understanding of medical error, and possibly less likely to pursue legal action in the event of a medical error.

Exemplifying the pediatric surgical patient, a recent 2007 analysis focusing on malpractice claims alleging morbidity or mortality after tonsillectomy, reviewed both public records of national court trials and the records of a large private New York medical liability insurance company. A total of 156 cases were identified, and despite tonsillectomy being one of the most common surgical procedures performed by otolaryngologists, malpractice after tonsillectomy was concluded to be uncommon. Interestingly, the majority of lawsuits following tonsil surgery are dismissed or settled, with reportedly 15% of claims proceeding to trial. Surprisingly little research exists outlining the events leading to those malpractice claims which are settled or dismissed. Furthermore, literature describing factors which result in successful litigation is likewise scant. As a result, the majority of medical errors or adverse events leading to litigation in this patient population are poorly documented, and, as a whole, are poorly understood by the medical community. Because tonsillectomy is one of the most common surgical interventions in this patient population, factors associated with litigation involving less frequently performed operations is likely to be exceedingly unclear to most physicians.

When considering the minority of cases which proceed to trial, some trends in the litigation process have been recognized. Not surprisingly, and consistent with previous studies, those cases in which the plaintiff is compensated are more likely to be associated with the presence of a defined medical error. Delays in diagnosis, intraoperative complications, and dissatisfaction with results are frequent claims leading to trial.[5,33]

A common thread revisited in all reports is the emphasis on good communication, thorough record keeping, and appropriate and adequate clinical assessments. Although these key factors are a common component of everyday practice and heavily emphasized in medical training, their absence is a frequent occurrence in the cases reviewed here. As expected, the absence of these elements in conjunction with an adverse event is more likely to result in a decision favoring the plaintiff.[2,34] A 2008 American College of Surgeons (ACS) review of closed claims against general surgeons discusses several deficiencies in physician behavior which were associated with preventable errors or adverse events. Failure to communicate was reported to be the most salient deficiency and accounted for 22% of complications in the study.[35] The report goes on to emphasize the necessity for communication skills to be a targeted component of continued medical education (CME), and for the development of systems care at an institutional level.

Undoubtedly, despite the current literature, more research is required to better understand events surrounding medical errors which contribute to malpractice litigation in the pediatric patient population.

## CONCLUSION

Medical error is an underreported phenomenon and a significant contributor to morbidity and mortality. An understanding of both the origins of medical error, as well as those behaviors which inhibit the reporting of adverse events, are important steps toward the effective reduction of error. Continued improvement therefore requires the constant recognition and interpretation of errors when they occur, thus allowing for the successful prevention of similar errors in the future.

## REFERENCES

1. Shah RK, Lander L, Forbes P *et al.* Safety on an inpatient pediatric otolaryngology service: many small errors, few adverse events. *Laryngoscope* 2009;119(5):871–879.
2. Rothschild JM, Landrigan CP, Cronin JW. The critical care safety study: the incidence and nature of adverse events and serious medical errors in intensive care. *Crit Care Med* 2005;33:1694–1700.
3. Mattioli G, Avanzini S, Pini-Prato A, *et al.* Risk management in pediatric surgery. *Pediatr Surg Int* 2009;25:683–690.
4. Kohn L, Corrigan J, Donaldson M. *To Err is Human: Building a Safer Health System.* Washington DC: National Academy Press, 2000.
5. Morris LGT, Lieberman SM, Reitzen SD *et al.* Characteristics and outcomes of malpractice claims after tonsillectomy. *Otolaryngol Head Neck Surg* 2008;138:315–320.
6. Engum SA, Breckler FD. An evaluation of medication errors — the pediatric surgical service experience. *J Pediatr Surg* 2008;43(2):348–352.
7. Wu AW, Pronovost P, Morlock L. ICU incident reporting systems. *J Crit Care* 2002;17:86–94.
8. Proctor ML, Patore J, Gerstle JP *et al.* Incidence of medical error and adverse outcomes on a general pediatric service. *J Pediatr Surg* 2003;38:1361–1365.
9. Garbutt J, Brownestein DR, Klein EJ *et al.* Reporting and disclosing medical errors: pediatricians' attitudes and behaviors. *Arch Pediatr Adolesc Med* 2007;161:179–185.
10. Taylor JA, Brownstein D, Chistakis DA *et al.* Use of incident reports by physicians and nurses to document medical errors in pediatric patients. *Pediatrics* 2004;114:729–735.
11. Leape LL. Reporting of adverse events. *New Engl J Med* 2002;347: 1633–1638.
12. Hevia A, Hobgood C. Medical error during residency: to tell or not to tell. *Ann Emerg Med* 2003; 42:565–570.

13. Loren DJ, Klein EJ, Garbutt J *et al.* Medical error disclosure among pediatricians. *Arch Pediatr Adolesc Med* 2008;162(10):922–927.
14. Mill DH. Medical insurance feasibility study. A technical study. *West J Med* 1978;128(4):360–366.
15. Leonard MS, Cimino M, Shaha S *et al.* Risk reduction for adverse drug events through sequential implementation of patient safety initiatives in a children's hospital. *Pediatrics* 2006;118(4):1124–1129.
16. Leape LL, Cullen DJ, Clapp MD *et al.* Pharmacist participation on physician rounds and adverse drug events in the intensive care unit. *JAMA* 1999;282(3):267–270.
17. Catchpole K, Mishra A, Handa A *et al.* Teamwork and error in the operating room analysis of skills and roles. *Ann Surg* 2008;247:699–706.
18. Makary MA, Sexton JB, Freischlag JA *et al.* Operating room teamwork among physicians and nurses: teamwork is in the eye of the beholder. *J Am Coll Surg* 2006;202:746–752.
19. Woods D, Patterson E. How unexpected events produce an escalation of cognitive and coordinative demands. In: Hancock PA, Desmond PA, eds. *Stress Workload and Fatigue.* Hillsdale, NJ: Lawrence Erlbaum, 2004, pp. 290–304.
20. Lingard L, Regehr G, Orser B, *et al.* Evaluation of a preoperative checklist and team briefing among surgeons, nurses, and anesthesiologists to reduce failures in communication. *Arch Surg* 2008;143(1):12–17.
21. Khoshbin A, Lingard L, Wright J. Evaluation of preoperative and perioperative operating room briefings at the Hospital for Sick Children. *Can J Surg* 2009;52(4):309–315.
22. Haynes AB, Weiser TG, Berry WR. A surgical safety checklist to reduce morbidity and mortality in a global population. *N Eng J Med* 2009; 360(5):491–499.
23. Roberson DW, KJentala E, Healy GB. Quality and safety in a complex world: why systems science matters to otolaryngologists. *Laryngoscope* 2004;114:1810–1814.
24. Schweingurth JM. Lifelong learning in otolaryngology: self-directed learning. *Otolaryngol Clin N Am* 2007;40:1323–1330.
25. Kolb DA. *Experiential learning: experience as the source of learning and development.* Englewood Cliffs, NJ: Prentice-Hall; 1984.

26. Russell T. Safety and quality improvement in surgical practice. *Ann Surg* 2006;244:653–655.
27. Hutul OA, Carpenter RO, Tarpley JL *et al.* Missed opportunities: a descriptive assessment of teaching and attitudes regarding communication skills in a surgical residency. *Curr Surg* 2006;63:401–409.
28. Chisholm CD, Croskerry P. A case study in medical error: the use of portfolio entry. *Acad Emerg Med* 2004;11:388–392.
29. Lynch DC, Swing SR, Harowitz SD *et al.* Assessing practice-based learning and improvement. *Teach Learn Med* 2004;16:85–92.
30. Cox ED, Raaum SE. Discussion of alternatives, risks and benefits in pediatric acute care. *Patient Educ Couns* 2008;72:122–129.
31. Merenstein D, Diener-West M, Krist A, Pinneger M, Cooper LA. An assessment of the shared-decision model in parents of children with acute otitis media. *Pediatrics* 2005;116:1267–1275.
32. Young B, Dixon-Woods M, Windridge KC, Heney D. Managing communication with young people who have a potentially life threatening chronic illness: qualitative study of patients and parents. *Br Med J* 2003;326:305–308.
33. Studdert DM, Mello MM, Gawande AA *et al.* Claims, errors and compensation payments in medical malpractice litigation. *New Eng J Med* 2006;354:2024–2033.
34. Savage JR, Weiner GM. Litigation in otolaryngology: trends and recommendations. *J Laryngol Otol* 2006;120:1001–1004.
35. Griffin FD, Stepehens LS, Alaxander JB, *et al.* Violations of behavioral practices revealed in closed claims reviews. *Ann Surg* 2008;248:468–474.

# Index